On the Heels of Ignorance

On the Heels of Ignorance

Psychiatry and the Politics of Not Knowing

OWEN WHOOLEY

The University of Chicago Press
Chicago and London

The University of Chicago Press, Chicago 60637
The University of Chicago Press, Ltd., London
© 2019 by The University of Chicago

Published 2019
Printed in the United States of America

28 27 26 25 24 23 22 21 20 19   1 2 3 4 5

ISBN-13: 978-0-226-61624-7 (cloth)
ISBN-13: 978-0-226-61638-4 (paper)
ISBN-13: 978-0-226-61641-4 (e-book)
DOI: https://doi.org/10.7208/chicago/9780226616414.001.0001

Library of Congress Cataloging-in-Publication Data

Names: Whooley, Owen, author.
Title: On the heels of ignorance : psychiatry and the politics of not knowing /
    Owen Whooley.
Description: Chicago : The University of Chicago Press, 2019. |
    Includes bibliographical references and index.
Identifiers: LCCN 2018036447 | ISBN 9780226616247 (cloth : alk. paper) |
    ISBN 9780226616384 (pbk. : alk. paper) | ISBN 9780226616414 (e-book)
Subjects: LCSH: Psychiatry—United States—History. | Ignorance
    (Theory of knowledge)
Classification: LCC RC443 .W46 2019 | DDC 616.89—dc23
LC record available at https://lccn.loc.gov/2018036447

♾ This paper meets the requirements of ANSI/NISO Z39.48-1992
(Permanence of Paper).

To Erin,
for the wonder and madness you bring to my life

"Not ignorance, but ignorance of ignorance, is the death of knowledge."

ALFRED NORTH WHITEHEAD

"The definition of insanity is doing the same thing over and over and expecting different results."

ATTRIBUTED TO ALBERT EINSTEIN . . . AND BENJAMIN FRANKLIN . . . AND MARK TWAIN . . . AND NARCOTICS ANONYMOUS, SO UNKNOWN FOR NOW

CONTENTS

ACKNOWLEDGMENTS

It is often assumed that researchers choose to study topics that somehow relate to their personal experiences. Of course, this is not necessarily so, but in this case, the assumption holds. I spent my childhood in the shadow of my father's mental illness, forced to grapple with its mysteries before I possessed the tools to do so. One could say I have lived the ignorance that surrounds mental illness. The influence of that experience on this book is a number of degrees removed, undetectable to most except those who know me best, but it certainly drove my desire to write it. The book's seeds were planted years ago in the mind of a young boy trying to walk the minefields of mental illness daily. As such, this book, and its themes, are not merely academic to me.

My father, Jim, was charming, intelligent, and perpetually overwhelmed by a black melancholy that cast an omnipresent pall over his days. He suffered from what would be diagnosed today as major depressive disorder comorbid with a drug addiction. Such diagnostic labels, when affixed, appear to suggest an understanding of his inner world. Instead, they strike me as superficial and inadequate. They could not bridge the chasm of misunderstanding that came between me and my father. I had no idea what was going on, where he was, why he was in such pain, and why he couldn't get out of bed. Consequently, I approached our interactions with apprehension and worry, not because he was violent or volatile—I've never met a gentler man—but because he was inscrutable. I never understood him. Neither did the well-meaning mental health professionals who tried to help him. I am indebted to my dad for many things, but his greatest gift might be the lesson that he would have liked *not* to pass on: The world brims with uncertainty and is shot through with questions we cannot answer. This uncertainty invites examination and spurs exploration, yes, but, most important, it forces upon us humility. This book is the product of that hard-won wisdom.

Thinking is an eminently social endeavor. My thoughts, as presented in this book, are my own (as are the errors), but they have been helped along by the generosity of others. To these people I owe a debt of gratitude that a brief mention here cannot possibly repay. For the past six years, the Department of Sociology at the University of New Mexico has been a stimulating home. Kristin Barker is a dear friend and mentor, who always delights and inspires me with her razor wit and intelligence. As chairs, Sharon Erickson Nepstad and Rich Wood have generously shepherded me through the tenure process. My fellow Med Heads—Jessica Goodkind, Kimberly Huyser, and Brian Soller—have offered their insights along the way. Rose Rohrer helped with some archival research for the book, and Natalie Fullenkamp lent her keen editing eye to some of the pages that follow.

This project originated during my NIMH postdoctoral fellowship at the Institute for Health, Health Care Policy, and Aging Research at Rutgers University. Allan Horwitz has been an invaluable source of insight and support; he is the model of a generous scholar to which I aspire. Deborah Carr, Gerald Grob, Ken MacLeish, David Mechanic, Tyson Smith, and Zoë Wool encouraged this project during its early stumbling days. Many others have offered feedback and timely encouragement along the way: Gabi Abend, Rene Almeling, Amy Almerico-LeClair, Claudio Benzecry, Ruth Braunstein, Bruce Cohen, Mariana Craciun, Andrew Deener, Annemarie Jutel, Sarah Kaufman, Donald Light, Erin Madden, Noah McClain, Richard Noll, Aaron Panofsky, Teresa Scheid, Jason Schnittker, Sandra Sulzer, Stefan Timmermans, Jerome Wakefield, and Jonathan Wynn. The book's analysis was refined in response to invaluable feedback gained during presentations at the UNM Sociology Department, the Health Working Group at UCLA, the Rotman Institute of Philosophy at Western University, and the Sociology of Mental Health section of the American Sociological Association. As with all my research and writing, Jane Jones has been indispensable, as an editor, a critic, and, most important, a friend.

I am indebted to all the psychiatrists who agreed to be interviewed; they helped me understand the often opaque practice of constructing psychiatric diagnoses. Like all historical sociologists, I lean heavily on the work of historians who have preceded me in slogging through the archives. These include too many to name, but especially influential were Gerald Grob, Nathan Hale, Elizabeth Lunbeck, Jack Pressman, Charles Rosenberg, Andrew Scull, and Edward Shorter. Doug Mitchell, my editor at the University of Chicago Press, has been a wise and witty interlocutor through two books now. That such a giant in the field would take me on as a project is one of the more unlikely and lucky developments of my career. Also at the Press, I'd like to thank Tamara Ghattas, Kyle Adam Wagner, and Susan Karani, as well as Marianne Tatom, who worked with Press staff. Kay Banning created the wonderful index.

Essayist and bibliophile Logan Pearsall Smith states, "People say that life's the thing, but I prefer books." As an avid bibliophile myself, I couldn't disagree more; I prefer the charmed life with which I have been blessed. My mother, Candie, and brother, Michael, have navigated my father's challenges with grace and grit. I cherish being on their team. Over the course of this book project, my two kids, Colum and Ayla, were born. These monsters infuse my days with that special kind of imagination and insanity gifted only to the very young. They make my world magical. Thanks to Jibbs for literally always being around. My wife, Erin, to whom this book is dedicated, is the fucking best, full stop. How I found such a loving, supportive, and weird partner, I'll never know.

Introduction

The history of American psychiatry is a history of ignorance. Underlying psychiatry's curious past—its repeated crises and dramatic transformations, its faddish theories and epistemic somersaults, its occasional achievements and egregious abuses—is a stubborn, inconvenient fact. Psychiatrists lack basic knowledge regarding mental illness. Madness evades articulation. Charged with the quixotic, perhaps doomed, mandate to impose reason on madness, psychiatrists have searched for an understanding of the mechanisms that produce mental distress, be they psychological, neurological, genetic, or social. These searches have been in vain. The most fundamental questions regarding their object remain unanswered.

Psychiatry's critics have been more than happy to point out its knowledge gaps. But to their general credit, the most consistent chroniclers of this ignorance have been psychiatrists themselves. One might think that psychiatrists would try to suppress their ignorance through conspiracies of silence, campaigns of misinformation, and sweepings under the rug. Indeed, such attempts have been made. However, psychiatrists have long balanced denial with sober acknowledgments of all that they do not know.

Confessions of ignorance resound throughout American psychiatric discourse. The establishment of American psychiatry as a profession dates to 1844, with the founding of the Association of Medical Superintendents of American Institutions for the Insane (AMSAII). Armed with a reforming ethos and inflated statistics, superintendents justified their new profession on the curative promise of the asylum. But a mere thirteen years after the founding of AMSAII, John Charles Bucknill, an English superintendent, threw cold water on the hyperbole of his American peers. Comparing psychiatry to other branches of medicine, Bucknill found it wanting: "The widely differing opinions which have been entertained by the ablest physicians respecting the pathology of Insanity, clearly show that there is some difficulty at the bottom of the question, greater than that which has existed with regard to the nature of other classes of disease."[1] Eight years later, John E. Tyler urged his fellow superintendents to admit a troubling lack of consensus regarding the nature of insanity. "Without doubt, any person who has read as much and thought as much upon the subject of insanity as each one of you, gentlemen, has done, realizes fully how difficult a thing it is to enunciate, in any short formula of words, or to make it clear by any brief description, what insanity is," Tyler told his colleagues. "And you cannot have failed to feel that the definitions which have been given by various and learned writers, have by no means been perfect definitions; that is, they have by no means distinguished insanity from everything else."[2]

Were it not for their persistence, these early admissions of ignorance might be shrugged off as the growing pains of a young field. But they have continued ever since. Over the next five decades, the comparisons between psychiatry and the rest of medicine grew even less favorable. In response to the laboratory revolution that swept medicine proper, psychiatry could offer only frustrating stasis. In a 1900 paper to the now rechristened American Medico-Psychological Association (AMPA), New York superintendent August Hoch expressed pessimism regarding psychiatry's future: "But while we infer the existence of different diseases, we have little knowledge of their real processes. Indeed, such a knowledge seems to be very remote."[3] Twenty years later, the prognosis remained just as grim. Dampening the puffed-up pretensions of psychiatry after World War I, Harold Gosline cautioned that "in the matter of psychopathology we are still in a maze."[4] In 1924, Thomas Salmon, the influential president of the once again rechristened American Psychiatric Association (APA), admitted that decades of study had "failed to illuminate the darkness that enshrouded the essential nature of disorders of the mind."[5] Near the end of World War II, during the acme of psychiatry's prestige, George Sprague, a prominent New York psychiatrist, voiced his disappointment at psychiatry's enduring difficulties in cracking mental illness. With so many factors to consider, "thousands of possibly relevant items," psychiatrists were still unable to identify the "exact causes" of mental diseases.[6] Even knowing *where* to look for insight was unclear.

By the 1970s, psychiatric ignorance was on full display. A chorus of criticism, unleashed in damning exposés, best-selling novels, and frank memoirs by former patients, threw into sharp relief all that psychiatrists did not know. An emboldened antipsychiatry movement questioned the very existence of mental illness, imperiling psychiatry's existence like never before. Psychiatrists were unable to mount an effective response to this challenge, hamstrung as they were by the obviousness of their failures and an atrophying psychoanalytic paradigm. In response to Thomas Szasz's provocative book *The Myth of Mental Illness*, psychiatrist Stephen Reiss conceded that while Szasz's critique had gone too far in calling mental illness a myth, the term "mental illness" "is best considered as a hypothetical construct," and that "basic psychiatric concepts are imprecise."[7] In a 1982 address to the APA, Roberto Mangabeira Unger warned that psychiatry would never "progress without confronting certain basic theoretical problems that it has habitually minimized or dismissed."[8] Chiding his colleagues for long neglecting these conceptual issues, Unger called upon them to reconsider "the basic explanatory structure of psychiatry: psychiatry's image of the relationship between biological and psychological accounts, its background conception of the fundamental reality of passion and subjectivity, and even its tacit assumptions about what it means to explain something."[9]

Responding to the antipsychiatry movement, a new generation of reformers, deeming themselves Neo-Kraepelinians, sought to reassert psychiatry's medical identity in the 1980s. Wielding a new diagnostic system, they would be the ones to resolve psychiatry's ignorance by grounding it in the biomedical sciences. Martin Roth and Jerome Kroll begged their fellow psychiatrists to "take scrupulous care to avoid overestimating the scope of the knowledge [psychiatry] possesses and the hypotheses it can formulate."[10] They did not listen; like generations of reformers before them, they got caught up in the hype, this time surrounding the efficacy of psychopharmaceutical drugs. But these reforms too have failed to illuminate the essence of mental illness. Genetic science and neuroscience have proven to be far more complicated than reformers anticipated. Psychiatry "has thus far failed to identify a single neurobiological marker that is diagnostic of a mental disorder."[11] Summing up the current state of psychiatric knowledge, Kenneth Kendler observes, "We have hunted for big, simple neuropathological explanations for psychiatric disorders and have not found them. We have hunted for big, simple neurochemical explanations for psychiatric disorders and have not found them. We have hunted for big, simple genetic explanations for psychiatric disorders and have not found them."[12]

From the founding of the APA in 1844 to today, psychiatrists have struggled with ignorance. What was unknown before is unknown now. An understanding of the causal mechanisms of mental illness, what historian Gerald Grob calls psychiatry's "holy grail,"[13] remains beyond psychiatrists' grasp. The hunt goes on.

The fruitless search for answers has placed psychiatry in an ever precarious position. Professions are granted authority on the basis of their ability to convince others that they possess the requisite knowledge and skill to intervene in well-defined problems.[14] They are accorded monopoly over work, mainly by state authorities, by staking claim to specialized expertise inaccessible to those outside the profession.[15] Ignorance threatens this professional authority. It strikes at the very justification for professional authority. It erodes trust and undermines vouchsafing. The problems posed by ignorance are most immediate for consulting professions, like psychiatry, which are tasked with not just developing knowledge, but also *doing* something.[16] They are judged on both the content of their knowledge claims, as well as the "good results" they obtain in solving practical problems for their clientele, often under conditions of great urgency. If knowledge is the "currency" of professional power,[17] ignorance reflects something akin to a system of credit. Professions borrow credibility on the promise of repaying this trust in the future. Support a profession today and tomorrow one's trust will be rewarded when it fills its knowledge gaps and, in turn, improves its efficacy in solving problems under its jurisdiction. But should a profession violate these terms—should its ignorance persist or become glaring—these debts can be called in for collection.

All professions must manage the threat of ignorance. But perhaps no other profession has suffered its slings and arrows more so than psychiatry. For this reason, confessions of ignorance in psychiatric discourse are often joined with forecasts of professional calamity. Psychiatrists find themselves regularly at a "crossroads"[18] or in "crisis."[19] The hoped-for resolution of its ignorance focuses psychiatrists' dreams, but their minds are ever preoccupied by nightmares of never obtaining it.

Psychiatry's ignorance comprises two related, but distinct, dimensions. First, there is its *ontological* dimension, namely, psychiatry's inability to pin down the essence of its object. Psychiatry struggles with what mental distress actually is. Are mental disorders equivalent to medical diseases or something distinct altogether? What causes mental distress? Where is the line between normal and abnormal behavior? Tentative, temporary agreements over ontological assumptions have emerged on occasion, but consensus has never been reached and any agreement has been fragile and precarious. As such, psychiatry's ontological assumptions have shifted over time, regularly. This shifting ontology is evident in the ever-changing nomenclature and labels that psychiatrists have affixed to their object over time. They have called it "madness," "insanity," "maladjustment," "neurosis," "mental illness," "mental disorders," and so on.[20] Mental distress appears ever ripe for reinterpretation. The second dimension of psychiatry's ignorance is *epistemological*, involving concerns over the nature of psychiatric knowledge. Epistemological assumptions are ancillary to knowledge claims. These assumptions involve second-order issues like the criteria by which communities discriminate between true and false claims, their definition of what constitutes knowledge, and their understanding of what an acceptable theory should look like.[21] Upon these assumptions, communities develop the taken-for-granted conventions (e.g., what constitutes "good" data, sound methods, legitimate kinds of questions and explanations, etc.) that enable the production and adjudication of knowledge claims. Psychiatry, however, has been unable to settle on the appropriate way of knowing its object. Instead, it has vacillated between drastically different *visions* of knowledge, or "styles of reasoning."[22] It is hard to build a knowledge base when research methods, evidentiary standards, and modes of argumentation are transformed by each generation of reformers.

The ontological and epistemological elements of psychiatry's ignorance are self-reinforcing. How one conceives of an object shapes how one goes about investigating it, and conversely, how one studies something shapes the very construction of that object. Unable to reach enduring consensus on questions related to either of these dimensions, psychiatry descends into deep confusion.

The result is perpetual insecurity and precariousness, a profession that is "always, so it seems, but a step away from a profound crisis of legitimacy," observes sociologist Andrew Scull.[23] Other medical specialties can make more credible claims to progress; they have accomplishments to point to as indicators of the accumulation of knowledge. Psychiatry, however, has amassed a frustrating record of failure, of false starts and dead ends. With progress so slow, insights so few, and uncertainty so tenacious, psychiatry is propelled less by the accumulation of its knowledge and more by the stubbornness of its ignorance.

And yet, despite the intransigence of its ignorance, psychiatry survives.

This book addresses a simple question: Why do we have psychiatry? It does not pose this question flippantly or disparagingly. There are plenty of antipsychiatry screeds out there.[24] This is not one of them. To the contrary, I ask this question as a serious puzzle in need of explanation. My intent is not to condemn, but to explain the resiliency of American psychiatry. Faced with a perplexing object, psychiatry has developed some compelling working hypotheses and even some effective treatments. Patients sometimes get better; their suffering is sometimes relieved. On balance, however, the psychiatric project has been a curious endeavor riddled with contradiction and conflict, one with few triumphs and many setbacks. Psychiatrists have committed horrifying abuses and then turned a blind eye to these horrors. They have also sat with patients in the throes of delusions and offered an empathetic hearing. They have joined an air of quackery with expressions of genuine sympathy for society's most marginalized. They have been prone to hyperbolic optimism toward the newest fads and then shock when such fads prove empty, or, worse, harm those under their care. Psychiatry endures lurid exposés of its abuses, surges of antipsychiatry sentiment, the abandonment of allies, withering institutions, and regular declarations of its impending death. Still, it perseveres.

To comprehend this perseverance, we must do more than lament the limits of psychiatry's knowledge or criticize the expansiveness of all that it does not know. We must understand how psychiatry has dealt with its ignorance.

The Many-Faced Profession

While the persistence of its ignorance is the most notable feature of psychiatry, there is another striking aspect of its history. American psychiatry has undergone numerous radical transformations over its nearly two-century existence. Over time, psychiatry's core identity has mutated in fundamental ways. Mid-nineteenth-century superintendents fancied themselves to be benevolent fathers who calmed the frayed nerves of their patients in the regimented environment of the asylum. This identity gave way to early twentieth-century eclectic pragmatists, who under "psychobiology" sought to integrate the mind and body to assuage maladjustments. Psychobiology engendered a subsequent era of division. In the next generation, psychiatry became a divided profession, composed of crude, lobotomizing somatists, on the one hand, and Freudian psychoanalysts, on the other. Today, psychiatry has been reconstituted as an aspiring medical science. Contemporary psychiatrists fancy themselves as correcting chemical imbalances in the brain through the prescription of psychopharmaceutical drugs. This contemporary version of psychiatry dates only to the 1980s, and even it is fraying.

Taken together, psychiatry's changing identities manifest a disjointed, cyclical history "that has alternated between enthusiastic optimism and fatalistic pessimism."[25] Crises give birth to entirely new paradigms, new identities, and new ways of thinking about mental distress. When the various promises lead to dead ends, a professional crisis erupts. In response, psychiatric reformers shift gears and, fueled by often ostentatious hype, pursue another course. As before, when the promised breakthroughs never materialize, malaise sets in. Disappointment and nihilism are followed by another crisis, and eventually, another reinvention. The cycle repeats anew every few decades.

These drastic transformations create challenges for those trying to make sense of psychiatry *as a whole*. Are there commonalities running through psychiatry's many faces and metamorphoses? Beyond sharing a professional organization—itself often reformed and renamed—psychiatry has lacked the consistency of other professional projects. Its history is messy, unwieldy, and resistant to neat narration. Narrative coherence is hard to come by when one's protagonist keeps changing character.

Psychiatry is hard to pin down. The historical scholarship on psychiatry is contentious and fractured. It consists of many different psychiatries, rival depictions so divergent from one another that they can appear to be of different professions altogether. Among these many depictions, one encounters psychiatrists as: managers of stultifying "total institutions"; beleaguered but ennobled humanitarians; indecisive inheritors of the Cartesian dualism who are divided by "two minds"; members of a "psy" discipline constituting a modern soul in order to govern it; and agents of social control, wielding the label of mental illness to police deviance.[26] Some of this bewildering diversity can be explained away by the different eras under study. Because psychiatry's identity has changed so fundamentally over its different eras, it is not surprising that the period a historian selects for examination colors her characterization of the profession. Some incarnations of psychiatry, like the asylum era or the current period, are more amenable to sympathetic renderings. Others are more obviously condemnable, like hospital psychiatry and its callous lobotomies. Still others are ripe for mocking ridicule, like psychoanalysts and their prattling dream analyses. But the lack of historical consensus of psychiatrists runs deeper. Historians of the same period, often using the very same data, can arrive at wildly different portrayals. For example, take one of the most studied periods of psychiatry—the asylum era. In the historical scholarship of this period, asylum superintendents assume a variety of identities that often contradict one another. They are variously depicted as well-intentioned reformers; disciplining agents denying madness its voice; bearers of utopian dreams that a well-organized asylum could meliorate the disruptions brought upon by modern society; administrators who inspired a "generous confidence" in the families of the mentally ill that went unfulfilled; professionals imposing controls congruent to the imperatives of modern capitalism; misogynists affixing designations of madness to subordinate women; and flawed advocates for the mentally ill undone by social forces beyond their control.[27]

The confusion over the basic character of psychiatry is compounded by the unusually polemical and contentious nature of the historical scholarship on psychiatry. Broadly speaking, the histories tend to congregate along two poles. On one end of the spectrum sit a small band of laudatory, "meliorist" depictions. While not necessarily Pollyannaish, meliorist historians paint a generally positive picture; psychiatrists are portrayed as intrepid scientists trying their best to carry out an impossible task, sometimes waylaid, but over time making incremental progress. On the other end of the spectrum resides a larger group of critical, "revisionist" accounts, inspired by philosopher Michel Foucault and social control theorists. Revisionist historians deem psychiatrists as agents of repression imposing a narrow view of normality upon individuals that respectable society deems deviant. Such polarization leaves little common ground for anyone trying to suss the moral of psychiatry's story.[28] Psychiatry's essence, it seems, is in the eye of the historian beholding.

Today, the historical pendulum has swung toward critical revisionist accounts. While psychiatry retains its boosters and sympathizers, most contemporary analyses trade on psychiatry's conspicuous abuses to frame it in a critical light. For better or worse, psychiatry has become a low-hanging fruit for those stressing the unscientific nature of much of medical practice and seeking to draw the links between knowledge and power.[29] Such critical depictions have merit. Psychiatry *has* served the interests of those in power. It *has* granted oppressive actions an air of legitimacy and a veneer of scientific respectability. It *has* been used to dismiss and dismantle resistance by pathologizing it and labeling it as crazy. Psychiatrists have transformed fleeing slaves into mad sufferers of drapetomania, nonconforming women into irrational neurotics beset with "penis envy," and homosexuals into deviants in need of reprogramming, to cite but a few examples. Legion and undeniable, these abuses demand historical accounting. But still, one wonders, do these morality tales of psychiatry as wicked capture the profession in all its complexity? After all, if things were so straightforward, if psychiatry were abjectly evil, its endurance would be nothing short of miraculous.

Most histories of psychiatry, be they of the meliorist or revisionist variety, share a common problem. They imbue psychiatry with too much coherence. One comes away from these histories with the misperception that psychiatry has had a clear program and agenda, as well as the capacity and discipline to carry out this program—for good or bad. In other words, the various histories of psychiatry give the impression that psychiatrists (1) know what they are doing; and (2) do it effectively, however honorably or nefariously. This gives psychiatry far too much credit. It elides its perpetual insecurity, its internal contradictions, and, most importantly, its basic ignorance. Psychiatrists grope in the dark for answers that elude them. Our histories of the profession should reflect this.

In this book, I uncover the thread that holds psychiatry's many faces together. My intent is not to heap yet another psychiatry upon the mountain of existing ones. Rather, I intend to overcome existing problems in the historical scholarship on psychiatry discussed above. I discard any pretense that psychiatry possesses, or has possessed, some grand program. Instead, I emphasize psychiatry's pattern of what I call "muddling through," its drifting through uncertainty, confusion, and crises. Instead of suppressing psychiatry's contradictions to fit some prefab narrative, I elevate them to a central place in the analysis in a way that eschews easy answers and pat explanations. Psychiatrists have been agents of power plagued by real impotence. They are marginalized among medical professions, and yet, they have traded on the prestige of medicine to solidify their own authority. Psychiatrists have performed horrendous treatments in the name of compassion. They have made brash claims while maintaining an inferiority complex. At root, psychiatry is an insecure profession, asserting its authority on the basis of its expertise, all the while knowing that such claims are built on the shakiest of intellectual foundations.

A Study in Ignorance

To capture psychiatry in all its shades and contradictions, I take a step back from its various incarnations to observe the bigger picture. Doing so allows me to home in on the animating force driving psychiatric reforms, the problem to which its recurrent transformations have become the de facto solution.

The continuity in all this seeming discontinuity is a profession plagued with and trying to negotiate that which it does not know. Ignorance is *the* consistent driving force behind the history of American psychiatry. The resilience of psychiatry is a testament to its more or less successful management of its basic ignorance, its ability to mitigate its effects and stave off a final reckoning. Consequently, understanding psychiatry requires a sophisticated analysis of ignorance.

We have a knotty relationship with ignorance. This is manifest in our aphorisms, be they religious, academic, or popular. Common sense treats ignorance as a problem, a lack or void that needs to be filled. We might recognize some of its blessings (e.g., "ignorance is bliss"), but generally we are coached against ignorance and warned of its dangers.

Such warnings have broad roots in Western culture. In Proverbs (19:2), the Bible preaches that the soul "without knowledge" is "not good"; ignorance hastens one's feet toward sin and mortal corruption. Still, these ancient aphorisms were often balanced by an appreciation of awe in the face of an unknowable divine, the sense of wonder that comes with the recognition of the limits of one's knowing. This balance was thrown out of whack in response to intellectual trends in the seventeenth century. Amid the tumult of religious wars, European thinkers jettisoned religious mysticism, now derided as superstition, as well as the messy humanist tradition that accommodated uncertainty. These were supplanted by an uncompromising commitment to rationality, embodied in Cartesian thought and the subsequent philosophical quest for certainty.[30] In so doing, Enlightenment thinkers constructed a rigid opposition between knowledge and ignorance.[31] Knowledge became associated with light, virtue, and mastery; ignorance was tied to darkness, incivility, and moral failing. Shorn of most of its wonder, ignorance became bad. It was to be avoided at all cost, dispensed with when possible, repressed when not. As inheritors of these Enlightenment ideals and residents of a disenchanted modernity, we cast a leery eye on ignorance, often glossing over the chasm of that which we do not know with false bravado and an insatiable will to accumulate more knowledge. If, as noted by Francis Bacon, "knowledge is power," ignorance is weakness to be conquered in its pursuit.

Having lost some of ignorance's more charming and beneficial features, contemporary Western common sense merges ancient wisdom, Enlightenment thought, and current axioms to tell a consistent tale of ignorance. And it plays the villain. Ignorance is "the mother of all evils" (François Rabelais). It emerges from sloth, deception, and delusion. Yet, despite these origins in weakness, ignorance is itself "bold" (Thucydides); it "more frequently begets confidence than does knowledge" (Charles Darwin). "Nothing is so firmly believed as that which we least know," observes Michel de Montaigne. False confidence, born from ignorance, can secure misbegotten and illegitimate achievements. Mark Twain sardonically quips, "All you need in this life is ignorance and confidence, then success is sure." Friedrich Nietzsche is less sure that ignorance breeds worldly success. For him, the "firm dome of ignorance" keeps people docile, blinking, conforming sheep. But whether ignorance is seen as powerful or weak, its general effects are depicted as catastrophic. Ignorance is "the most violent element in society" (Emma Goldman). Evil "almost always comes of ignorance" (Albert Camus), and "nothing in the world is more dangerous than sincere ignorance and conscientious stupidity" (Martin Luther King Jr.). When joined with the mechanisms of power, ignorance is "the most ferocious enemy justice can have" (James A. Baldwin); if we allow it to become our master, "there is no possibility of real peace" (Dalai Lama). The cultural message comes through clear as day; ignorance must be eradicated. Or, as Cotton Mather, never one for subtlety, cried, "Ah! destructive Ignorance, what shall be done to chase thee out of the World!"

The hegemonic notion of ignorance as bad, however, is not total. One can still find glimmers of contradictions. As inconsistent beings, we hold aphorisms that work at cross-purposes. Below the cacophony condemning ignorance is a quieter countertradition, whispered by those who go against the negative grain. This provides the raw materials for a reclamation of ignorance. Confucius and Socrates held that the height of knowledge was an appreciation of one's own ignorance. Religious thinkers have long valorized the virtues of awe and humility, what one anonymous Christian mystic referred to as the "cloud of unknowing," in the face of the incomprehensible divine. Nicolas Cusanus, German theologian and humanist of this apophatic tradition, sings of "learned ignorance" as the highest ideal of faith. For aesthetes like Oscar Wilde, ignorance is shot through with romanticism. Its childlike awe needs to be protected and incubated, not eliminated and murdered: "I do not approve of anything that tampers with natural ignorance. Ignorance is like a delicate exotic fruit; touch it and the bloom is gone." Even today, ignorance is a tool for conceiving a more just and ethical society à la the useful thought experiment of "the veil of ignorance."[32]

Nevertheless, the scales of Western culture tip decisively toward the negative. The minority voices, the contrarians for ignorance, are overwhelmed. Ignorance is something bad to be overcome.

The general condemnation of ignorance—and the understanding of it as a simple lack—has stultified research on it. Philosophers, historians, and social scientists have said far less about ignorance than they have about knowledge. Harboring deep uneasiness toward ignorance, they duck it altogether, relegating it to irrelevance, as a topic unworthy of serious scholarship. Knowledge is exalted and examined; ignorance is denigrated and disregarded.

Recently, however, some researchers have taken up the banner of ignorance, embracing ignorance as an object of analysis in its own right. Coming from a variety of disciplines and operating under diverse banners—"agnatology," the "sociology of the non-knowledge," the "sociology of ignorance," or simply "ignorance studies"[33]—these researchers share the common goal of correcting our collective ignorance of ignorance by subjecting it to rigorous study.[34] They view ignorance as something more than an empty negative. It has a presence in its own right, which, while related to knowledge, operates according to its own distinct dynamics.[35] Moreover, ignorance is neither deviant nor exceptional, but omnipresent. The universe of ignorance is far vaster than that of knowledge. We swim in its sea. In order to accomplish anything, we must navigate its swells, its ebbs and flows. Because all human endeavors invariably run up against the vicissitudes of ignorance, people are always "negotiating, calculating, or playfully experimenting with what is known and what is not known."[36] Consequently, the study of ignorance is essential to any account of human action.

By resisting the tendency to reduce ignorance to the mere lack of knowledge, ignorance researchers reveal the distinct features and contours of ignorance as well as its prominent role in shaping human action. They have opened up opportunities for identifying and exploring different *kinds* of ignorance. Indeed, much of the initial research in ignorance studies has focused on categorizing and cataloging the array of ignorances. In doing so, researchers have produced a dizzying proliferation of terms and typologies constructed around a handful of key distinctions.[37] They differentiate ignorance on the basis of its recognition, or ignorance that is known and acknowledged versus ignorance of which people are unaware. Related to the issue of recognition, researchers categorize ignorance according to the motivations behind it: intentional, willful ignorance versus unintentional ignorance. Ignorance can also be differentiated according to perceptions regarding its potential scrutability, or ignorance that is temporary and conquerable versus ignorance that is permanent as a matter of property. Finally, some researchers distinguish ignorance according to its effects: ignorance that is functional and yields valued effects (e.g., as "a prelude to problem-solving"[38]) versus ignorance that is dysfunctional and problematic. This impetus to draw distinctions between types of ignorance has even found its way into popular discourse. In an infamous press conference on the Iraq War and the issue of weapons of mass destruction, US Secretary of Defense Donald Rumsfeld stated: "There are known unknowns; that is to say there are things we know we don't know. But there are also unknown unknowns—there are things we do not know we don't know." In the politically charged context of the Iraq War, Rumsfeld was mocked for his comments. He was prevaricating. But in delimiting different types of ignorance, the man had a point.

The unpacking of different kinds of ignorance is not just an exercise in classification and description. It has deeper analytical implications in that it primes researchers to pay attention to the distinct political dynamics that follow from certain types of ignorance. We need to explore the different uses to which ignorance is applied as well as the differing effects ignorance can have. And it turns out that some of these uses and effects are counterintuitive, running contrary to the prevailing common sense of ignorance as bad. Indeed, much of most insightful and provocative work coming out of ignorance studies focuses on cases of so-called strategic ignorance, or ignorance that is embraced and cultivated for political gain.[39] Ignorance researchers also highlight the productive role of ignorance in driving scientific inquiry.[40] Such counterintuitive analyses stress that ignorance's effects are not inherently negative to those who bear it. Ignorance interacts with, and affects, social action in complicated ways. Moreover, its effects in any given case are shaped by the particular perceptions of it, perceptions that emerge from the dynamic struggle over how ignorance is defined, framed, and understood.

The analysis in this book falls under the purview of ignorance studies but examines ignorance from a slightly different angle. Whereas much of ignorance studies has focused on atypical, counterintuitive ignorance, I examine a more prevalent (and perhaps more prosaic) form of ignorance, one that resonates more with our popular conception of ignorance as bad. In examining the history of psychiatry, I focus on ignorance that is unintentional and unwanted but nevertheless acknowledged, or, in other words, a "known unknown." Ignorance is a problem for psychiatry, one that has threatened its very existence. The response to this problem is what most interests me. Psychiatric ignorance is not outright denied or ignored; psychiatrists think about it, talk about it, and mold and massage it in order to maintain their professional authority. The endurance of psychiatry despite its visible and persistent ignorance reflects a measure of success in these efforts.

Psychiatry's survival underscores that ignorance is not destiny, that the ramifications of ignorance are determined, *not by the state of being in ignorance but in the machinations and actions that follow in its wake.* It is to these machinations that I turn, focusing on what I term the "collective management of ignorance." Once identified, people attempt to interpret their ignorance so as to mitigate its negative effects. How ignorance is represented—as temporary, as necessary, as damning, and so on—shapes the consequences that follow from it. And this representation is an emergent property of the struggle between interested parties. Thus, I am not interested in judging psychiatric ignorance, but rather in examining how *psychiatrists* have managed it so as to achieve professional success.

Throughout its existence, psychiatry has been haunted by a known unknown, its inability to comprehend the basic essence of its object. But the implications of this ignorance have never been settled or obvious. Instead, they have arisen from the unfolding efforts on the part of subsequent generations of psychiatric reformers to define this ignorance as temporary. Faced with the potential professional fallout from its ignorance, American psychiatrists have responded by depicting it as temporary, a negative to be sure but not damning. They have framed their ignorance as a problem in need of remedy, but have held fast to the belief that the remedy exists. In other words, mental distress is deemed a known unknown that is knowable. Psychiatrists have waited for this eventual insight, sometimes resolute, sometimes wavering, but ever expecting its arrival.

Managing Ignorance via Reinvention

Ignorance complicates knowledge-producing endeavors. This is especially true for professions where the marriage of expert knowledge and the pressure to act can make the challenges posed by ignorance acute. And yet, despite the centrality of ignorance as an issue, most histories and analyses of professions focus myopically on knowledge. This oversight must be addressed. Professional authority is not a result of knowledge accumulation alone; it stems the interplay between knowledge and ignorance and how professions negotiate and balance the tensions between the two.

While all professions grapple with non-knowledge, no struggle is as profound as psychiatry's. Psychiatry is steeped in ignorance. Attempts to pin down a basic understanding of its object have been in vain. Moreover, the problem faced by psychiatry is not just the absence of knowledge, but the apparent surfeit of its ignorance. Its ignorance has been uniquely evident. Psychiatry's failings have been exceptionally public, splashed as they often are on the front pages of major news outlets. Ignorance, therefore, is inescapable for psychiatrists, an ever-present concern, always lurking and threatening to expose them.

Given the depth and breadth of psychiatric ignorance, it is no wonder then that psychiatry has not followed the typical professional trajectory. When compared to the modern medical profession generally—the archetype for theories of professionalization—psychiatry's path to professionalization has been fraught. Other medical specialties have obtained tremendous clout. Psychiatry, on the other hand, has been perpetually insecure, always on the precipice of a crisis and ever at a crossroads, scrambling to ward off challengers and to defuse recurrent antipsychiatry sentiments. In other words, its professional authority has been shot through with heavy uncertainty. Thus, while the trappings of psychiatric power are similar to other professions (professional organizations, specialized training, certification, government policies, etc.), how it secured these trappings—and how it maintains them—are not.

How has psychiatry achieved professional success in the face of its ignorance? To answer this question, we must turn to its collective management of ignorance. One obvious way to manage ignorance is to deny its existence. But, contrary to what we might expect, psychiatry has not ignored its ignorance. There is an extensive and ongoing discussion of ignorance within psychiatric discourse. While psychiatrists might downplay their ignorance and/or exaggerate their knowledge, psychiatry's known unknowns have never been denied or outright suppressed. The reasons for this are many and complicated. In part, denial is not an option because psychiatry's critics have been so successful in drawing attention to its ignorance. In part, it is because psychiatry's scandals have been uncommonly public and recurrent. And in part, the lack of recourse to denial reflects a degree of intellectual humility by psychiatrists. Psychiatrists deserve credit for being forthcoming about what they do not know, whatever their motivations for doing so. Regardless of the cause, however, outright denial has never been a tenable strategy for psychiatrists. Perhaps effective in the short term, it has always been accompanied by a short expiration date.

Rather than deny their ignorance, psychiatrists have tried to tame it. Once ignorance has been identified, it is incumbent upon bearers of that ignorance to frame it in a way that mitigates its effects (or at least defers them). The solution that psychiatrists have hit upon in response to ignorance is reinvention. Reinvention is a process, containing cultural and organizational dimensions, by which reformers have transformed the fundamental purpose and character of the profession, so much so that it appears to be something new altogether. Psychiatry's reinventions have been comprehensive. They have involved reconstitutions of psychiatry's identity under entirely new guises. New styles of reasoning take hold. New organizations are created. And new hopes are conjured from the ashes of the old ones.[41] It is crucial to note that these reinventions are driven less by developments in knowledge, and more by a desire to mitigate the deleterious consequences of ignorance.

In resorting to reinvention often, psychiatry has created a cyclical, repetitive history. When a crisis emerges and psychiatry's ignorance is exposed, psychiatric reformers frame these failures as stemming not from unattainable knowledge but from the improper conceptualization of its object and misguided assumptions underlying its research agenda. Given the insolvable problems with this agenda, the solution proposed is complete reinvention. By reformulating its foundations and assumptions, psychiatric reformers transform their profession. And these transformations happen regularly. Unlike the medicine generally, which has undergone a single revolution once over the past two hundred years, psychiatry regularly undergoes them, to the tune of one roughly every thirty to forty years. The cyclical reinventions of psychiatry have been sweeping, involving a wholesale reimaging of the identity of the profession, the nature of its knowledge, and the working conceptualization of what constitutes its object. Indeed, psychiatry's cyclical reinventions have been so all-encompassing that one generation's understanding of the psychiatric project would be unrecognizable to prior or subsequent generations.

Therefore, while psychiatry's foundations have been altered extensively, ever shape-shifting, the professional playbook has remained remarkably consistent. Reinvention is the through line of psychiatry's curious history. The very transformations that vex historians and thwart a consistent picture of psychiatry from emerging turn out, in a curious way, to be the very source of psychiatry's continuity. What looks like chaos is rendered coherent when seen as a consistent professional response to recalcitrant ignorance. Faced with its persistent ignorance, psychiatry reinvents itself, over and over.

At its core, reinvention serves a central function for psychiatrists looking to maintain their authority in the face of their ignorance. It allows psychiatrists to frame their ignorance as *unknown but knowable* rather than *unknown and unknowable*. Psychiatrists recognize and acknowledge their ignorance, but neutralize it by framing it as temporary in nature. In doing so, ignorance is treated as an epistemic problem, one that requires better knowledge or better intellectual programs, as opposed to an ontological problem, or ignorance that is a result of the property of its object. This is a crucial distinction; the implications of drawing it are monumental professionally, involving nothing less than the maintenance of professional power. If its ignorance is temporary, we might be frustrated by psychiatry's failures and dead ends, but still hold out hope for the future. We might even admire psychiatry's doggedness in the pursuit of knowledge. But if we understand its ignorance to be permanent, that there is something inherently unknowable about mental illness, psychiatry becomes something of a Sisyphean task, destined to end in failure. We might react with pity or scorn, but either way, permanent ignorance compromises psychiatry's claims to expertise, its professional authority, and its entire legitimacy.

Playing the Expectations Game

Drawing the distinction between psychiatric ignorance that is permanent versus ignorance that is temporary has depended on the construction and dissemination of certain expectations. Reinvention plays the expectations game, because psychiatrists' management of ignorance is an intensely future-oriented business. If one anticipates the endurance of ignorance, of more of the same, then the justification for psychiatry is compromised. But if one has reason to expect that things will be different—that the future will indeed be brighter—then psychiatry can secure some benefit of the doubt and a deferral of final reckoning. Given enough patience, hard work, and the appropriate reforms, insight is posited as just around the corner.

Increasingly, social scientists[42] are becoming attuned to the ways in which social action is shaped by expectations. It turns out that what we do, the courses we pursue, are determined in great part by the expectations we cultivate, our projections into the future. The future, of course, is fundamentally unknowable, but this does not mean that people do not speculate and project into it. In doing so, the future can be "mobilized in real time to marshal resources, coordinate activities and manage uncertainty."[43] Such future projections entail the social construction of expectations through processes social scientists call "promissory practices" or "techniques of prospection."[44] These expectations have generative dimension, in that they guide and coordinate activities in the present aimed at securing the articulated future.[45] They are "forceful fictions."[46] Expectations lay out promises and incentives for particular courses of action. In doing so, they secure the investments and obligations for such an action, which, in turn, can bring about the very vision of the future being predicted.

In the study of expectations, particularly the role they play in technological innovation, researchers have identified what they term the "hype/disappointment cycle."[47] Essentially, to create expectations and win a hearing, advocates of change must generate a certain amount of hype for their proposals.[48] Hype engenders the excitement necessary to overcome the status quo. Of central importance to the dynamics of the hype/disappointment cycle is that hype itself can have significant social effects, regardless of whether it is ever realized. Expectations do not have to be actually fulfilled to achieve a measure of success; they can be enough in and of themselves to secure resources, mobilize actors, induce action, and change the course of history.[49] This is because by the time expectations come up for assessment, they have already achieved the reforms needed to bring about something akin to the future articulated (even if in a bastardized form). In other words, expectations can accomplish much even if they ultimately disappoint. And, once instituted, such changes take on their own inertia. Sunk costs become justification for staying the new course in the face of growing disappointment. As such, the specter of disappointment is not much of a check on the tendency to overpromise. In fact, disappointment is almost inevitable because hype has to be so exaggerated in order to gain attention and momentum. Results rarely achieve the grandiose expectations by which they were initially sold. Over time, this hype/disappointment dynamic can damage the credibility and reputation of a field; there seems to be an inherent limit to the number of times a field can overpromise and dissatisfy. But in the short term, in the face of present uncertainty and indeterminacy, a hyped future of certain success, however illusory, can work masterfully in prompting changes that can have widespread ramifications. In this way, expectations mold the future in their image.

This dynamic between hope and disappointment has played out countless times in the history of psychiatry. On a small scale, every proposed innovation of psychiatry, every new treatment, succumbs to its logic. For example, lobotomy was introduced to great hype in the 1940s, promising a cure for the most intractable cases of mental illness. Advocates of the procedure generated expectations that it would solve the vast problems in hospital psychiatry. Many bought what these advocates were selling and altered their treatment accordingly. The hype, as we now know, proved to be wrong, but it alone altered the course of the profession in a disturbing way (see chapter 4 for more discussion). On a larger scale, the hype/disappointment cycle undergirds every reinvention. Psychiatric reformers have tapped hype to advocate for wholesale transformations of the profession. Given the depth of psychiatry's ignorance and the existential nature of its regular crises, this hype has conveyed the sense of decisive action, when tinkering on the margins would not suffice. Every generation of reformers indulges in hype and has "gone big" to generate the expectation that psychiatric ignorance would be resolved if their proposed reinvention were embraced. Gaining support and instituting changes, they have been able to reconstitute their profession on the basis of an imagined future. Once secured, reinvention staves off psychiatry's reckoning; the expectations buy time and provide reformers with the breathing room to rebuild psychiatry's knowledge base anew. Gradually, however, clouds of disappointment gather as the reality fails to mesh with the reinvention's shiny promises. Ignorance rears its head yet again, leading to another professional crisis to be assuaged by yet another reinvention secured by brash hype.

Thus, playing to the future by constructing expectations is a core feature of psychiatric reinventions. But reinvention also entails addressing the past. Reformers reinterpret the past in such a way as to justify dramatic reforms. The construction of a bright future is accompanied by, and juxtaposed with, a dark reconceptualization of the past. The framing of ignorance as "unknown at this time but knowable" (given the proper reforms, of course) locates the responsibility for ignorance at the feet of reformers' misguided forebearers. Rather than an inherent property of mental distress, psychiatric ignorance is depicted as the by-product of bad psychiatry—and bad psychiatric thinking—that must be relegated to the dustbin of history. The only solution is to move on and not look back. In this way, reformers reset psychiatry's "historical chronometer at zero."[50] Current and future generations of psychiatrists are not to be held accountable for the sins of their fathers. This reframing of the past is conspicuous throughout psychiatric discourse. Psychiatrists regularly discuss their history, not in a triumphalist way, but to hold the past up as an "other" against which the current era is defined.

Thus, reinvention inserts a useful discontinuity into the trajectory of the profession. It redirects attention away from the ignorant past and the confused present, toward a hyped future of promise.[51] Clinging to future expectation, reformers have rescued psychiatry from irrelevance, over and over, only to repeat the cycle anew when the promised payoff fails to arrive.

A Habitual Response to a Habitual Problem

It would be wrong to think of reinvention as a conscious, *general* strategy that psychiatrists draw upon time after time to dupe the public and mute their critics. Certainly, at the level of individual reforms of any particular era, reformers pursue a *particular* reinvention consciously. These are planned reforms secured via strategic thinking. Each generation of reformers sought out to shift the course of the profession in a particular direction. They might not have conceived of their plans in grandiose terms, but the plans were undertaken with this aim. Still, reformers have understood their actions in a circumscribed fashion, as a *specific* solution to a time-bound problem in front of reformers, and *not as* part of a cumulative history of reinventions or a patterned response to the ongoing problem of managing ignorance. And each reinvention has been posited as the *last* reform, the one that will finally overcome ignorance.

The repeated recourse to reinvention *over the long term*, however, reflects something less conscious, something more instinctual, default, knee-jerk. One reinvention is a planned endeavor. Multiple, repeated reinventions are a pattern reflecting something altogether different. Rather than viewing these reinventions as a single overarching strategy—an idea that carries connotations of deliberate planning or even cynical scheming—I understand reinvention as an engrained collective habit, acquired and cultivated over time in psychiatrists' response to their fundamental ignorance.[52] Through experience and socialization, people acquire "predisposition[s] to ways or modes of response" to their environment and the challenges presented therein.[53] These habits entail a low level of conscious reflection.[54] They are akin to the default settings by which social actors respond to challenges. Through them, the past gets encoded in the present, leaving traces through the repetitions of particular responses.

Reinvention has become the habitual reaction of psychiatrists to their ignorance in times of crisis. This habit is the legacy of psychiatry's history, its formative experiences, and its core challenges, which, over time, has hardened into a reflex that persists despite its apparent defects. Although it occasionally becomes an object of overt discussion in psychiatric discourse, more typically it remains a predilection than a deliberate strategy.

This is not to suggest that reinvention is fixed or rote. The hues and character of this habit change and evolve. Each subsequent reinvention changes and adapts in response to the failures of the past and the particular demands of the present. Each is pursued by different means, using different tactics, by reformers wielding different styles of reasoning, different understandings of mental illness, different suites of concepts, and even different conceptualizations of what it means to be a psychiatrist. Nevertheless, while the *content* of each particular reinvention maintains its own specificity, its *form*, as a response to ignorance, remains the same, playing out in a repeated pattern. Crisis, reinvention, crisis, reinvention, crisis, reinvention, on and on and on.

The end result is a profession whose entire trajectory is shaped by its persistent problem of ignorance and the habit of reinvention that it enacts in response to this problem. Asylum superintendents, once offering utopian dreams of managed mental illness, gave way to eclectic psychobiological electric reformers, attempting to merge psychiatry with neurology, modern medicine, and public health to escape the provincial naïveté of superintendent forbearers. Psychobiology, which yielded clutter and confusion, was supplanted by psychoanalysis, which promised to unveil the subterranean drives of humanity's consciousness. Again these promises went unfulfilled, and ignorance remained. A new generation of reformers stepped into the breach, armed with a new diagnostic system and new drugs, promising (once again) to achieve a valid understanding of mental disorders. Thirty years in, this has produced little progress. It is being challenged by yet another new vision, this time constructed around neuroscience, in which the unlocking of the brain through new imaging technologies will—you guessed it—secure true understanding of the basic mechanisms of mental distress. The expectations for this neuro-turn are high, the eventual outcome to be determined.

Psychiatry never overcomes its fundamental ignorance and its perpetual precariousness. Instead, it bides its time. The benefits it accrues from reinvention—namely, its survival—do not come without significant costs, costs that have become manifest in psychiatry's worst abuses. First, the desire to embrace the next new thing can lead to premature enthusiasm for unproven methods and treatments. In promoting its newest reinvention, psychiatrists can start to believe their own hype and get carried away in experimenting on the mentally ill with untested treatments. Egregious abuses like lobotomies, which seem unfathomable from today's perspective, are an unintended, but perhaps unsurprising, by-product of hype. Second, in positing a break with the past, reformers can be too quick to set aside useful insights from the past. These insights are rarely lost altogether, but they can lie dormant for unnecessary periods of time. In the interim, important lessons get lost. Psychiatry learns them, forgets them, and must relearn only to forget them again. Finally, over time, reinvention risks running afoul of its inherent limits. At some point, one would think, the lurchings from identity to identity would become unacceptable to the audiences they are meant to convince. Why should people continue to believe that this time will be different? Reinvention, therefore, is no panacea, no perfect solution to psychiatry's ignorance. It affords perseverance rather than flourishing.

Despite its limits, however, reinvention has staved off a more conclusive assessment of psychiatry's ignorance—that is, that mental distress is unknowable. As long as psychiatry can sell itself as possessing a viable means by which to resolve its ignorance, it retains a social function. It survives.

What Follows

Combining intellectual and professional history with the sociology of the professions, this book examines the dynamics between knowledge, ignorance, and politics to account for American psychiatry's peculiar trajectory, from its establishment to the present. In a habitual response to ignorance, psychiatric reformers have returned to reinvention over and over. As a result, psychiatry has staggered from vision to incommensurable vision. It never achieves its promises, but it does stay one step ahead of attempts to dismantle it. In a strange way, then, ignorance and reinvention comprise the consistent features of psychiatry's seemingly disjointed eras. They connect asylum superintendents and Freudian psychoanalysts, lobotomies and psychotherapy, Oedipal complexes and chemical imbalances, electroconvulsive therapy (ECT) and selective serotonin reuptake inhibitors (SSRIs), the drab campuses of mental hospitals and the buttonless couches of the psychoanalytic office, the frazzled neurotic and the deluded schizophrenic.

Before laying out my argument, it is important to note that the observation of these cycles of reinvention does not require taking a firm stance as to the actual status of the knowability of mental distress. Madness is an elusive thing. Psychiatry is tasked with explaining boundary conditions, social and emotional dilemmas that may be conceptualized as diseases, but are not quite diseases.[55] Mental distress has been, and remains, unknown. Of course, this could change tomorrow with some groundbreaking discovery. This possibility cannot be rejected out of hand, although psychiatry's track record would suggest it is unlikely. And neither can its opposite—that mental distress is fundamentally unknowable—be dismissed. A final reckoning on the stakes of psychiatry's central problematic—whether its ignorance is temporary or permanent—cannot be made. For this reason, I leave the issue as to the essential nature of mental disorders to the unfolding of time or to others more brazen than myself.[56] I am not interested in pinning down this essence, but in exploring how psychiatrists, in search of answers and authority, have negotiated their ignorance, with their livelihoods on the line, and in doing so, created ways for patients to be mentally ill. Whether mental illness is knowable matters less in understanding the history of American psychiatry than the fact that it is a known unknown that the profession has had to manage.

The story told in the following pages has been reconstructed from multiple data sources. Because I am concerned with how psychiatry sells its wares and manages its ignorance, I focus my attention on the official discourse by which leaders of the profession have done so. The backbone of the analysis is the *American Journal of Psychiatry* (*AJP*), the official organ of the profession that has been deemed the "best single source reference for tracing the development of organized psychiatry over the years."[57] I analyzed the *AJP* over its entire run from 1844 to the present as a means to index psychiatric thought as well as its professional politics. In terms of its content, I analyzed both programmatic statements (e.g., presidential addresses), for their overt assessments of psychiatry and articulations for future directions, as well as "typical" journal articles. The latter I examined less for their particular research findings and more as embodiments of a particular vision of psychiatry.[58] This record reveals not only the discourse on ignorance but also discussions on how to deal with it.

While the *AJP* grounds my exploration of psychiatric discourse, to capture the full breadth of this discourse, I supplemented this data with additional documentary evidence. These diverse materials include articles from other professional journals (e.g., *American Journal of Psychoanalysis, Archives of General Psychiatry, Journal of the American Medical Association*), influential books and textbooks, and institutional documents (e.g., annual reports from the state lunatic asylum in Utica, NY; reports from federal task forces). The final empirical chapter on contemporary psychiatry makes use of interviews I conducted with thirty mental health professionals involved in the revision to DSM-5, either as direct participants or as public critics.[59] The book also draws on a large secondary literature, mainly historical and sociological analyses of psychiatry. This impressive body of scholarship has been invaluable. It helped me fill out my own history and provided much-needed context for my discursive analysis of texts, often doing the difficult leg work that allowed me to home in on reconstructing the foundations for each reinvention.[60] Therefore, while much of the material in this book will be familiar to scholars interested in psychiatry and mental health, I provide an innovative framework to understand the history of psychiatry in all its complexity.

In selecting these materials for analysis, I have privileged what historian Richard Noll deems the "literary elite" of American psychiatry, the leaders of the profession who are the prime producers of psychiatric discourse and who, in turn, shape public opinion on matters related to mental distress.[61] This is intentional. The book is driven by questions pertaining to the professional politics of psychiatry and the collective response to its ignorance. My objectives led to an emphasis on what is sometimes referred to as "aspirational psychiatry," those who are concerned with "what psychiatry will look like in the future, about what will be contained in a 'final' psychiatric textbook, so to speak."[62] In psychiatry's encounters with ignorance, it has been the aspirations of elites that have ruled the day, determined the way forward, and justified the reinventions. Those who articulate and set the visions of the psychiatric project are therefore at the center of the analysis.

Every research decision comes with trade-offs. Achieving a depth of focus often involves foregoing breadth of coverage. In this case, my analysis has a tendency to de-emphasize two important groups. First, the focus on elite leaders of the profession leaves the experiences of countless working psychiatrists mostly unexamined. There is good reason to believe that this aspirational elite has often constituted a universe unto itself, and that the actual practice of psychiatry has diverged from the blueprints laid out by professional elites. I have tried to remain sensitive to the practices of psychiatry on the ground, but in detailing the aspirations of elite psychiatrists, the rank and file can get lost in the shuffle. Their hopes, joys, and disappointments are largely absent from this analysis. Second, the story recounted here is an internal one attuned to the inner workings of the profession of psychiatry in the United States. Of course, these workings have been influenced by outside forces and nonprofessional actors. I discuss these in relation to the internal dynamics of the profession, but they remain largely in the background.

Each chapter examines a particular reinvention of psychiatry and its implications for psychiatry's politics of ignorance. The chapters all open with a significant event that distills the particular challenges facing psychiatry during the period under discussion. Following this, the first half of each chapter describes the vision of psychiatry purported by reformers championing the reinvention, highlighting the expectations they proffered and the interventions they undertook to deliver on these expectations. Here, I discuss key facets of each reinvention: the tactical decisions by which reformers secure the reinvention, its ontological assumptions regarding the nature of mental distress, its epistemological commitment, its dominant modes of treatment, and its institutional and organizational infrastructure. The second half of each chapter examines the course of the reinvention and its culmination in a professional crisis. At their core, every crisis is born of the persistent problem of psychiatric ignorance, but each takes on its own flavor.

Thus, while the problem of ignorance traverses the entire history of psychiatry, each chapter recounts a distinct cycle within psychiatry's cyclical history of crisis–reinvention–crisis. Such a history reveals an unnerving lack of progress. However, this is not to suggest that psychiatry has not progressed at all, that it has been static, entombed in its own inescapable ignorance. Psychiatry has evolved, particularly in the means by which subsequent reformers have achieved their reinventions. The overall habit of reinvention has endured as the means by which psychiatry has achieved professional success despite its intellectual failures. But reinvention takes on a particular character during each period. Not only do the core assumptions, suites of concepts, and understandings of mental distress change, but so do the tactics and targets of these reform efforts. These changes are revealed in the chronological unfolding of the book's chapters.

Chapter 1 examines the emergence of ignorance as a problem out of the feigned certainty of the asylum era. It discusses the origins of psychiatry in the asylum, revealing psychiatrists' roots as superintendents charged with caring for those with serious mental illness. The chapter concludes with psychiatrists' first crisis—one that focused on the dissolution of the cult of curability—and their early conflict with neurologists. Chapter 2 explores the eclectic, pragmatic reinvention of psychiatry in the first decades of the twentieth century. Coming out of the failure of the asylum, reformers, led by Adolf Meyer, sought to overcome ignorance by investing in the broad program of psychobiology. The solution to ignorance that they proposed was an eclectic, multipronged psychiatry that pursued potential insights wherever they might lead. Under psychobiology, psychiatry spun out in multiple directions, and eventually fragmented into silos that undermined any sort of coherent vision. Chapter 2 reveals the pitfalls of trying to overcome ignorance through a broad program that refuses to cut off any possible avenues of exploration.

Chapter 3 recounts the rise and eventual fall of psychoanalysis in the United States. Coming out of the heady experiences of World War II, psychiatric leaders redefined psychiatry according to a distinct version of psychoanalysis based on ego psychology. Psychoanalytic reformers tried to manage ignorance by obscuring psychiatric knowledge; they constructed an elaborate, byzantine theoretical edifice and confined psychiatric knowing to physical/conceptual spaces accessible only to psychiatrists. Psychoanalysis maintained its dominance until the 1970s, when a fervent antipsychiatry movement emerged and spurred calls for greater transparency. Chapter 4 overlaps with chapter 3, in that it examines concurrent developments within institutional psychiatry. It focuses on the decades of the 1960s and 1970s and the emergence of psychiatry's brief and ill-fated attempt to pivot to the community. Community psychiatrists attempted to manage ignorance by diluting it, spreading it around to various arenas so as to mask its full extent. But while diluting ignorance, community psychiatry also diluted psychiatric authority and encouraged its competitors. For this reason, it was quickly jettisoned.

Chapter 5 brings the history of psychiatry up to the present. It explores the emergence of "diagnostic psychiatry" and the embrace of a more avowedly medical identity in the 1980s under what is called the Neo-Kraepelinian revolution. Interpreting psychiatry's problems as stemming from a lack of diagnostic reliability, reformers harnessed the revision to DSM-III to induce a "paradigm shift" toward a biomedical model of mental disorders. Classification became the means to manage ignorance; by carving up the universe of mental distress, reformers sought to signify mastery over that universe while simultaneously establishing a foundation for the scientific resolution of psychiatric ignorance. These reforms raised expectations of a psychiatry grounded in biomedical science. However, the recent failed

DSM-5 revision has revealed the limits of nosological reforms. The politics of this period have led to a growing consciousness among psychiatrists regarding the accumulated failures of reinvention, thus jeopardizing what has long been psychiatry's primary response to ignorance.

Here, a word of caution and a caveat are in order. The first regards the organization of the book around distinct eras. Periodization has the benefits of bringing a measure of coherence to the historical record. But it risks overstating the boundedness of each period and eliding heterogeneity within given eras. The reader should be cautioned against drawing too firm boundaries around each period discussed here. They are to be treated as trends in the evolution of aspirational psychiatry rather than discrete eras. In reality, periods bleed into each other and, within each, diversity abounds. Second, the story recounted here is an American story. While there has been some convergence in psychiatry across national contexts, the specificities of professional trajectories are shaped by their distinct national contexts. The ignorance of mental illness is a global phenomenon, but different political and cultural contexts have led to different negotiations with this ignorance. Any parallels observed between the American psychiatric profession and their peers in other countries should therefore be drawn cautiously.

In the concluding chapter, I turn to the implicit question nagging the analysis throughout the book. Given its persistent ignorance, why do we continue to recognize and defer to psychiatry? This question warrants an entire book on its own, but I use the opportunity of the conclusion to formulate an initial response. This discussion is by necessity more speculative than other parts of the book. In the first part of the conclusion, I elaborate on my conceptual framework for understanding reinvention and the tactics it encompasses. Here, I draw out insights from the case of psychiatry applicable to other cases, specifically in regard to the tactical maneuvers available to collective actors in negotiating ignorance. The conclusion ends in a reflection on the long-standing societal failure to hold psychiatry to proper account. Psychiatry does not have a monopoly over the ignorance of mental distress. We all share in it. But, unlike psychiatry, most of us ignore this ignorance and are keen to delegate it to others. Psychiatry, therefore, survives on the basis of a combination of inertia and indifference. Psychiatry benefits from a lack of viable alternatives and from a collective fear toward the patient population over which it maintains unchallenged jurisdiction—individuals with serious mental illness. This indifference has a long history with well-known effects for patients—stigma, marginality, straitjackets, lobotomies, incarceration, homelessness, underfunding, and lack of political clout. It does not take an astute social observer to recognize the horrors accompanying the sad marginality of those with serious mental illness. Less acknowledged, however, is the positive effect of this indifference on psychiatry. The malevolent neglect of the mentally ill translates into a type of benign neglect toward psychiatry. The benefit of this neglect is nothing less than psychiatry's continued existence.

On the Heels of Ignorance recounts the cyclical history of crisis–reinvention–crisis of American psychiatry. Narrating the risings and fallings of visions, it offers a frustrating history of frustrated reforms, occasional triumphs, but ultimately recurring failures. It lacks the satisfaction of a narrative of progress. It contains no dénouement, no climax, just a profession constantly circling back to its fundamental ignorance. It highlights how far the profession has traveled only to return to the same place. It is a not quite hopeless tale, but it is by no means a hopeful one.

It is, however, a tale that brings with it harsh lessons. We have long relegated those with serious mental illness to "zones of abandonment,"[63] and in doing so, have abandoned our obligation to them, leaving it in the hands of psychiatrists to deal with them. Faced with madness, we bury our heads and willingly pass off the problem to psychiatrists so we need not confront the challenges it poses. But well-founded criticisms of psychiatry should not distract from our collective culpability and our societal apathy. It is wrong to pin all of our failings on psychiatry.

In the end, this book is not an indictment of psychiatry, although it maintains a strident criticism of it. Historian Jack Pressman eloquently states, "Put simply, psychiatry is the management of despair. This is the heart of the psychiatrist's social function: to care for those whose problems have no certain cure or satisfactory explanation."[64] The larger professional politics should not obscure the profundity and difficulty of this task. We must not lose sight of the hard job we have placed at psychiatrists' feet, the intense suffering we have turned over to their care, and the vexing puzzles we have left to them to explain. Thus, psychiatrists emerge from this book not as cynical schemers, nor innocent dupes, nor admirable advocates. Rather, they are revealed to be individuals struggling to make sense of complex phenomena with imperfect tools, subject to enthusiasms, overexcitement, and dismay, achieving the rare insight but mostly succumbing to confusions, capable of startling acts of kindness and disturbing acts of violence.

In other words, I reveal a profession that is decidedly and tragically human.

As are we who enable it.

ONE

The General Superintendence
of All Their Departments

In the United States, psychiatry[1] was fortified not by a psychiatrist or the Association of Medical Superintendents of American Institutions for the Insane (AMSAII), but by an indefatigable former schoolteacher who traversed the eastern seaboard promoting the mental asylum. Insofar as the asylum ensured a place of prominence for psychiatrists in the management of madness, it is to Dorothea Dix that they owe a debt of gratitude. Dix did not invent the asylum. The model that underwrote her efforts, she got secondhand. But more than anyone else, she was responsible for the American system of publicly funded asylums. The institutions that she fought for would become strongholds of psychiatric authority and refuges to which psychiatrists could retreat during periods of crisis.

Dix's childhood was marred by sorrow and neglect. Her father was an abusive alcoholic. Her mother was likely mentally ill herself. Dix was forced to endure the wrath and fallouts of their troubles, essentially burdened with the responsibility of raising her younger brothers. The precariousness of her youth left a lasting mark; Dix would suffer bouts of anxiety and melancholy throughout her life. Still, her inner demons had their benefits; they begat a deep empathy for the insane. This empathy would propel her to become, in the words of her biographer, "the most productive woman in nineteenth century American politics."[2] But if it was Dix's fate to become the voice of the mad, destiny had to wait.

Dix began her career as a schoolteacher, one of the few fields open to educated women of her day. She gained a measure of notoriety for her educational book for young girls, *Conversations on Common Things*.[3] But her attempted move from the classroom to education reform was waylaid by a nervous collapse in 1836. Unable to work, Dix left the United States to convalesce in England at the estate of William Rathbone III, a wealthy reformer sympathetic to Dix's plight. There she encountered the ideas of English asylum reformers, specifically those of Samuel Tuke, a friend of the Rathbones and grandson of the founder of the famous York Retreat, William Tuke. The York Retreat was *the* model of moral treatment in the English-speaking world, and Dix "instinctively responded to the Retreat's therapeutic program."[4] Moral treatment resonated with her Unitarian religious beliefs and paralleled with own recovery at the serene Rathbone estate. She would carry the message of moral treatment back to her home country.

Upon her return to Massachusetts in 1837, Dix found herself drawn to the plight of the insane. An inheritance from her grandmother's estate gave her financial security and freed her to pursue her reforming drive. In 1841, Dix departed on an eighteen-month tour to study the condition of the mentally ill in Massachusetts. This tour changed her life. It changed her country as well.

Compared to other states, Massachusetts was generous when it came to mental health. One of the first private hospitals for the insane, McLean Hospital, was founded in Charlestown in 1811. Two decades later, in 1833, the legislature established the state-run Worcester State Lunatic Hospital. When demand outpaced space at Worcester, in 1839, the legislature built a new hospital for the insane poor, Boston Lunatic Hospital, in the state's most populous city. Yet, despite the state's relative attentiveness to the mentally ill, Dix's tours revealed the inadequacies of the available services. Throughout the state, she witnessed abject suffering among the insane. With encouragement from friend and reformer Samuel Gridley Howe, Dix published her findings in her *Memorial to the Legislature of Massachusetts* in 1843.

The *Memorial* seethed with quiet indignation as Dix described the miserable situation of the mentally ill in Massachusetts. Claiming to only "tell what I have seen," she reported brutal tales of "the *present* state of Insane Persons confined within this Commonwealth, in *cages, closets, cellars, stalls pens! Chained, naked, beaten with rods,* and *lashed* into obedience."[5] Some of her anecdotes were lengthy, with fleshy humanizing details. In Danvers, Dix discovered

. . . a young woman, exhibiting a condition of neglect and misery blotting out the faintest idea of comfort, and outraging every sentiment of decency. She had been, I learnt, "a respectable person"; industrious and worthy; disappointments and trials shook her mind, and finally laid prostrate reason and self-control . . . She had passed from one degree of violence to another, in swift progress; there she stood clinging to, or beating upon, the bars of her caged apartment, the contracted size of which afforded space only for increasing accumulations of filth, a *foul* spectacle; there she stood with naked arms and disheveled hair; the unwashed frame invested with fragments of unclean garments, the air so extremely offensive, though ventilation was afforded on all sides save one, that it was not possible to remain beyond a few moments without retreating for recovery to the outward air. Irritation of body, produced by utter filth and exposure, incited her to the horrid process of tearing off her skin by inches; her face, neck and person, were thus disfigured to hideousness. . . .[6]

Other anecdotes drew their power from their jarring succinctness. In Lincoln, Dix found "a woman in a cage."[7] In Medford, she encountered "one idiotic subject chained, and one in a close stall for 17 years," and in Bridgewater, "three idiots; never removed from one room."[8] The *Memorial* linked quaint Massachusetts towns—Springfield, Northampton, Brookfield, Granville, Plymouth, Scituate—to stories of misery and suffering. In the process, Dix exposed the collective guilt of the state. When accumulated, these stories painted an overwhelmingly bleak picture of "human beings, reduced to the extremest states of degradation and misery."[9] Such wretchedness was rendered all the more stark when juxtaposed with the figure of demure femininity that Dix struck.[10] To exhort the legislature to act, she joined a moral appeal to their Christian humanity with an economic argument—it would be cheaper to humanely cure the insane than to house them in indefinite squalor—that spoke to legislators' more pragmatic instincts.

The response to Dix's *Memorial* was electric. Although some towns refuted her claims, the public firestorm she ignited forced the state legislature to act. And while the victory in Massachusetts was a modest additional $25,000 of funding for the mentally ill, it crystallized Dix's passion. She extended her investigations into New York, then New Jersey and Pennsylvania, before departing on a tour of the South. The southern tour was capped by a trip to Washington, DC, to convince the federal government to grant land for the treatment of the insane, a plan that was eventually vetoed by President Franklin Pierce. Wherever she went, Dix followed a similar course. She toured the state, recorded her observations of the woeful treatment of the insane, composed a memorial to the state legislature,[11] and lobbied the legislature unrelentingly. In the end, she was responsible for founding, or enlarging, over thirty mental hospitals in the United States and abroad. Her work ended in a poetic manner rarely afforded by life's vicissitudes; she died as a guest in the New Jersey State Lunatic Hospital—an institution that she not only founded but designed, an institution that she called her firstborn child.[12]

Despite her herculean efforts, Dix always had a complicated relationship with the very psychiatric superintendents whose interests she was advocating. For her part, Dix maintained a deep admiration of superintendents. She absorbed their reports, spread their understanding of mental distress, and translated their ideas into concrete policies. Her memorials articulated their concerns. In them, she parroted superintendents' inflated claims about the curability of the insane, for example writing to the Illinois state legislature:

> Insanity is no longer regarded as the extinction of the mind; a disease hopeless and incurable; but proceeding from the physical causes, which disable the brain for a time from the correct exercise of those functions through which the mind is represented: And this malady is subject to successful physical treatment, as surely as a fever, or other common bodily disease.[13]

Dix's unwavering (some might say naïve) support, however, was rewarded with indifference from superintendents. Despite the outsized role she played in establishing the institutional infrastructure for their profession, psychiatrists dedicated scant attention to Dix in their flagship journal, the *American Journal of Insanity* (*AJI*). When they did mention her, it was mostly to express misgivings about her tactics. They worried that she conflated asylums and prisons in her lobbying efforts and thereby tainted superintendents by associating them with prisoners and unscrupulous wardens. Such complaints were colored by prevailing gender ideologies and patriarchal dismissiveness; superintendents chafed at the fact that the most prominent voice for their profession was not just an outsider, but a woman.

Superintendents' wariness toward Dix reflected their concern that she was saddling them with unrealistic expectations. Dix won support for asylums through a hard sell that promised sweeping cures at low costs. This put superintendents on notice, and many of them pinned the responsibility for these unrealistic expectations on her. But this was unfair. After all, Dix, who had "no feel for numbers,"[14] reiterated the inflated curability rates, often upward of 90%, that superintendents themselves published. Dix might have been a convenient scapegoat when the stark realities of the asylums contradicted the optimistic hype used to justify their existence, but superintendents had no one to blame but themselves. They were the ones who published the misleading statistics that fostered an impression of success when there was little.

For a profession that would become so steeped in ignorance, psychiatry was reared in the warm glow of certainty. Superintendents created great expectations that they would cure insanity. These expectations would end in disappointment, but not before a new profession was born.

This chapter covers the asylum era of American psychiatry, from the establishment of the profession in the 1840s to its first crisis at the turn of the twentieth century. No other period of American psychiatry has received as much scholarly attention.[15] And perhaps no other period has elicited as much controversy. For some, the asylum, with its grand facades, serene grounds, rich programming, and benevolent care, marked a period of all-too-rare kindness in the history of psychiatry.[16] Freed of the fetters of religious strictures, psychiatry loosened the fetters binding the insane and embraced a gentler approach to treatment, the effect of which, while never obtaining the hype, was positive nonetheless.[17] Other scholars counter that the asylum is better characterized as a technique of social control par excellence; moral treatment replaced ineffectual external constraints with a more effective and insidious form of control that operated on the soul. Through "great confinement" of the insane in asylums, psychiatrists "domesticated" madness, transforming nonconforming deviants into docile, tractable, and even productive members of society.[18]

Despite the controversy regarding the essential *character* of the asylum, consensus has emerged as to the *details* of its history, including the factors leading to its establishment, the philosophical foundations of its operation, and the causes of its decline. Building on this consensus, this chapter recounts the birth of psychiatric ignorance as a professional problem, thus establishing the dynamics for the subsequent politics of psychiatry, dynamics that endure to this day. Superintendents built their profession upon a foundation of deep certitude. Confident in the asylum and moral treatment, they made grand promises to state legislators, raising expectations that they could cure insanity and do so affordably. On the basis of these promises, they generated support and mobilized resources from legislatures to build up a network of asylums over which they maintained unencumbered authority. For a time, superintendents' inflated statistics of cure rates obscured their ignorance and masked the daily difficulties they encountered. However, the exposure of these statistics as fraudulent revealed the superintendents' promises as empty. Accused of bad faith and, worse, ignorance, psychiatrists succumbed to crisis when finally forced to confront all that they did not know.

The asylum era may have yielded psychiatry's first crisis, but it would not be its last. Its hype/disappointment trajectory would become the cyclical template that all subsequent reinventions would play out. To this fraught future, the asylum left two legacies that would shape psychiatry for the next century. The failure of the asylum raised the specter of ignorance with which psychiatrists still struggle and for which reinvention would become the solution. But it also created its organizational foundation and infrastructure from which subsequent generations of reformers launched their reinventions. The network of asylums that dotted the countryside became fortresses of psychiatric authority that, for a century, helped psychiatrists weather ignorance's assaults. Psychiatry can thank the asylum system for both its existence and the existential crisis that it is still negotiating.

The Rise of the Asylum

That Dix was the catalyst for the expansion of the asylum system in the United States was an anomaly only in the fact of her gender. Her nonmedical background would not have struck contemporaries as strange. Indeed, the initial momentum for the asylums was driven primarily by lay reformers.[19]

Asylum reforms were part of a larger response to the bewildering social changes of the early 1800s and the problems that followed in their wake. During the Jacksonian period, Americans experienced profound upheaval resulting from population growth, urbanization, capitalism, industrialization, and democratization.[20] The effects of these disruptions on the problems posed by the mentally ill were manifold. Madness, long interpreted through a religious lens, came to be viewed as an unfortunate side effect of modernization, or "part of the compensation for our progress and refinement," as the famous neurologist George Miller Beard put it.[21] The frenzied pace of social change produced what the astute American observer Alexis de Tocqueville described as a kind of mental agitation.[22] Urbanization and revolutions in transportation increased mobility and social dislocation that exacerbated this agitation.[23] As people migrated from isolated communities to the city, they came into more regular contact with strangers. The increased anonymity made daily interactions more fraught, uncertain, and possibly treacherous.[24] Disruptions caused by the insane threatened an already fragile social cohesion. Modernization, it seemed, produced more madness, while eroding the communal bonds that traditionally handled the problems of the insane.

In response to these changes, reformers began to lobby state legislatures to take control of madness. Early reformers were inspired by an activist model of religious life, born of the Second Great Awakening that emphasized good works.[25] The philosophy undergirding the asylum—moral treatment—resonated with these beliefs. More than isolated buildings with walls to contain, the modern asylum's true innovation lay in its humane, psychosocial approach to treating mental illness. This approach eschewed the use of force and violent "heroic" medical therapies for a calming therapeutic milieu and a retreat-like atmosphere. The new institutions would not just confine the insane; they would cure them by means that resonated with reformers' Christianity.

Moral treatment was not an American creation. Instead, two international figures provided much of the inspiration for the early American asylum movement. The first was William Tuke, grandfather to Samuel Tuke, under whose spell Dix had fallen. Tuke's concern for the mentally disturbed was driven by his religious convictions. The deprivation and squalor of Bethlehem Hospital (aka "Bedlam") in London offended Tuke's Quaker sensibilities. He condemned the imprisonment of the insane as well as their physicians, who performed violent, depletive treatments, like blistering and bleeding, on those with mental illness. While such treatments were consistent with medical practice of the day, they were applied with particular aggression to the mentally ill, who were perceived as uncivilized and thus less sensitive to physical pain. Marrying his Quaker beliefs with his business acumen, Tuke developed a more humane alternative, opening the York Retreat in 1796. He promised York would be a place where "neither chains nor corporeal punishment are tolerated."[26] Here the insane were to be treated with dignity. Kindness replaced violence. The influence of the Retreat on American asylum reformers was direct. It served as the model for the Friends' Hospital in Philadelphia, founded in 1813, one of the first institutions in the United States dedicated to the treatment of the mentally ill.[27] Tuke's gentler approach was promoted by his American adherents as an effective means of cure.

If Tuke embodied the lay and religious wing of the asylum movement, his French contemporary, Philippe Pinel, represented its medical wing. Pinel's ideas regarding treatment were formed from observation and study he conducted in the infirmaries at Hôpital Général (later renamed Bicêtre Hospital), which was located in a Parisian suburb. He combined these with the revolutionary political ideologies permeating Paris in the late 1700s. In his "Memoir on Madness," read before the Society for Natural History in 1794, Pinel refuted the widespread perception of madness as intractable: "To consider madness as a usually incurable illness is to assert a vague proposition that is constantly refuted by the most authentic facts."[28] The raving, irredeemable lunatic of the madhouse was a creation of the harsh treatment therein. In place of the madhouse and their ignorant managers, who "have been permitted to exercise towards their innocent prisoners a most arbitrary system of cruelty and violence," Pinel proposed treating the insane with "an intelligent mixture of affability and firmness."[29] In his experience, this kind of moral therapy "affords amply and daily proofs of happier effects of a mild, conciliating treatment, rendered effective by steady and dispassionate firmness."[30] Pinel's legacy was not just his ideas regarding madness or his institutional accomplishments, but also his symbolic act of unchaining the insane—famously depicted in the 1876 painting *Pinel a la Salpêtrière* by Tony Robert-Fleury—to which he is given credit (wrongly, it turns out).[31]

American reformers drew inspiration from Tuke, Pinel, and other international models of moral treatment to advocate for the creation of asylums by state legislatures. Adopting a strident, "utopian language,"[32] they promoted the asylum as *the* solution to the problem of insanity. The asylums would provide solace and promote stability at the historical moment when the problems stemming from the insane were pressing and growing and when traditional ideas seemed outmoded.[33] The founding of the Friends' Hospital in 1813 was accompanied by other private asylums inspired by moral treatment: McLean Asylum for the Insane in Massachusetts (1811), Bloomingdale Insane Asylum in New York (1821), and the Hartford Retreat in Connecticut (1824). The first public institution, Worcester Insane Asylum, was founded in 1833, and by 1860, largely because of Dix's efforts, twenty-eight out of thirty-three states had at least one public hospital for the insane.[34]

Capturing the Asylum

In 1847, Amariah Brigham, the first editor of the *AJI*, laid out the rationale behind the asylum's therapeutic innovations. Speaking for the *AJI* editorial board, Brigham stated: "The removal of the insane from home and former associations, with respectful and kind treatment under all circumstances, and in most cases manual labor, attendance on religious worship on Sunday, the establishment of regular habits and of self-control, diversion of the mind from morbid trains of thought, are now generally considered as essential in the Moral Treatment of the Insane."[35] Moral treatment, inherited from Tuke, Pinel, and other European reformers, formed the crux of the asylum's stated purpose, and all superintendents avowed their commitment to its tenets. Yet, very little of moral treatment's features seemed to suggest a particular need for *medical* expertise. Indeed, Brigham admitted "that in a majority of cases of insanity, the moral treatment is of more importance than the medical."[36] This posed a problem for the nascent profession of psychiatry. The initial asylum reforms had been accomplished primarily by lay reformers like Dix. Moreover, moral treatment had arisen in explicit opposition to prevailing medical treatments of the insane. If they wanted to secure their professional existence, American psychiatrists somehow had to transpose a commitment to "benevolence" into "a medical key."[37] How did physicians reposition themselves from adjunct advisors to the controlling figures of the asylums?

Before addressing this question, it is important to contextualize it historically. That lay individuals initiated and led the early asylum reforms should not mislead one into thinking, as some have argued, that the asylum system was a social reform rather than a medical one.[38] This imposes a categorical distinction—lay versus medical—on a period in which things were more muddled. First, given the fledgling state of medical professionalization in the United States, the distinction between lay leaders and the medical profession itself was neither as stark nor as clear as it is today. The formal trappings of a modern profession—standard education, certification, licensing laws, and so on—did not exist for medicine during much of the nineteenth century.[39] Second, while lay driven, physicians were involved in asylum reform efforts from the start. Drawing on the work of Benjamin Rush, American physicians professed a somatic account of mental illness, with its cause "seated primarily in the blood-vessels of the brain, and that it depends upon the same kind of morbid and irregular actions that constitute other arterial diseases."[40] While asylum reformers challenged the heroic treatments the somatic account inspired, they did not reject medical input altogether. Instead, within the asylums, a division of labor emerged. Lay administrators supervised and managed the institutional regimen but consulted with physicians, whose job was to decide whether medical intervention was required.

Still, the question remains: If the moral treatment required no obvious medical training, and if prevailing etiological accounts of insanity emphasized its social origins as "part of the price we pay for civilization," as put by physician and medical reformer Edward Jarvis,[41] how did superintendents convince others that they, as physicians, should be the primary agents responsible for the insane?

Superintendents' takeover of the asylum, in part, involved a successful reframing of mental distress as a problem rooted in the brain. Rather than altering or rejecting popular understandings, superintendents co-opted them and subsumed them under a brain-based account. While insanity might spring from diverse sources, at its core it involved a somatic corruption of the brain caused by nervous irritation. Whatever its cause, madness corrupted the brain. Thus, superintendents folded prevailing ideas about insanity into a medical rationale by positing a deeper somatic cause underlying its surface causes. This view was conjured by combining two contemporary ideas regarding the mind. First, superintendents subscribed to an understanding of the mind inherited from Lockean philosophy. John Locke's famous notion of the mind as a "tabula rasa" held that humans were not born with innate ideas, but rather acquired them through experience mediated by sense perception. The mind was thought of as comprising distinct faculties that enable this acquisition.[42] Locke's view of the mind was revolutionary in that its empiricism moved away from supernatural conceptualizations of the soul.[43] It also posited that the corruption of the mind's faculties could proceed through false impressions that lead to faulty thinking.

Lockean philosophy only got superintendents halfway; its understanding of the mind did not entail a somatic grounding in the brain. Superintendents still needed to connect mind to brain, to articulate a physical basis of mental illness that would justify medical control of it. For this, superintendents combined Locke's with ideas from phrenology, a psychological theory first espoused by Franz Joseph Gall and later popularized in the United States by George Combe and brothers Orson and Lawrence Fowler. Derided today as an exemplary pseudoscience, phrenology gained a significant following in the United States around the 1840s, especially among the upper classes. Phrenologists argued that the brain was the organ of the mind, that certain areas of the brain correspond to localized functions, and that measurements of the head and skull could yield information regarding which functions were developed or underdeveloped in a particular brain.

Phrenology was a popular topic among superintendents. Early articles in the *AJI* situated superintendent thought squarely within this tradition. Brigham, who in addition to being the editor of the *AJI* was the director of the Utica State Asylum, drew on phrenology to "infer that the brain is not a single organ, but a congeries of organs, as maintained by the illustrious Gall and his celebrated successors, Spurzheim and Combe."[44] Brigham went on to articulate a somatic account of mental illness: "We consider insanity a chronic disease of the brain, producing either derangement of the intellectual faculties, or prolonged change of the feelings, affections, and habits of an individual."[45] Plainly, insanity was "the result of diseased brain."[46] While most American superintendents did not accept phrenology wholesale (they were skeptical of craniometrics), it provided the crucial link between the faculties of the mind and the structures of the brain, positing an ontology of mental illness that necessitated medical expertise.[47]

The somatic basis of madness became an article of faith among superintendents. This belief was reinforced by a conviction that "the examination of tissues in an autopsy would reveal organic lesions, clear evidence of physical damage, in every insane person."[48] But such revelations were not forthcoming. Brain autopsies rarely revealed lesions, and even when they did identify abnormalities, it was difficult, if not impossible, to correlate these with specific behaviors.[49] Autopsies were expected to confirm superintendents' faith in the somatic basis of insanity, but their findings never paid off in the way superintendents envisioned. In a series of articles on "The Pathology of Insanity" appearing in the *AJI*, John Charles Bucknill, a respected English psychiatrist, admitted, "A large number of brains of the insane I have diligently investigated with a first-rate microscope. The results appear to me to have afforded no distinction between the sane and the insane brain."[50] Research was slow and frustrating:

> To the pathologist the substance of the brain is as yet practically structure-less. Although the microscope reveals cells and tubes and intervening stroma, up to the present time it is unable to indicate when these are in a normal or abnormal state; and although it may prove that in some cases the smaller arteries are diseased—that in a few others there are exudation corpuscles, or an increase of fatty particles in the substance itself—it has not yet been able to distinguish between states of the whole organ which must be diametrically opposite, for instance, between the states of hypertrophy and atrophy.[51]

Despite these frustrations, superintendents maintained their faith. Perhaps imminent discoveries would come from anticipated technological developments. Even though "a first-rate microscope" of the day might not be able to detect these problems, future technological improvements, coupled with advances in research techniques, would. Present empirical uncertainty, therefore, was explained away by appeals to future promises. Through such promises, superintendents neutralized the disruptive potential of their negative findings and put off their assessment to another day. In the meantime, the somatic basis went unquestioned, enduring as a commonsense assumption to which all superintendents subscribed. As Isaac Ray, one of the original founders of AMSAII, insisted, it "is an undoubted truth, that the manifestations of the intellect, and those of the sentiments, propensities and passions, or generally, of the intellectual and affective powers, are connected with and dependent upon the brain."[52]

This somatic assumption thus supplied an ontological account of insanity necessary for superintendents' professional aspirations. It could be flexibly applied to popular notions of madness, by ensuring that the myriad potential causes of insanity could be traced back to a somatic origin, at least theoretically. Environmental and social dislocations might foster mental agitation, but these external factors acted on the brain. All the possible causes of insanity were thus perceived as operating *through* the brain, frazzling a patient's nerves and manifesting in madness. And these potential causes were dizzyingly diverse. For example, in its first report, the Utica State Asylum listed the causes of madness among its patient population, in order of prevalence, as

> religious anxiety (50); ill health (46); unknown (40); puerperal (20); Loss of property (17); doubtful (15); excessive study (12); intemperance (10); death of kindred (10); fright (7); "Millerism" (5); abuse of husband (5); perplexity of business (3); disappointed ambition (3); Epilepsy (3); Seduction (3); blows on the head (3); disappointment in love (4); masturbation (3); political excitement (2); jealousy (2); neuralgia (1); malformation of head (1); excessive labor (1); inhaling carbonic acid gas (1); exposure to excessive heat (1); exposure to fumes of charcoal (1); excitement from sea voyage (1); opium eating (1); irregular decay of faculties from old age (1).[53]

This census includes cases of insanity stemming from social factors, like loss of property, political excitements, and disappointed ambition, as well as those rooted in physical causes, like "masturbation, blows on the head, malformation of the head, excessive labor, inhaling carbonic acid gas, exposure to the fumes of charcoal, opium eating, and exposure to the sun."[54] Superintendents were willing to accept almost anything as a probable source of insanity, provided that these surface causes were understood as operating on and through the brain. This reasoning offered a fundamental causal argument that legitimated their medical authority. Any uncertainty or ignorance regarding the source of insanity was either deflected by a promise of future research gains or obscured by a flexible understanding of madness that allowed for multiple accounts of causality to seem as if they were participating in the same conversation.

Organizing themselves into a professional association, superintendents produced a flood of treatises that reiterated the somatic view of insanity. The wave of writing convinced lay leaders and state legislatures to defer to them. By these means, superintendents converted their initial, ancillary foothold in the asylum into complete and utter control. The asylums were more than just benevolent institutions; they were instruments of cure that acted upon the brain.

The Nature of Psychiatric Expertise

Beyond justifying the professional control of medical superintendents, these medical ideas shaped little of psychiatrists' practice, discourse, or workaday world during its founding period. In 1844, thirteen superintendents gathered in the Jones Hotel in Philadelphia to form AMSAII. The primary goal of the professional association was to exchange practical know-how on running asylums. "The medical gentlemen connected with the lunatic asylums," asserted Pliny Earle of the Bloomingdale Asylum, "should be better known to each other, should communicate more freely the results of their individual experience, should cooperate in collecting statistical information relating to insanity and above all should assist each other in improving the treatment of the insane."[55] For its first fifty years, AMSAII membership was based on institutional affiliation and restricted to superintendents. The particular kind of expertise that AMSAII sought to cultivate was one rooted in managing asylums, rather than in any specialized training or specific scientific credentials. Its annual meetings, as well as the content of its official organ, the *AJI*, were filled with practical discussions on the construction, organization, and general arrangements of the asylum.[56]

Early psychiatric expertise was posited as a managerial expertise. As members of an administrative specialty, superintendents' identity and purpose revolved around the asylum, their "professional showcase, their most effective public advertisement."[57] The asylum was not just a building or an institution but an instrument of cure. It performed an array of "custodial, disciplinary, educational, and medicative" functions, which if given "proper degree of prominence" would lead to cure.[58] Because the asylum was *the* therapeutic entity itself, no aspect of its functioning was too small or insignificant for the attention of the superintendents. "It is a great error to suppose that there is any detail about the management of a Hospital for the Insane, beneath the dignity, or unworthy the attention of its Chief Medical Officer," claimed Thomas Story Kirkbride, superintendent of the Pennsylvania Hospital for the Insane.[59] Superintendents reflected upon, attended to, and oversaw every aspect of the asylum, from the size of the windows to the content of the cultural programming, from the organization of the wards to the planning of the menu. These responsibilities demanded herculean attention to detail. Consequently, superintendents poured their energies into developing the managerial acumen in order to exercise "a general superintendence of all their departments."[60]

Superintendents drew on diverse sources of knowledge and inspiration to develop their managerial expertise. These were woven together to construct a distinct kind of expertise that went far beyond the claims to medicine. One major source of inspiration was architecture. The mental agitation of the brain was to be assuaged by removing individuals from the tumult of modern civilization—and their families, who more often than not exacerbated things—and relocating them to a meticulously crafted healing environment. Believing that the societal transition from rural to urban life had produced mental distress, superintendents tried to reverse this process for their patients. They removed them to the countryside and an institution that reproduced the salubrious features of rural life. The moral architecture of the asylum was to offer a retreat from the hectic trappings of modernizing America.

Nothing preoccupied superintendents more than architectural design, and nothing would come to frustrate them more than compromises they had to make on these designs, which were forced upon them by legislatures in the name of financial prudence. Between 1851 and 1853, AMSAII codified the architectural standards for the asylum. These were developed by Kirkbride and elaborated in his treatise *On the Construction, Organization and General Arrangements of Hospitals for the Insane*. One of the original founding members of AMSAII, Kirkbride held numerous offices in AMSAII over his career, serving eight years as secretary, seven as vice president, and another eight as president (1862–1870). In his biography—he was a physician with a Quaker religious background—and intellectual influences—he was greatly taken with the York Retreat—Kirkbride embodied early American asylum reform. And he dedicated much of his career to spelling out in fine detail how the asylum should be built. For at stake in his architectural plans was nothing less than the cure of insanity: "Of the recent cases of insanity, properly treated, between 80 and 90 percent recover. Of those neglected or improperly managed, very few get well."[61]

According to what became known as the Kirkbride Plan, a proper asylum displayed certain characteristics. First, it had to be located "on a plot of land no smaller than one hundred acres, to enable it to have the proper amount for farming and gardening purposes, to give the desired degree of privacy and to secure adequate and appropriate means of exercise, labor and occupation to the patients, for all these are now recognized as among the most valuable means of treatment."[62] Set back from the road and surrounded by greenery—"to protect the patients from the gaze and impertinent curiosity of visitors"[63]—a proper asylum consisted of a single main building with a staggered-wing design. The central building was to house the administrative offices with the two wings flanking it reserved for patients, one wing for males, the other for females. In all, the asylums were intended to house no more than 250 patients. The edifice "should have a cheerful and comfortable appearance, everything repulsive and prison-like should be carefully avoided, and even the means of effecting the proper degree of security should be masked, as far as possible, by arrangements of a pleasant and

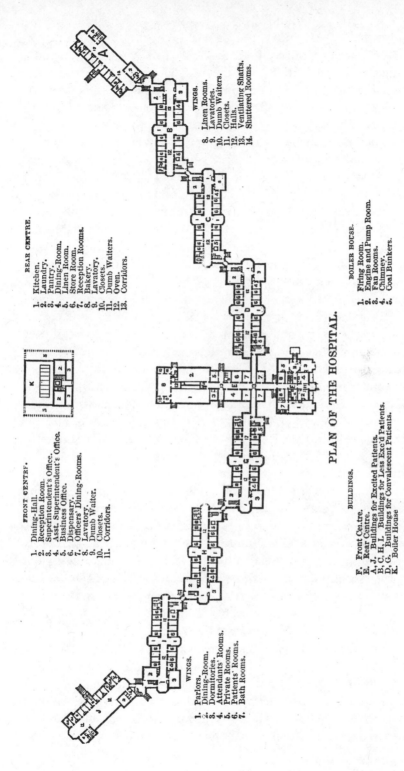

PLAN OF THE HOSPITAL.

FRONT CENTRE.

1. Dining-Hall.
2. Reception Room.
3. Superintendent's Office.
4. Asst. Superintendent's Office.
5. Business Office.
6. Dispensary.
7. Officers' Dining-Rooms.
8. Lavatory.
9. Dumb Waiter.
10. Closets.
11. Corridors.

REAR CENTRE.

1. Kitchen.
2. Laundry.
3. Pantry.
4. Dining-Room.
5. Linen Room.
6. Store Room.
7. Reception Rooms.
8. Bakery.
9. Lavatory.
10. Closets.
11. Dumb Waiters.
12. Oven.
13. Corridors.

WINGS.

1. Parlors.
2. Dining-Room.
3. Dormitories.
4. Attendants' Rooms.
5. Private Rooms.
6. Patients' Rooms.
7. Bath Rooms.

WINGS.

8. Linen Rooms.
9. Lavatories.
10. Dumb Waiters.
11. Closets.
12. Halls.
13. Ventilating Shafts.
14. Shuttered Rooms.

BOILER HOUSE.

1. Firing Room.
2. Engine and Pump Room.
3. Fan Rooms.
4. Chimney.
5. Coal Bunkers.

BUILDINGS.

F. Front Centre.
E. Rear Centre.
A. J. Buildings for Excited Patients.
B. C. H. I. Buildings for Less Exc'd Patients.
D. G. Buildings for Convalescent Patients.
K. Boiler House

1. Floor plan for the Danvers State Insane Asylum in Massachusetts, modeled after the Kirkbride Plan. Courtesy of the Danvers Archival Center, Danvers, MA.

attractive character."[64] Above all else the façade had to reflect the asylum's curative function. These were not to be custodial warehouses to segregate and hold, but therapeutic instruments to effect cure. By housing the entire patient population under a single roof, the plan placed all under the watchful eye of the superintendent.

Accompanying the building specifications were extensive recommendations for the interior design down to the minutest detail. No decision was arbitrary. Doors to patient rooms "should be about 6 feet 8 inches by 2 feet 8 inches";[65] walls should be sturdy in order to insulate sound. Keys "for the male and female wards should be so entirely different that it will be impossible by any slight alteration to make those for one side open the locks for the other," and urinals "should be made of cast iron, well-enameled, with a downward current of air through them, and have a steady stream of water passing over their whole surface."[66] Kirkbride's consideration of every structural aspect of the asylum included deliberate assessments of practical building issues, economic costs, the special needs of the insane, and organizational imperatives to maintain control.

This attention to detail was by no means unique to Kirkbride. During its first decades, the *AJI* functioned as a clearinghouse for practical tips on constructing and managing the most effective asylum environment. It brimmed with articles on ventilation, appropriate construction materials, and similar topics. Conversely, there was a dearth of what we would deem medical articles. Consumed with the demands of creating, maintaining, and running these asylums, superintendents had neither the time nor the inclination to conduct much in the way of medical research.

The buildings were the physical embodiment of a vision for a curing environment. But for this nurturing vision to work, superintendents had to embody a certain role. A second source of superintendents' authority was derived from prevailing cultural understandings of the family, specifically patriarchal authority. Given the multifaceted causes of insanity, the asylum and moral treatment demanded the "removal of the insane from home and former associations."[67] This removal required cooperation from families, who traditionally had been responsible for their insane relatives. In convincing relatives to commit their loved ones, the asylum was pitched as a surrogate family, with the superintendent assuming the "role of the stern, authoritarian, yet loving and concerned father."[68] Superintendents promised to govern the daily life of the asylum as if it were an extended household by acting the role of benevolent but firm fathers. In drawing from cultural expectations regarding familial power, superintendents were able to induce a "generous confidence" from patients as the unquestioned authority of the asylum household.[69] Their caring discipline would guide their patients back to sanity.

Superintendents' authority as architects and benevolent fathers dovetailed with another key aspect of their power—that of establishing a well-ordered regimen. With so many responsibilities placed at their feet, it was incumbent upon superintendents to institute a "system of internal organization and the general arrangements [based] on correct principles and carried out with judicious liberality."[70] This system was structured according to the dictates of moral treatment. In its broadest formulation, moral treatment was conceived as the "attention to the mental peculiarities and everything relating to the personal management of the insane, exclusive of medical treatment."[71] Patients needed a regimented and consistent environment to improve, and it was incumbent upon superintendents to create a milieu governed by routine, where daily life was organized around the dictates of moral treatment.

To achieve this, superintendents had to first sort patients in a particular way. Rather than classifying patients according to mental disorders or types of insanity, superintendents classified patients in terms of their potential to upset the asylum order:

> The hospital for the insane is not merely a structure with rooms for the reception of a certain number of persons, but a building internally so arranged as to classify the inmates in wards according to their influence upon each other and their power of self-control . . . The physician is to direct his skill, not simply to the application of medical remedies to disordered bodily conditions, and to the necessary sanitary measures, as in other diseases, but also to such classification as will secure the best possible control and adjustment of the innumerable morbid mental manifestations, and the various personal habits and peculiarities of patients.[72]

Classification became a tool to maintain control, to impose consistency and regularity on asylum life, and to stave off the potential disruptions to which their patients were prone. The architecture of the building, with its center and peripheries, mapped the distinctions between "the excited and the noisy" and those able to more fully participate in the regimen.[73] The wards of each wing were organized according to the severity of the cases of insanity. The more excitable and unruly patients were housed in the farthest ends of the wing, with the more rational patients placed near the central building. This division and allocation of space kept the disrupted noisy "at a distance" to ensure the proper functioning of the asylum and the general tranquility so necessary for treatment.[74] Ward placement was folded into an incentive structure to get patients to cooperate in their cures. As a patient's condition improved, he or she would be moved to a more settled ward, closer to the heart of the asylum. Consequently, the conceptual and spatial organization of patients was dictated less by the characteristic features of their insanity, and more by the imperative of ensuring the controlled, efficient running of the asylum.

Having organized patients according to their potential for disruption, superintendents set to work on managing patients' days. Regimentation sought to counteract the uncertainty of modernizing America outside the asylum walls, uncertainty that patients could not manage, as evident by their insanity. Patients did not need to concern themselves with what they should be doing; all their daily comings, goings, and activities were structured for them by superintendents. Idleness was a threat, not only to the environment being cultivated by the asylum, but also to the minds of the insane, and a full regimen was established to combat this threat. Earle asserted:

> The hospital, no less than the college, should have its established curriculum; and this should comprehend a course of exercises, hygienic, laborious, disciplinary, amusing, recreative, instructive and devotional. The patients should go from exercise to exercise as students from lecture to lecture. They would then be subjected, during a large part of the day, to restraining, diverting, and hence curative influences, instead of being left to lounge, apathetically, or to wander to and fro in their rooms or halls, subject to the wayward impulses of their disorder, as is now too generally the case with a large proportion of them.[75]

Beyond its calming effects on patients, regimentation accomplished two other goals. First, superintendents folded it into an incentive system in which activities and privileges could be granted and confiscated according to a patient's conformity to the routine. By these sticks and carrots, superintendents asserted control over their patients, imposing a rigid order without having to resort to constraints. Second, the activities socialized the insane into productive and healthy behaviors. In addition to structuring basic tasks like eating and sleeping, superintendents constructed elaborate schedules of activities aimed at improving the character of the insane. Central to this was labor. Kirkbride argued that labor "is one of our best remedies . . . one of the best anodynes for the nervous, it composes the restless and excited, promotes a good appetite and a comfortable digestion, and gives sound and refreshing sleep to many who would without it pass wakeful nights."[76]

Patient labor had the added benefit of helping maintain the functioning and self-sufficiency of the asylum.

Extensive cultural programming provided another means to build the character of patients. According to humanities professor Benjamin Reiss, the asylum "was something of a laboratory for the purification of culture and the production of useful citizens who could live in modernity without being unstrung by its temptations, agitated rhythms, and destabilizing messages."[77] Superintendents believed that the proper consumption of culture could induce patients into regaining their reason. Through lectures, guided readings, dances, concerts, and other cultural programs, they sought to cultivate right thinking among patients, to steer them toward healthy habits and away from bastardized and inappropriate cultural influences of modern society. By these means, superintendents established themselves as cultural curators. This dimension of their expertise became manifest in a seeming curiosity of early psychiatric discourse—the repeated exegeses on Shakespeare that filled the pages of the *AJI*. In the first two decades, the journal published no fewer than thirteen articles on Shakespeare. Superintendents spoke of "the wonderful sagacity of Shakespeare," treating him as an authority whose discussions of insanity "may be ranked with the highest triumphs."[78] Through these exegeses, superintendents developed their thinking on madness, while demonstrating their cultural *bona fides*.

In the day-to-day management of the asylum, superintendents demonstrated a multifaceted managerial authority, little of which drew explicitly on medical science. The asylum stood as the crowning achievement of psychiatry and the promise of its future. Within the asylum walls, psychiatric power was defined, cultivated, and expanded. Unfortunately for psychiatrists' professional aspirations, only two decades into this grand experiment, it became all too evident that the curative dream of the asylums was a mirage.

Exposing the Cult of Curability

Weaving together diverse strands of authority—medical, architectural, cultural, organizational, managerial—superintendents established a unique type of expertise, a bricolage that helped them manage the uncertainty and disruptions they encountered in the asylum. However, this internal authority—and the space within which to create it—was dependent upon the claims that the asylum effectively and economically cured the insane. Desperate legislatures assumed a pragmatic stance toward the asylum. If it worked, they would fund it. But their support was contingent on demonstrable results, not on the philosophy that undergirded the asylums' operations. Despite the certainty superintendents displayed (and in many cases, believed) regarding the promise of the asylum, psychiatric knowledge was limited. The somatic origin of insanity or a demonstrated connection between mental distress and the structure of the brain remained elusive, an expected, much pined for, but heretofore unrealized dream.

To mask this ignorance and stave off its negative effects, superintendents turned to statistics. Although they engaged in little medical research, superintendents did compile reams of statistics.[79] The effort and emphasis that superintendents placed on statistical rhetoric—and the eventual trust legislatures placed in their curative statistics—reflected the high status of statistical reasoning during the nineteenth century. At this time, statistics, and numbers generally, were viewed as pre-evaluative and non-interpretive.[80] They gave off a veneer of objectivity. As seemingly transparent data, they became a solution to the problems of trust created by a diversifying and growing society.[81] For this reason, state legislatures, tasked with managing the fallouts and dilemmas of modernization, became early adopters and accumulators of statistical data. During a period of minimal state activity, one of the few tasks legislatures undertook was to gather and produce statistical reports.[82] Given statistics' privileged status—along with the often unsophisticated and primitive understanding of statistical modeling and data collection—there was a tendency to take statistical information at face value, to "trust in numbers."[83]

Superintendents took advantage of this trust, legitimating their authority on statistics that were, in fact, less than transparent. Superintendents claimed the tremendous efficacy of moral treatment in inflated curability statistics. They cited cure rates of 75%, 85%, even 95%. These seemingly hard numbers were highlighted in the annual reports that superintendents sent to legislatures. And they were cited by superintendents in justifying the construction of more asylums, additional funding, and more autonomy from meddling state oversight. When accumulated, these cure rates amount to an avalanche of favorable data that confirm the asylum's efficacy and, by extension, superintendents' worth. Thus, statistical claims performed a critical rhetorical function for superintendents and their professionalizing aspirations. They reduced the confounding reality of asylum practice into tidy numbers that appeared to speak for themselves. They absorbed and concealed the uncertainty of working with the insane by translating it into numbers, and good numbers at that. In short, superintendents were able to mask their ignorance behind glowing statistics.

Given the extent to which superintendents depended on statistical hyperbole, it would not be a stretch to say that the asylum system was built on this "cult of curability."[84] Initially this rhetoric worked magically. Not only did these numbers persuade legislatures to invest tremendous and often scarce resources into the asylums; they also helped convince family members to commit their sick relatives.[85]

It is important to note that, for superintendents, the risk of fostering unrealistic expectations via such statistical exaggerations was mitigated to a degree by the nature of moral treatment itself. The sheer comprehensiveness of moral treatment left a possible out, a ready-made excuse for any exposed disappointment. If reality did not meet the statistical hype, superintendents could claim that at least some aspect of their efforts had been thwarted by external meddling and forced compromises. In the minds of superintendents, legislatures, out of avarice, ignorance, or miserliness, imposed financial constraints on asylums that decreased the efficacy of their moral treatment. Maybe the legislatures cut corners in the construction of the building. Or perhaps they failed to provide the requisite funding for sufficient cultural programming. With so many elements involved in moral treatment, it was not hard to find at least one excuse, one area of need that had not been met by the legislature. Provided that the superintendents maintained a measure of demonstrable efficacy, they could deflect responsibility for failing to live up to their promises onto those who controlled the purse. Moreover, they could turn failure on its head to justify even more support from legislatures that lacked the will or capacity to interrogate the annual reports closely. Cloaked in their inflated statistics, superintendents were given wide berth to carry out their efforts.

Over time, however, the realities of the asylums began to diverge too extensively from the rosy statistics. As superintendents attempted to one-up each other in order to curry favor with their home legislatures, the inflated numbers grew bolder. Expectations were elevated to absurdly unrealistic heights, setting the bar unreachably high. They also began to stretch credulity. Hiding behind them became less tenable, as the mismatch between the statistical depictions and the on-the-ground reality grew wider.

This mismatch was first exposed by overcrowding, a problem that more than any other would come to vex inpatient mental health treatment. According to the Kirkbride model, which was adopted by AMSAII, asylums should house no more than 250 patients. Any more and the asylums ran the risk of overwhelming the building, fostering disruptions, and undermining moral treatment. A superintendent could not cultivate working relationships with the patients under his charge if the asylum census grew too large. But once established, demand for asylum treatment outpaced supply. Superintendents, believing their inflated cure rates, underestimated how many intractable cases they would encounter. This set off a pernicious sort of math. If even a few beds became occupied by chronic cases, these beds got taken out of circulation. Over time, as more intractable cases accumulated, more beds were taken out of circulation, impairing superintendents' ability to appropriately incorporate new cases. This "silting up" led to overcrowding.[86] Asylums intended to house a maximum of 250 patients were by 1870 housing two to four times as many.[87] The pressures from silting up were compounded by increasing demand that appeared unrelenting. The asylums, established as institutions to heal, also appealed as a place to stash unwanted and problematic individuals. Families and states started sending patients that superintendents never intended to treat. Asylum halls became overrun by poor, elderly, often immigrant patients with chronic conditions like general paresis, dementia, and insanity related to alcohol.[88] There was little superintendents could do to stem this demand, as they had no control over who was sent their way.[89] Overcrowding began to crack the façade created by superintendents' statistics, giving lie to their glowing annual reports. The fact that asylum superintendents kept returning to the legislatures with petitions for more asylums and more funding to expand current ones started to speak louder than their exaggerated claims of cure.

Superintendents' statistics, previously accepted at face value, became objects of scrutiny, then contention, and finally derision. The critique of psychiatric statistics was led by an unlikely gadfly. Pliny Earle was a superintendent and one of the original thirteen founders of AMSAII. In 1876, after some soul-searching prompted by a tour of forty-six institutions in Europe, Earle published a series of studies that eviscerated the statistical claims of his peers.[90] The studies assumed a confessional tone; having once engaged in the statistical manipulations, Earle was coming clean after a crisis of conscience. Using data from tables publicly available in asylum reports, he showed that superintendents, whether out of deception or plain ineptitude, adopted a number of problematic practices when calculating cure rates, the sum of total of which was a thoroughly misleading picture of what was happening in the asylums. First, patients who died under care in the asylum were either not counted or counted as cured. This artificially decreased the number of failed cases. Second, superintendents inflated cure rates by the "fallacious methods of calculating the proportion of recoveries upon the number of patients discharged, instead of the number admitted."[91] The denominator, represented as the number of discharged patients, was much smaller than if it were the number of total patients admitted. And finally, superintendents treated each admission as a separate *case* even if it was a readmission of a relapsed (read, not cured) patient. Earle observed:

> The deceptive nature of the word cases was thus exposed. The superintendents reported the recovery of cases. The unprofessional readers of the reports, thoughtless of the technical use of the word, believed that case is equivalent to person, and, consequently, that the number of cases represented an equal number of persons. When the Bloomingdale Asylum reported, without explanation, six recoveries in one year, all of which were furnished by one woman, who was again brought to the asylum before the report was in print, and who finally died there, the public necessarily inferred that six different persons had recovered. . . .[92]

By operationalizing a case in this favorable way, superintendents systematically misled legislatures and readers of asylum reports. Under such accounting, a hypothetical patient could come and go six times within the course of a year and be counted as six cured cases.

This statistical chicanery set off a race to the bottom. Superintendents, under pressure from state legislatures, jockeyed with each other to claim ever higher cure rates so as to look good in comparison to their peers. They had a perverse incentive to deceive. And whether they did so consciously or not, Earle laid the responsibility for this dishonesty at the feet of the superintendents:

> The medical officers of institutions for the insane can claim no exemption from the common weaknesses of human nature. They are men "with like passions as other men." Self-interest, in some instances, and ambition in perhaps all,—that ambition, at least, which is manifest in the desire to show as fair a record and as favorable results as are exhibited by colleague in the specialty,— have probably not been wholly inoperative in the reporting of recoveries from insanity, even though unconsciously to the persons producing those reports.[93]

Out of self-interest and/or professional concern, the "zeal and rivalry" of superintendents "gave to the public mind a false impression, from which sprang hopes and expectations that could never be fulfilled."[94]

The responses to Earle's exposés were swift. AMSAII's critics rallied around them to convince legislatures to impose more oversight. But it would be misleading to portray the exposés as the sole cause of the loss of faith in the asylum. Rather, they served to confirm already bubbling suspicions that the asylums were not yielding the returns promised. The legislatures already suspected that something was amiss. Earle's reports confirmed their suspicions. In response, legislatures asserted more control over the asylums and, in the process, challenged the heretofore unchallenged authority of superintendents when it came to their management. The increased oversight of asylums was part of a more general push to rationalize public charities. Many states established Boards of Charities, whose power, while limited, nevertheless demanded greater accounting from superintendents. At the same time, the state spigot of funding dried up. Under the economic scarcity of the post–Civil War period, legislatures were less willing to entertain more funding for the asylums, or even to maintain existing levels. State legislatures retrenched into a more general indifference toward the insane and, by extension, psychiatry.

Superintendents buckled under the weight of this new reality. To assuage legislative concerns and cope with the decreased funding, some superintendents began to fiddle with the sacrosanct Kirkbride model. Alternative plans for the asylum, anathema to the AMSAII, were floated and gained some support. A cottage system, promoted by superintendents like John M. Galt, argued that instead of housing all patients under a single roof, asylums should be composed of a series of cottages, with the most insane and disruptive relegated to cottages on the fringes, free to go about their madness without causing too much disruption.[95] The cottage plan was sold as cheaper and easily expandable (or contractible). The ensuing debate over "congregate" versus "separate" models, which divided the profession during a vulnerable time, encompassed more than just technical architectural differences. The Kirkbride asylum had been the basis for psychiatric expertise. As such, alternative plans posed an almost existential challenge and were vehemently opposed by the AMSAII leadership. In the end, only a handful of asylums adopted the cottage system, but overcrowding often led to peripheral expansion that de facto duplicated its form.

Superintendents lost another debate over the model asylum more decisively. To alleviate overcrowding in existing asylums, some legislatures proposed creating separate, alternative facilities for the chronically insane. AMSAII objected to these plans, arguing that separate institutions for more difficult cases would succumb to neglect, abuse, and the erosion of moral treatment. Against these objections, state legislatures went ahead anyway and established institutions designated for the chronically insane, which, unsurprisingly, over time became plagued by the very problems superintendents warned of.[96]

Superintendents had built a profession on the asylums and justified it via statistical rhetoric that hid the troubling realities on the ground. The asylums that dotted the countryside throughout the United States were constructed upon a foundation of "funny numbers."[97] By these means, superintendents obscured their own ignorance—perhaps even to themselves—and made grand, utopian promises of cure. For a time, these promises played a crucial generative role. They garnered state support, led to the erection of a system of asylums, and gave birth to a new form of professional authority. But when called to account, these expectations proved hollow.

Conclusion

The asylum era commenced in earnest utopianism and cocksure certainty. Its advocates, both lay and medical, hyped the asylums as *the* solution to insanity. Dix traversed the country, singing the praises of moral treatment. Superintendents captured the imagination of state legislatures by cultivating ambitious expectations. Upon these promises, they constructed a network of asylums, within which they ruled with unquestioned authority. Any lingering questions or uncertainty regarding the nature of mental illness, its effects on the brain, and the mechanisms of cure were swamped by overconfidence, absorbed in tidy statistics, deflected by appeals to ever forthcoming insight, and displaced by the alluring vision of a future in which madness was a fixable problem. Ignorance was whitewashed, hidden behind puffed-up certainty. But psychiatrists' ignorance regarding mental distress never went away. It lay dormant, always below the surface. When it was revealed—when the hype of the asylum was exposed as fraudulent—this ignorance came back with a vengeance to threaten the fragile edifice upon which psychiatric authority was built.

The asylum era bequeathed a complicated legacy to subsequent generations of psychiatrists. On the one hand, its failure, when compared to its grand promises, forced psychiatrists to come face-to-face with all it did not know, with how little they understood the object they so confidently believed they could control. For the first of what would become many instances, psychiatrists had to confront the problem of their own ignorance. And over the next century and a half in dealing with this ignorance, they would never recover the confidence and optimism of its salad days, however misplaced they were. On the other hand, the initial hype of the asylum led to the creation and institutionalization of psychiatry as a profession, no matter the disappointing results it yielded. Psychiatry was built on false promises, but it was built nonetheless.

Superintendents assumed that insanity was somatic in character and that it could be cured by moral treatment. But these assumptions amounted to mere beliefs, reinforced by creative accounting. When interrogated, they crumbled. By the 1880s, the cult of curability had been exposed and asylums were overrun. Legislatures lost interest, leaving superintendents to fend for themselves. The asylums, overcrowded and underfunded, fell into disrepair. The physical deterioration of asylum conditions came to embody a profession in crisis. Asylums entered a new era as custodial institutions for society's unwanted. What were once instruments of cure transformed into warehouses of despair. And superintendents, exiled to these overcrowded and crumbling custodial institutions, suffered from their association with an incurable clientele. Thus, in the last decades of the nineteenth century, a malaise took hold as their profession descended into crisis. They were assailed on all sides, under attack from other physicians, social activists, lawyers, state regulatory agencies, and former patients.

No threat was as great as that of neurologists, who themselves aspired to be the authorities of madness. Wrapped in the banner of positivism and scientism, neurology organized in the decades following the Civil War—the American Neurological Association (ANA) was founded in 1875—into a medical specialty based on an uncompromising somatic view of nervous conditions. As neurology grew in influence, an uneasy division of mental labor with asylum superintendents emerged. Neurologists treated an assortment of minor conditions in office-based settings, while the more severe and chronic cases accumulated in the overcrowding asylums. Still, the two professions continued to jockey for control over madness.

The contest between superintendent-psychiatrists and neurologists was punctuated with great drama. On May 16, 1894, Silas Weir Mitchell delivered an address before the now renamed American Medico-Psychological Association (AMPA) in celebration of the association's fiftieth anniversary. Mitchell was the most prominent neurologist of the day. Like many of his peers, Mitchell cut his medical teeth in the Civil War, where, as a contract surgeon, he became interested in the brain injuries of wounded soldiers.[98] Famous for his "rest cure,"[99] Mitchell became one of the most vocal advocates of neurology.

Rather than use the occasion of its anniversary to celebrate psychiatry, Mitchell seized it to deliver a scathing rebuke of asylum medicine. Comparing psychiatry to other medical specialties like neurology, Mitchell chided superintendents' lack of scientific acumen. "It is to be feared that you also have cause to recall the fact that as compared with the splendid advance in surgery, in the medicine of the eye and the steady approach to precision all along our ardent line, the alienist has won proportion little," he told his audience.[100] While acknowledging that this lack of scientific progress was "partly due to the nature of the maladies with which you have to deal,"[101]

Mitchell pinned most of the responsibility on superintendents' lack of curiosity. Superintendents failed "to keep treatment or scientific product on the front line of medical advance."[102] Their geographical isolation reflected an intellectual isolation: "You soon began to live apart and you still do so. Your hospitals are not our hospitals; your ways are not our ways. You live out of range of critical shot; you are not preceded and followed in your ward work by clever rivals, or watched by able residents fresh with the learning of the schools."[103] "Cloistral lives" gave rise to "certain mental peculiarities."[104] These peculiarities were evident in the "research" that graced the pages of its journals, or as Mitchell described them, "odd little statements, reports of a case or two, a few useless pages of isolated post-mortem records, and these are sandwiched among incomprehensible statistics and farm balance-sheets."[105] When it came to science, psychiatry was found wanting.

Mitchell's speech caused quite an uproar. The medical press pounced on it to paint superintendents as retrograde laggards who were missing out on the revolution sweeping medicine. The "words fitly spoken" exposed "the least progressive of all elements constituting the medical profession of America."[106] The speech also established the template for the neurologists' critiques of asylum psychiatry for the next few decades. For example, in 1912, William Norton Bullard, president of the American Neurological Association, mocked psychiatrists, joking that they were adept at "direct[ing] the building and heating of their buildings, the buying of coal and groceries, the making up of accounts even to minute details."[107] Likewise, Edward Charles Spitzka, another prominent neurologist, described superintendents as scientifically inept "gardeners and farmers."[108]

Yet lost in the drama of the speech was the surprisingly muted response to the criticism by psychiatrists.[109] By 1894, many psychiatrists acknowledged their ignorance and held many of the very same criticisms of their profession. Walter Channing, a Harvard-trained physician and respected founder of a private mental hospital in Massachusetts, argued that Mitchell's speech did little than restate many of the concerns that superintendents themselves had long identified:

> Nearly every point taken up by Doctor Mitchell has in some form been discussed by those having the care of the insane, and given rise to very serious consideration. At every stage of progress of the association, there have been anxious and able men in its ranks, alive to the problems and duties of the hour. They have not sat blind-folded, or played puss-in-the-corner, or milked the cows. This is a veritable fact, strange and impossible as it may appear to those ignorant of insane-hospital history.[110]

Some psychiatrists, like Channing, blamed these problems on the demands of the "insane-hospital management."[111] Superintendents had neither the time nor the energy to conduct scientific research. After all, "no man can do everything."[112]

Others, however, took ignorance as a motivator and saw an opportunity for reform. Long before Mitchell's speech, even before Earle's exposés on asylum statistics in the 1870s, a new generation of psychiatrists, inspired by European medicine, expressed similar misgivings to Mitchell regarding the inadequate knowledge base of the profession. An 1861 editorial in the *AJI* observed that psychiatry "is hardly yet permitted to take rank as a formal science."[113] Four years later, in an article discussing the process involved in determining insanity for legal purposes, psychiatrist John E. Tyler acknowledged how hard it was to enunciate "what insanity is."[114] In 1873, Earle admitted that superintendents "all know that the pathological anatomy of the brain has thus far furnished no grounds whatever, for a rational theory of insanity."[115] And in 1891, three years before Mitchell took the dais, AMSAII president Henry P. Stearns observed psychiatry falling behind.

> Within the year passed, a criticism has been advanced to the following effect: that while new discoveries have been made relating to the etiology and treatment of several of the genera of disease . . . there has not been any corresponding advance made in the specialty of insanity; that, notwithstanding the fact that large sums of the public money have been expended in the construction of hospitals and asylums for the treatment of the insane, and that they have been consigned to the more especial care of physicians with large opportunities for study and observation; yet there have not been corresponding results in the way of increased knowledge; that, in fact, we are still involved in the mists of hypotheses, and really know very little more regarding the aetiology of insanity than we did twenty years ago; while the percentage of recoveries remains lamentably small.[116]

As these admissions of ignorance reveal, nothing Mitchell said that day in 1894 was news to the profession. That the criticisms came from an outsider and a neurologist may have increased their sting and inflamed professional defensiveness, but they were not revelatory. Indeed, superintendents had already begun to initiate reforms aimed at promoting research and de-emphasizing the managerial elements of their expertise. This was symbolically reflected in the name change of the "Association of Medical Superintendents of American Institutions for the Insane" to the "American Medico-Psychological Association."

Fifty years into the association's existence, psychiatrists were well versed in their own ignorance. They had identified and acknowledged ignorance as a problem, something that needed to be managed and overcome. Psychiatry would never again be able to wrap itself in false certainty. Any attempts to do so would always be countered by sobering assessments of its uncertain knowledge base. In this way, the failure of the asylum shaped the subsequent trajectory of psychiatry. Henceforth psychiatrists would have to address their ignorance if they were to maintain their authority and uphold the justification for their profession. This ignorance would be accompanied by existential dread. It became the professional albatross with which future generations of reformers would struggle. Thus, this first brush with ignorance set off the cycle of crisis–reinvention–crisis-reinvention in which psychiatry remains to this day. More than anything, this was the legacy of the asylum era.

But the problem of ignorance was not the only legacy of the asylum era. Streaked within psychiatry's first fall was a silver lining. The asylum had given birth to a new profession, with a corresponding organizational infrastructure, that would prove resistant to dismantling. Though compromised and aggrieved, the asylums did not disappear. Rechristened as mental hospitals, they continued to perform a crucial function. They became places of confinement for society's most disrupted, most insane members. And as the de facto keepers of the asylum, superintendents became the custodians of patients with serious mental illness. Psychiatry had little to offer these patients, but these patients had much to offer psychiatry in terms of justifying its existence. Subsequent generations expressed ambivalence and misgivings about tying their fate to such a marginalized population, but at the very least, the association ensured psychiatry a place at the table of those charged with addressing madness. Moreover, the institutional infrastructure built by superintendents provided a fortress to which it could retreat in periods of crisis and a stronghold from which future psychiatrists would make incursions into professional contests over less serious, more treatable patients. As long as these institutions endured, however degraded they became, psychiatrists remained relevant. A custodial function was not what superintendents intended, nor were they happy about the marginalization that came with the role, but it ensured the profession's perseverance in the near term.

Hobbled, psychiatrists met the new century with trepidation. Yet, their pessimism carried a faint glimmer of hope. Their ignorance had been exposed, but so too had the way forward; psychiatrists had to reinvent themselves.

TWO

Unruly Ignorance and Pragmatic Eclecticism

On a humid July morning in 1881, an unkempt stranger approached President James A. Garfield as he boarded a train in Washington, DC. The stranger, Charles Guiteau, drew his English bulldog pistol and shot, striking Garfield twice, once in the back and once in the arm. The wounds were not immediately fatal. Garfield would languish for months, suffering under the care of a team of physicians schooled in the inadequate medical treatments of the day. On September 18, he died, succumbing to an infection he likely caught from his doctors.

Guiteau's motives for the assassination were murky, incomprehensible to those of sound mind and body. Prone to delusions of grandeur limited to those who perceive themselves as divinely chosen, Guiteau felt called by God to kill the corrupt Garfield. But his vendetta was also fueled by a sense of personal betrayal. During the 1880 election, Guiteau had delivered a single, unsolicited speech in support of Garfield. Convinced that his oratory had swayed the election, Guiteau felt he was due the requisite political spoils for his efforts in the form of an ambassadorship. After his entreaties were rebuffed by the administration, Guiteau concluded that Garfield was corrupt, irredeemable, and needed to be killed to save the Republic.

For months, as Garfield suffered, Guiteau languished in prison. Meanwhile, the grieving country struggled to make sense of the assassination. The press speculated endlessly about Guiteau's mental health, raising "a Babel of voices that would naturally be ambitious to make themselves heard."[1] At issue were seemingly straightforward questions: "Was he sane or insane; and if insane, was he responsible or irresponsible?"[2] Guiteau appeared mad, but the deliberateness with which he acted suggested a mind capable of reason. Perhaps he suffered from "moral insanity," a form of monomania in which an individual was incapable of resisting the impulse to harm others but was otherwise normal. If so, would this diagnosis preclude his due punishment, which everyone agreed should be death?

The sensationalist media coverage was stoked by a farcical trial. During the trial, Guiteau indulged in bizarre, disruptive antics. Insisting on conducting his own defense, he interrupted proceedings, denounced witnesses, challenged his own counsel, and made grand speeches at random moments. The judge, Walter Cox, gave Guiteau "extraordinary latitude"[3] to act out, reasoning that since Guiteau's sanity was on trial, he should have ample opportunity to display his mental state. This freedom provided the rope with which Guiteau hanged himself.

The intrigue of the trial was not the product of Guiteau's antics alone. Expert witnesses also contributed to the circus-like atmosphere. The trial exposed the disconcerting state of knowledge on insanity. The public demanded an account, some sort of sober assessment of Guiteau's mental state, some reason for his actions. Instead, what they got was more confusion. The experts gathered, and the experts disagreed. Despite Guiteau's odd behavior, the thirty-six psychiatrists and neurologists called to testify could not reach consensus on the most fundamental issues regarding Guiteau's mental state. Was he insane and therefore culpable? On the one hand, Guiteau's motives were delusional and irrational. Only a broken mind could conjure such ravings. On the other hand, the planning involved in the crime implied a degree of reasoning that did not square with the prevailing legal notions of insanity. If Guiteau was insane, what condition did he have? Proposed diagnoses proliferated. Did Guiteau suffer from mania without delirium? General paralysis? Something called "chronic subacute mania of a recurrent or paroxysmal type?"[4] Or something else altogether? And, while all agreed Guiteau's behavior was strange, experts offered up competing causes for his bizarre behavior. Some insisted that they were proof of hereditary madness, an inborn state of insanity that had degenerated over time. Others argued that they were the outcome of a life of vice and corruption, that his bad character resulted from "nothing more than devilish depravity," for which he was responsible.[5] Compounding matters were the differences between legal definitions of insanity, which focused on a binary, either/or determination, and medical definitions, which left room for insanity absent deficiencies in reasoning. Indeed, Guiteau himself played to this difference in his own muddled defense. He insisted, "I believe I was insane in law, but not in fact."[6]

The trial highlighted the general ignorance surrounding insanity. As such, it took on a curious air. With the outcome all but inevitable, the trial became a proxy for adjudicating professional claims to mental health expertise. Sides traded mocking barbs, as expert witnesses aired their professional grievances in the courtroom. While these grievances were complex,[7] they tended to map onto a dispute between neurologists and superintendents. The nature of this dispute was captured in the contrasting testimonies of two luminaries representing different sides of the neurology/psychiatry divide. Dr. Edward Spitzka, a well-regarded young neurologist and prominent member of the New York Neurological Society, testified for the defense. He proclaimed that Guiteau was insane: "There is not a scintilla of doubt in my mind that, if Guiteau, with his hereditary history, his insane manner, his insane documents, and his insane actions, were to be committed to any asylum in the land, he would be unhesitatingly admitted as a proper subject for sequestration."[8] Embracing a hereditarianism that was becoming fashionable in scientific circles, Spitzka insisted that because Guiteau's insanity was caused by a congenital predisposition, he should not be held responsible for his crime.[9] In his testimony, Spitzka displayed great disdain for psychiatrists, who he had once derided as experts in gardening, farming, roofing, engineering, "experts at everything except the diagnosis, pathology, and treatment of insanity."[10]

The prosecution, for their part, leaned on the testimony of Dr. John B. Gray. As a superintendent of the New York State Lunatic Asylum and influential editor of the *AJI*, Gray represented an endangered breed of psychiatrist. After multiple interviews with Guiteau, Gray determined that he was depraved, not insane.[11] Attuned to environmental and behavioral causes of insanity, Gray argued that Guiteau's state was a by-product of a life misled. A "life of moral degradation, moral obliquity, profound selfishness and disregard for the rights of others"[12] had deteriorated Guiteau's moral capacity and led to the assassination. For this, Guiteau was legally responsible.

Despite the professional pandemonium it unleashed, the trial was a foregone conclusion. The grieving country simply would not tolerate an acquittal, no matter what the experts said. After deliberating for just over an hour, the jury returned a guilty verdict. On June 30, 1882, Guiteau was hanged.

The professional effects of the trial, however, lingered long after Guiteau's execution. It had left a pox on both the houses of neurology and psychiatry. The trial exposed how little was known about insanity. In an editorial assessing the case, one doctor admitted, "We are sadly ignorant of the various types of human character, especially those abnormal ones which border on the region of well-recognized mental aberration."[13] Presented with an opportunity to display their mastery to the public, the experts had failed. The contentious back-and-forth, despite the egos so assured, gave public testament to the fundamental ignorance of knowledge of insanity.

For psychiatrists in particular, the fissures on display in the courthouse inspired little confidence in their authority. For half a century, psychiatrists had tied their fate to the asylum, laying claim to an administrative expertise justified by the supposed efficacy of moral treatment. By the turn of the twentieth century, this lay in ruins. The ignorance superintendents had hidden behind neat tables of statistics was thrown into sharp relief. Asylums fell into disrepair, the now rundown buildings buckling under the weight of growing patient populations. Censured by neurologists, other physicians, social activists, lawyers, state regulatory agencies, and former patients, psychiatry succumbed to a crisis with broad fibrous roots.

Psychiatry was adrift. Confronting their lack of understanding of the object they had once purported to have tamed, many surrendered to deep pessimism. The days of overconfidence were past; early twentieth-century psychiatrists were forced to acknowledge all that they did not know. Psychiatric discourse took on a confessional, apologetic tone as leaders admitted ignorance. August Hoch, director of the New York State Psychiatric Institute, summarized the situation:

> But while we infer the existence of different [mental] diseases, we have little knowledge of their real processes. Indeed, such a knowledge seems to be very remote; but what are accessible to us are the manifestations of these processes with all their great variety of differences. It is just here that we are at once confronted with the greatest problem, i.e., which of these differences are essential and which are not.[14]

Not only did psychiatrists have "little knowledge" of the "real processes" of different mental disorders; they were hard-pressed to identify which of the many manifestations of madness were relevant. Knowledge remained "remote." E. Stanley Abbot, psychiatrist at McLean Hospital in Massachusetts, was more blunt: "In fact, our present ignorance of the causes of insanity is largely due to our ignorance of what insanity really is."[15] This was ignorance of a profound kind.

At the beginning of the twentieth century, a handful of reformers, led by Adolf Meyer, recognized the need to regroup. But how? With the asylum in disrepair, a group of young reformers, some of whom were trained in Europe and thus less antagonistic to neurological ideas and laboratory science, schemed an escape from the asylum. While many of their peers reacted to psychiatric ignorance with dismay and even nihilism, these reformers saw the challenges facing psychiatry as an opportunity, a chance to tackle the complex problems that superintendents had long avoided. Instead of wallowing, they manufactured a reinvention out of the wreckage of the asylum era.

No figure embraced this challenge more than Adolf Meyer. Meyer's response to Silas Weir Mitchell's scathing critique was indicative of his understanding of psychiatry's predicament. Meyer felt the "storm" that Mitchell created was "a spur in more than one way" for psychiatry to evolve into a scientific endeavor.[16] Instead of rebutting Mitchell or denying his assessment, Meyer used it as an opening wedge for reform, going so far as to forward Mitchell's address to the governor of Illinois to justify improvements he wished to undertake.[17] In Meyer's hands, Mitchell's rebuke was transformed into a new start.

For reformers like Meyer, this start began with an acknowledgment of the complex nature of mental illness. Psychiatrists, argued Meyer, dealt with "the most unruly and willful part or aspect of man."[18] Rather than indulging in false certainty, like their superintendent forbearers, this new generation of psychiatrists would rebuild psychiatry upon an appreciation of the depth of their ignorance. In response to the challenges this ignorance posed, they promoted a wide-ranging program, one grounded in, but not reducible to, medical science. The protean character of mental illness—its composition of social, psychological, and biological facets—demanded a diverse research program. Put plainly, reformers articulated a new vision for psychiatry in which their ignorance was to be met head-on, not denied, by a wide-ranging and eclectic research program that refused to prematurely cut off any possible path to enlightenment. They dubbed this vision "psychobiology."

Covering the period from 1890 to 1940, this chapter recounts the reinvention of psychiatry under psychobiology. This was a fecund but confused period in which psychiatry was transformed from a narrow profession of asylum superintendents into a sprawling endeavor. Even the label of psychobiology is misleading, as it suggests a clear, delineated program when, in reality, it reflected more of a general ethos, an open-ended conceptualization for the psychiatric project. This open-ended character can defy neat narration. As such, it can be all too easy to minimize the importance of psychobiology, to reduce it to a muddled, vacuous mess. This was a time of flux, as psychiatrists grappled with basic questions of identity and epistemic commitments. But what reformers constructed out of this morass had lasting impact. In this chapter, I reclaim the historical importance of the psychobiological period as a key moment of experimentation in response to psychiatry's ongoing ignorance.

Psychobiology, as articulated by Meyer and his collaborators, refused to funnel psychiatry into a single system. Recognizing the immature state of psychiatric knowledge, it pursued an open-ended agenda that promoted pluralism. The reimagined psychiatry would pursue mental illness down multiple paths through all its manifold causes and characteristics. And it would draw on diverse sources of insight to do so. Under psychobiology, psychiatric reformers would try to merge the somatic with the psychological, exploring the neurological, biological, psychological, and social aspects of mental illness. Some reformers hewed closely to medicine proper, trying to reconstruct neurological mechanisms or positing genetic accounts of madness that intersected with the new science of eugenics. Others homed in on psychological dynamics and meaning-making, stressing the potential of psychotherapy. Still others sought to remedy madness through its social factors, drawing inspiration from successful public health campaigns on infectious diseases to posit a wide-ranging program of mental hygiene. New organizations were created, novel institutional alternatives to the deteriorating mental hospitals. As a result of this experimentation, psychiatry, once circumscribed to the realm of superintendents, sprawled and diversified. The psychobiological program promised to resolve ignorance by pursuing it in all directions in the expectation that these efforts would coalesce into a complete picture of mental illness. It promised that a widely cast net would clarify the nature of madness, that experimentation and diversification would evolve into a synthesis worthy of a medical science.

It did not. Instead of synthesis, psychobiology devolved into fragmentation. Over time what began as a cooperative division of labor, a parceling out of responsibilities in a "both/and" spirit, devolved into "either/or" competition. Pluralism brought forth a cacophony of perspectives, advocates of which jockeyed for supremacy. Moreover, problems that would plague psychiatry for decades—theoretical dogmatism, premature overzealousness, and a lack of caution when experimenting on patients—thrived in an environment in which psychiatrists grasped for any sign of progress amid few intellectual constraints. Eventually, psychobiology would be reduced to a mere signifier, one that conveyed a vague commitment to integrating the psychological with the biological, the brain and the mind. Eventually, it would be cast aside altogether.

Nevertheless, psychobiology left a legacy that reverberates to this day. For it was during this time that psychiatry developed its habit of reinvention.

The Dean of American Psychiatry

Psychiatry between 1890 and 1940 was an eclectic affair. During this period, psychiatrists embraced divergent understandings of the nature of mental illness, posited multiple causes and cures, and pursued different courses of action. This diversity presents distinct challenges for those trying to understand this period. Unlike the asylum era that preceded it or the psychoanalytic period that would follow, psychiatry under psychobiology lacked evident cohesion. It comprised an almost unwieldy multitude of perspectives and research programs, often operating with incommensurate assumptions. What, if anything, held this mélange together?

Fortunately, one can begin to comprehend how these disparate pieces fit together by examining a single psychiatrist. A real living Martin Arrowsmith of psychiatry,[19] Adolf Meyer's career brought him into contact with all the major strands of psychobiology. As a powerful figure looming over the most influential institutions of the period, he had a hand in creating most all of psychobiology's various offshoots.

A man of short stature and dark complexion, Meyer spoke with a Swiss-German accent that many Americans perceived as distinguished. He had the kind of European pedigree that elevated him in the eyes of his peers. Born in Switzerland in 1866, Meyer received his medical degree from the University of Zurich, where he trained under some of Europe's most renowned neurologists. In 1892, he immigrated to the United States. Well versed in the laboratory sciences, Meyer secured a position as a pathologist at Illinois Eastern Hospital in Kankakee, Illinois. In 1895, he left for Worcester State Hospital, where he instituted a number of important organizational reforms, most notably the creation of a pathological laboratory. In 1902, he became director of the New York Pathological Institute, an organization dedicated to psychiatric research. As only its second director, Meyer would be instrumental in shaping this novel kind of institution. Finally, in 1908, Meyer moved on to Johns Hopkins University, *the* model for a laboratory-based approach to medical education in the United States. Here, he established the Phipps Clinic in 1913, where he trained generations of psychiatrists until he retired in 1941.

Throughout his career, Meyer positioned himself as the fulcrum of American psychiatry. Holding in succession two of the most powerful posts in American psychiatry, first as director of the New York Pathological Institute and then as psychiatrist in chief at the Phipps Clinic, he was central in bringing about significant reforms in psychiatry. He stimulated fledgling research programs, introduced laboratory methods to mental hospitals and psychiatric training, and established the organizational template for independent psychiatric research institutes and university-based psychiatric hospitals. He was also involved in the training of almost every influential psychiatrist in the first half of the twentieth century.[20] Prominent neuropsychiatrist Elmer Ernest Southard declared that "no greater power to change our minds about the problems of psychiatry has been at work in the interior of the psychiatric profession in America than the personality of Adolf Meyer. If he will pardon me the phrase, I shall designate him as a ferment, an enzyme, a catalyzer."[21] More than anyone else, Meyer remade psychiatry's image and helped it regain a measure of respectability.

Meyer used his influence to promote a new vision for psychiatry, one that approached mental illness from multiple angles. This vision reflected Meyer's own personality, his distinct epistemic commitments, and his acute appreciation of the immature state of psychiatric knowledge. Meyer displayed an unwavering commitment to synthesizing diverse traditions. Compromise, not conflict, characterized his approach. In his own words, he had "a non-dogmatic and perhaps actually anti-dogmatic nature, and devoid of any messianic urge."[22] He gave all new ideas a respectful hearing, avoiding quick judgments concerning the legitimacy or illegitimacy of novel research programs, however eccentric or quixotic they might appear. Meyer was optimistic to a fault, and put his faith "on a search for the common ground."[23] Almost allergic to controversy—he acknowledged, "With me, there is some deep drive to attain unity"—he could be coy in taking sides in disputes.[24] This coyness, combined with his willingness to play with ideas, was often mistaken as endorsement. As a result, some of the most egregious abuses of psychiatry during this period, notably psychosurgery and eugenics, would be associated with his name. But if Meyer was sometimes naïve to these dangers, his failings reflected a conscious effort to construct a big tent for psychiatry, one that could accommodate diversity and promote a dialogue needed to comprehend the "multi-conditioned character of all the conditions with which we deal."[25]

Meyer dubbed this loose program "psychobiology." The name signaled his desire to eradicate "the dualistic tendency to speak in terms of 'psyche' and 'soma'" and join the biological and psychological strands of psychiatry that were often viewed as antagonistic.[26] Rather than circumscribing the psychiatric project, Meyer encouraged an experimental ethos in the face of psychiatry's ignorance. He never wavered in the belief that, over time, the diverse strands of psychiatry he encouraged would converge into a comprehensive understanding of mental illness.

While psychobiology reflected Meyer's tendencies as a thinker, it had intellectual roots in American pragmatist philosophy and the Paris clinical school of medicine, which Meyer mingled to create a distinctly American psychiatry.[27] From pragmatist philosophy, Meyer took his most fundamental epistemological commitments. As a school of thought, pragmatism arose as a response to the American Civil War, which, for a generation of thinkers, revealed the violent consequences of undue certitude.[28] Pragmatists championed pluralism and common sense in the face of dogmatic ideology. A diffuse philosophical school, all pragmatists shared an appreciation of the instrumental function of thought. Deriding the "spectator theory of knowledge," the search for immutable truth, and the "quest for certainty" as misguided, pragmatists sought to bring philosophy down from the rarefied air of abstraction by focusing on thinking's practical effects.[29] The purpose of thought was not to describe or represent reality, but to facilitate action and problem-solving in an ever-changing world. Ideas were treated as instruments for "coping," their "cash value" determined by what they allow people to accomplish.[30] As such, pragmatism linked the act of thinking to human adaptation and survival by focusing on the role of habit.

Meyer was first exposed to pragmatism at the University of Chicago, during his tenure at Kankakee and then through his close relationships with pragmatist thinkers John Dewey and William James. He selectively adopted some of pragmatism's tenets in developing his approach to psychiatric knowledge. First, he endorsed pluralism and openness "as liberating factors in throwing off dogmatic dualism and making unnecessary an ideal and forced monism which disregarded the specificity of many biological data."[31] The pluralism reflected an appreciation of the limits of any one individual to comprehend what James termed the world's "great buzzing, blooming confusion."[32] Second, Meyer took pragmatists' stress on experimentation, which they construed as a basic feature of human existence. The way to refine ideas over time was to test and challenge them, by courting new experiences, exposing oneself to new ideas, and exploring their practical implications. By this means, ideas would evolve toward closer reflection of reality. Just as pragmatists reclaimed the provisional and evolutionary aspect of knowledge production, so too did Meyer promote flexibility and experimentation in the face of psychiatric ignorance. As a communal endeavor unfolding over time, psychobiology would push provisional beliefs into agreement with each other and, in turn, closer agreement with the reality of mental illness itself. Finally, Meyer embraced pragmatists' emphasis on action. He insisted that psychiatrists never lose sight of the patient and the clinical imperative to heal. Because of this pragmatist-inspired instrumentalism, he chafed at academic psychology and abstract system-building, which he felt was too removed from the messy clinical world to be of much use. Instead, he applauded practical common sense as the key to science: "What is good in common-sense is the best part of science and if there is much need of correcting common-sense there is also plenty of opportunity to improve the scientific attitude."[33] Ideas were to be, in the words of James, things "upon which we can ride."[34] The measure of good psychiatric science must always be whether it helps patients get better.

Meyer combined these pragmatist ideals with a commitment to empiricism and inductive reasoning inspired by the Paris clinical school of medicine.[35] In the US imagination, the Paris School stood for an empiricism accrued via the careful observation of facts untainted by cumbersome theory.[36] This was juxtaposed to the speculative abstract systems of disease in vogue in the early decades of the nineteenth century. Departing from pragmatists like James who maintained a skepticism toward the accuracy of human observation, Meyer, inspired by the Paris School, maintained an almost fetishistic commitment to facts. Indeed, Meyer's conceptualization of science was not founded on a particular method or body of knowledge, but on an ethos dedicated to the rigorous accumulation of facts. Pre-interpretive facts were to be the material of psychiatric work: "We work the facts contained in the life history and family history and the results of our examinations, with the individual assets and maladjustments and the individual and social adjustments open to us."[37] This ethos was reflected in Meyer's lifelong efforts to reform administrative procedures related to data collection.[38] It was also evident in his skepticism toward classification schemas and diagnostic labels, which he derided "as [a] form of nosological dogma."[39] The way forward for psychiatry was to loosen its theoretical assumptions—especially its reductionist somatic theories—and to pursue the accumulation of the facts of the case. On this, the often equivocating Meyer did not mince words:

> Unfortunately, the intemperate craving for logical unity which our education teaches us to strive for as the only worthy resting place, and the habit of sacrifice of the concrete reality to the Moloch of simplicity at any price are apt to vitiate seriously our standards of moral responsibility in the presentation of facts. Psychiatric experience has sadly suffered from veritable debauches in unwarranted systematization. To this are added the effects of a common self-deception about the meaning and purpose of diagnoses. An orderly presentation of facts alone is real diagnosis.[40]

If the purpose of psychiatric knowledge was to help the patient, investigations should stay close to the individual and "the positive facts of life as found."[41]

Underwriting all this was a protean ontology of mental illness, one that appreciated its multidimensional character. At root, psychobiology rejected attempts to separate and dichotomize the biological and psychological aspects of the mind, what Meyer referred to as "a deadly parallelism between mind and body," or "an effete and impossible contrast between mental and physical."[42] Mind, argued Meyer, is a "sufficiently organized living being in action; and not a peculiar form of mind-stuff."[43] Psyche and soma were different dimensions of the same complicated thing. Stressing the interaction between the body and mind, psychobiology sought to liberate psychiatry from reductive somatic understandings of mental illness that had been an article of faith among most superintendents.[44] Mental illness thus assumed a more complicated form. Drawing on a Darwinian model of adaptation, Meyer held that mental illness resulted from the interaction between the individual and his environment. Mental activity was "understood in its full meaning as the adaptation and adjustment of the individual as a whole."[45] In turn, mental illness was conceived of as failed adaptation. "We do not think of disease entities but of processes, that is, miscarriages and deviations of functions," Meyer insisted.[46] Mental illnesses were reconceptualized as maladaptive responses on the part of the organism—the patient—to its environment, social or otherwise: "What is vaguely called insanity—a term which physicians would gladly leave to the lawyer if he can use it—is really a wide range of greatly differing conditions and diseases all playing havoc with our organ and functions of conduct and behavior."[47]

Consequently, psychobiology stressed not disease entities but the total patient in relation to his or her environment. Each maladaptation was understood as "involving defective habits" unique to the individual.[48] This was not to suggest that mental illness was entirely idiosyncratic. Developed in response to the patient's specific life experiences, "conditioned by a great variety of factors, none which can be safely neglected," these habits could be grouped into what Meyer termed "reaction patterns."[49] Nevertheless, the focus remained not on diagnostic labels or patterns, but on the individual, his or her distinct biological and psychological features, situated within a particular context. Treatment, thus, focused on understanding the emergence of maladaptive habits specific to the patient within his or her life course and the cultivation of better ones.

Psychobiology's multidimensional conceptualization of mental illness demanded a diverse knowledge base. To accumulate all relevant information, "a psychiatrist has to have a truly comprehensive knowledge of the human organism and also of its functioning in complex personal and social relations, past, present and future, and objective and subjective."[50] Meyer's was not a narrowed vision for psychiatric knowledge but a broad one that refused to reduce a case to one of its constituent parts. For this reason, he insisted that psychiatrists receive an "all-round training," for while "[n]obody can expect to govern all fields alike," those who were not well rounded were "likely to drift."[51]

Meyer's programmatic statements on psychobiology often displayed a high degree of ambiguity. This was in part a reflection of psychobiology's reach and complexity, and in part a consequence of Meyer's obtuse writing style.[52] To capture the spirit of psychobiology, it is often necessary to look elsewhere at the concrete forms and practices it assumed. And perhaps no other manifestation testified to this spirit than Meyer's life chart. Recognizing that the vast terrain of relevant facts threatened to overwhelm psychiatrists, Meyer introduced the life chart to organize and standardize the collection of information pertinent to the case. As a diagnostic tool, the life chart created a visual reconstruction of the entirety of a patient's mental and physical development. It was organized chronologically by year, starting with the patient's birth, listed down the left-hand side of the page. Biological information, gained from an extensive examination, was represented by growth curves for each organ system. This information was traced down the middle of the chart, with space on either side of the curves reserved for brief comments on the most important medical, sexual, social, and environmental facts.[53] Along the right-hand border, important life events were noted. Thus, the life chart sorted relevant facts in temporal relation to both the biological development of the organism and his or her biography. In doing so, it revealed the multiple factors that led the individual to deviate from his or her own normative development. The patient's mental state was assessed not according to some external referent, but in relation to the individual's own experiment in living. Once organized and set within this framework, the life chart mapped "a chain of cause and effect that Meyer analogized to the results of a laboratory experiment."[54] Having identified the chronological unfolding of the patient's unique maladjustment, treatment could be catered to the specific patient so as to reestablish his or her equilibrium.

The extent to which psychiatrists used the life chart in practice varied, but this does not detract from its usefulness as a representation of psychobiological thought. It embodied the spirit of psychobiology—the appreciation for the multiple relevant factors leading to distress, the need to embed these factors within the biological and social life of the individual, and the importance of temporality in sorting out the emergence of maladjustments to external stimuli. The life chart, along with Meyer's other data-collection reforms, established an understanding of mental illness grounded in the detailed reconstruction of the case. "The object then in recording a patient's history," insisted Clarence Farrar, psychiatrist and editor of the *AJP* for over three decades, "should not be to describe a cut-and-dried disease-picture made up of such and such stereotyped symptoms, to which a definite and final name can be assigned, but rather to furnish as complete a psychic

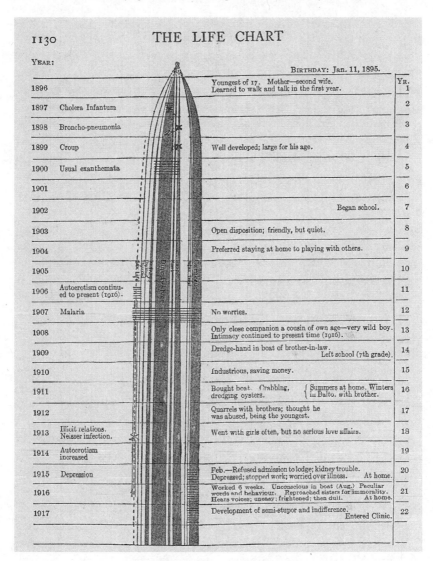

1130

THE LIFE CHART

YEAR:

BIRTHDAY: Jan. 11, 1895.

1896		Youngest of 17. Mother—second wife. Learned to walk and talk in the first year.	YR. 1
1897	Cholera Infantum		2
1898	Broncho-pneumonia		3
1899	Croup	Well developed; large for his age.	4
1900	Usual exanthemata		5
1901			6
1902		Began school.	7
1903		Open disposition; friendly, but quiet.	8
1904		Preferred staying at home to playing with others.	9
1905			10
1906	Autoerotism continued to present (1916).		11
1907	Malaria	No worries.	12
1908		Only close companion a cousin of own age—very wild boy. Intimacy continued to present time (1916).	13
1909		Dredge-hand in boat of brother-in-law. Left school (7th grade).	14
1910		Industrious, saving money.	15
1911		Bought boat. Crabbing, dredging oysters. { Summers at home. Winters in Balto. with brother.	16
1912		Quarrels with brothers; thought he was abused, being the youngest.	17
1913	Illicit relations. Neisser infection.	Went with girls often, but no serious love affairs.	18
1914	Autoerotism increased		19
1915	Depression	Feb.—Refused admission to lodge; kidney trouble. Depressed; stopped work; worried over illness. At home.	20
1916		Worked 6 weeks. Unconscious in boat (Aug.) Peculiar words and behaviour. Reproached sisters for immorality. Hears voices; uneasy; frightened; then dull. At home.	21
1917		Development of semi-stupor and indifference. Entered Clinic.	22

2. Line drawing of the life chart by Adolf Meyer
(Wellcome Collection, London, CC BY 4.1).

biography of the individual as possible, setting forth the manner and degree
in which the diseased psyche departs from the normal for the individual."[55]
Psychiatric assessments and the records based on these assessments had to
paint a complete picture of the patient, for this was the object of psychiatry's
scrutiny and treatment.

Through psychobiology, Meyer transformed the negative perceptions of psychiatry and its ignorance into a positive program of reform. In this, he assumed a particular stance vis-à-vis psychiatric ignorance. Meyer never shrank from ignorance. To the contrary, he displayed a great tolerance for uncertainty, acknowledging ignorance in the service of articulating his wide-ranging program to overcome it. Given the depth of psychiatric ignorance, psychiatrists could take nothing for granted. They could not cut off any possible avenue of insight. Multiple research programs needed to be cultivated. Each might focus on a particular aspect of mental illness. Meyer was not opposed to specialization or a division of labor. Yet, these diverse strands were always seen as part of a larger communal project evolving over time. Taking a cue once again from pragmatism, he believed that a process of elimination and survival of the truest ideas would ultimately bring these multiple strands together in agreement, a process that Charles Sanders Peirce called the "fated agreement of convergence through the process of inquiry."[56] This was the promise of psychobiology made in regard to ignorance. Psychobiology would lead to a future in which the diverse strands of psychiatry converged in a comprehensive synthesis. By these means, psychiatry's unruly ignorance would be tamed.

Assuming Our Position as a Medical Science

Psychobiology was pitched as a long-term collective project, consisting of diverse psychiatries. Meyer proposed it as a science "which brings together into the service of modern life both the humanistic and the natural sciences, claims for itself an active place within the study of man in health and disease and why it deserves a fundamental recognition in medical work, side by side with anatomy and physiology, as a natural foundation for all pathology and therapy."[57] Putting this broad, multifaceted program into practice, however, proved challenging.

Foremost in the minds of reformers was securing professional legitimation through an association with medicine proper. The historical fluctuations of American psychiatry are often characterized using the pendulum metaphor, whereby the profession is portrayed as swinging back and forth between a focus on the mind or the brain, the soma or the psyche, the psychological or the biological, the scientific or the humanistic. While possessing a crude accuracy, this metaphor imposes an artificial dichotomy on the perceptions of mental illness in any given era.[58] These elements have never been so neatly separated in practice. In the grip of this metaphor, there is a tendency among some to misread psychobiology as a program opposed to medicine, or at least in tension with it.[59] This misperception has been reinforced over time. In its contemporary usage, the term "psychobiology" has become reduced to something of a shibboleth indicating a critique of the medical model. Once again, there is a grain of truth here: psychobiological reformers were hostile to the notion that mental illness could be reduced to biological factors. But psychobiology always maintained a prominent role for medicine. Psychobiological reformers recognized the growing prestige of medicine and sought to capture some of its glow for themselves. Therefore, even though "a large part of psychiatric problems are not essentially medical," it was "in the best interests of psychiatry" to associate itself with medicine.[60] The question was how to reconceive psychiatry along medical lines, while still retaining a distinct identity. Reformers sought to reconstruct psychiatry, via psychobiology, as a non-reductionistic, humanistic medical science that maintained an appreciation for the kaleidoscopic character of mental illness.

During the latter decades of the nineteenth century, a revolution swept medicine, brought about by the laboratory sciences, the emergence of the germ theory of disease, and the development of effective vaccines. Psychiatry was excluded from most of these developments. Lewellys F. Barker, physician and laboratory reformer, spoke to the obstacles facing psychiatry. "We have as yet, it must be admitted, no pathology of mental diseases worthy of the name," observed Barker, "nor can we expect any very satisfactory psychiatric pathology until our knowledge of cerebral anatomy and physiology has been much extended."[61] Nevertheless, like many of those pushing psychiatry to adopt laboratory reforms, Barker did not let these challenges deter him: "Yet a beginning has been made, and we have every reason to believe that continued conscientious work will lead to important results."[62] The embattled medicine of the mid-1800s, which superintendents were content to keep at arm's length, had been revolutionized. And psychiatric reformers wanted in.

In one case, this revolution touched mental illness. Neurosyphilis became an exemplar of how psychiatry might be transformed by laboratory medicine. For decades, psychiatrists were responsible for treating a condition termed "general paresis," a disorder characterized by insanity or paralytic dementia. Contemporary analyses of asylum records show that patients with this condition comprised a substantial part of asylum populations. For example, between 1911 and 1919, 20% of all male first admissions to the New York State mental hospitals were cases of general paresis.[63] Although the discovery of syphilis is a complicated story,[64] the causative organism was first identified in 1905 by Fritz Schaudinn and Erich Hoffmann. Just as significant was the discovery of an effective treatment. In 1910, Paul Ehrlich developed Salvarsan, an arsenic compound that targeted the bacterial agent that caused syphilis. Treatment with Salvarsan could prevent syphilis from progressing into general paresis and insanity. This heralded victory provided a crucial link between psychiatry and the germ theory revolution. It suggested that psychiatry was amenable to the reforms along similar lines to those happening in medicine proper. And it fueled optimism that similar discoveries were on the horizon. This raised expectations that germ theory and the laboratory revolution would find their way into psychiatry. If one mental illness could be cured by the laboratory, perhaps all could.

The story of neurosyphilis, however, carried a professional warning, as the victory over general paresis was somewhat pyrrhic for psychiatrists. Once the bacteriological origin of the disease was identified, the disorder was removed from psychiatry's jurisdiction and became the property of other physicians. Therefore, while proving that mental illness could be made intelligible and manageable through the latest developments in medical science, general paresis also revealed that once a mental illness was reinscribed in more conventional medical terms, it could be taken away from psychiatrists. If other mental illnesses followed this trajectory, psychiatry risked becoming obsolete. This has been a long-standing tension in psychiatry's dealings with medicine proper—as disease entities become more responsive to medical reasoning and intervention, they exit the contested space of psychiatry and become the province of other medical specialties.

Aware of this dilemma, psychobiological reformers posited a psychiatry built upon medical science, but not reducible to it. Here, they attempted to walk a fine line. With the fortunes of medicine proper rising at the very time that psychiatry's were declining, reformers saw a stronger association with medicine enticing. Jealous of medicine's progress, they hoped to trade on medicine's growing prestige in pursuing their own professional aspirations. But they needed to carve out a distinct niche within medicine to ensure that psychiatry was not subsumed into other medical specialties, that it had a particular contribution to make. For psychobiological reformers, this meant retaining a framing of mental illness as something more than just medical. They promoted a conception of mental illness that stressed the relevance of *both* psychological and biological factors. Mental illness was uniquely complicated, far more so than infectious diseases like cholera and diphtheria. It thus required a medical specialty uniquely attuned to this complexity. For psychiatrists, the prestige medicine enjoyed, while not unwarranted, was seen not as an indication of its superiority over psychiatry, but rather reflected its easier subject matter. Mental illnesses were just more resistant to explanation. Of all the medical branches, argued Meyer, "[psychiatry] is the most subtle, the most complicated, the most refractory to simple and easy presentation."[65] Gerald Adler Blumer, superintendent of Utica and AMPA president from 1903 to 1904, asserted:

> In the whole medical hierarchy there is no specialty fraught with greater per-
> plexities, insomuch that it was natural and logical that, while we may our-
> selves claim to have approached and met its stupendous problems with no
> faint heart and with a reasonable measure of success, recognition should have
> come to us tardily under the slow but sure compulsion of achievement, while
> other branches of medicine, driving the ploughshare over easier and narrower
> fields of research—I say it not in disparagement—have seemed to advance by
> leaps and bounds and to permit their votaries to hold high the head in "pride,
> rank pride, and haughtiness of soul."[66]

Psychiatry's lack of progress was not from lack of effort or acumen, but the complexity of the object.

Under the ominous cloud of ignorance, medical science supplied psy-chobiological reformers a silver lining of optimism. By heeding its tenets, psychiatrists, in the words of southern superintendent James Thomas Searcy, were "assuming our position" as a medical specialty, "entering the field of scientific psychology and psychopathy."[67] To signify this reinvention, AMSAII changed its name twice, first in 1892, to the American Medico-Psychological Association, and then in 1921, to the American Psychiatric Association. In his 1922 presidential address announcing the second name change in two de-cades, Albert M. Barrett stated that it "marked the broadening of [psychiatry's] interests and a more specific statement of its concern with mind in medical relationships," heralding a new period in which psychiatry has "shaped for itself a definite position as a branch of medicine."[68] Psychiatrists could expect that insights, although perhaps harder won, would follow. "The past of psy-chiatry has been full of discouragement," argued Bernard Sachs, a New York neurologist, "the present is involved in a maze of uncertainty, but the future is full of hope."[69]

No name change, however, could gloss over the growing pains that the shift from an administrative specialty to a medical specialty entailed. Wit-nessing the gains laboratory medicine had made, and responding to cri-tiques of neurologists that psychiatry was isolated in asylums, reformers created new organizational reforms to encourage the very type of scientific research that critics argued psychiatry lacked. Led by Meyer, these reforms had mixed success. First, they attempted to reform the operations of asylum to allow more time and resources dedicated to research. For example, Meyer strove to encourage research cultures within the traditional asylums where he worked. He improved laboratory facilities, organized the collection of data, and standardized procedures for more in-depth medical examinations. These efforts, however, remained hampered by the administrative demands on hospital psychiatrists. They were also hindered by the geographic isolation of the asylums, which left "little hope of building up a regular division or a closely-knit group [of researchers], as the state hospitals have not wakened up yet to their responsibilities for doing investigative work."[70] Always at a disadvantage given that they were responsible for managing the most intractable cases of mental illness, the asylums, now rebranded mental hospitals, remained focused on containing mental illness, not researching it.

Recognizing that scientific psychiatry could not flourish in mental hospitals, reformers created two novel organizations to promote research. The first were state psychiatric research institutes. Justified as clearinghouses for psychiatric cases, these institutes coordinated research on mental illness. This research had two mandates: to study the causes and conditions that underlie mental disease and to offer instruction in brain pathology to state hospital physicians. The archetype for the research institute was the New York Pathological Institute, founded in 1895. When Meyer became head of the Institute in 1902, he sought to transform it into a nexus for laboratory research for the state. He increased its scientific productivity by expanding its facilities and creating a postgraduate program to train a new generation of psychiatrists in laboratory research methods. Yet, despite Meyer's accomplishments in New York, psychiatric institutes failed to catch on nationally.

Reformers also led efforts to create new mental hospitals, distinct from the traditional asylums. Here, reformers followed the cue of hospital reforms more generally. Once charitable institutions, biomedical reformers were in the process of transforming hospitals along the lines of laboratory science.[71] Psychiatric reformers proposed similar innovations for new mental hospitals—a program referred to as "the hospital ideal."[72] Targeting acute, short-term cases, the new hospitals, like the Boston Psychopathic Hospital (est. 1912) and Phipps Psychiatric Clinic (est. 1913), were to be located in urban centers and often affiliated with medical schools. Their smaller, temporary patient populations would allow for more time dedicated to research, creating places where "the laboratory comes in for an even greater share."[73] The hope was that the pursuit of psychiatric knowledge in such hospitals could unfold along a more scientific vein. While these urban hospitals spread more than research institutes, they were often too bogged down trying to attend to their patients to produce much in the way of research.

In addition to organizational innovations, the commitment to medicine brought about a slew of new medical "treatments" for patients, for better or worse (but mainly worse). Even as reformers shifted their attention away from traditional mental hospitals, psychiatrists in these settings, although isolated, were nevertheless developing new treatments. The population of chronic patients—defined as those hospitalized for five years or more—had increased from 39.2% in 1905 to 54% in 1923.[74] Hospital psychiatrists had to manage overcrowding populations of the most severely mentally ill, with few resources at their disposal. Circumstances forced them to improvise, and therapeutic experimentation, done under a loose imprimatur of science, thrived under these conditions.

Perhaps the most infamous case of experimentation was psychosurgery. Psychosurgery was developed by Bayard Taylor Holmes, a Chicago physician, and Henry Cotton, superintendent of the Trenton State Hospital in New Jersey.[75] Taking syphilis as a cue, Holmes and Cotton posited that mental illness was caused by focal sepsis, whereby chronic infections poisoned the brain. To excise these infections, they turned to surgery, which had undergone a recent renaissance. Holmes, viewing mental illness as the product of gastrointestinal infection, was the first to try abdominal surgery as a cure for mental illness. He performed surgery on his son, Ralph, after growing dissatisfied with the results of conventional psychiatric treatment. His son died four days later. Undeterred, Holmes continued to perform psychosurgery until his death in 1924.

Cotton's lengthier and more notorious career in surgical bacteriology began in 1916. Cotton believed the mouth was the source of infection and initiated treatment by removing patients' teeth. If mental illness persisted, he proceeded to remove their tonsils, stomachs, bladders, spleens, colons, ovaries, and other organs, cutting and extracting until he eliminated the infection and cured the insanity. Claiming a success rate of up to 85%, Cotton's psychosurgery intrigued many psychiatrists at first. Meyer, a mentor to Cotton, encouraged his experiments, going so far as to write a glowing foreword to a publication of Cotton's lectures. However, as Cotton performed more radical and dangerous surgeries, his peers became squeamish of his methods, which left his patients diminished, maimed, and often dead. The treatment caught the attention of the media and eventually the New Jersey State Senate, which commissioned an investigation in 1925. The investigation discovered statistical improprieties in Cotton's results that exaggerated the efficacy of psychosurgery. More damning, firsthand accounts painted an unnerving scene of "hundreds of people without teeth," starving and unable to chew the food that the hospital neglected to even even purée for them.[76] While the high-profile investigation did not result in a punishment, it drew sufficient negative attention to Cotton, and most psychiatrists distanced themselves from him. It is worth noting, however, that their abandonment of Cotton was driven as much by a professional calculus as it was by moral opprobrium. Not only was psychosurgery a black mark for the struggling profession; it could also hurt the cause of psychiatry, as psychiatrist William A. White noted, by reducing it to "an adjunct or the handmaiden of the gastro-enterologist, the genito-urinary surgeon and the dentist."[77]

Psychosurgery was no anomaly. Upon the altar of experimentation, hospital psychiatrists were all too willing to sacrifice their patients' well-being. The potential professional benefits of new treatments that acted on the body were too seductive to abandon.[78] Malarial therapy was developed in 1920s, insulin coma therapy and metrazol therapy followed in the 1930s, and electroshock treatment in 1940. Each new treatment followed a script similar to psychosurgery. Developed in isolation and tested on unwitting patients, each was introduced to great hype and exaggerated claims of efficacy. Over time, optimism gave way to skepticism, disappointment, and the eventual abandonment of existing treatments for the next new thing. Despite the repeated failures and accompanying horrors, the experiments did not cease, for, as sociologist Andrew Scull argues, they "were visible symbols of psychiatry's reconnection to scientific medicine and its break from early isolation and therapeutic impotence."[79] It did not hurt that in addition to giving hospital psychiatry a scientific patina, the treatments were often useful in controlling problematic patients. This ensured their continuing appeal even despite their poor results.

The organizational and therapeutic innovations introduced during the psychobiological period diversified the profession, providing psychiatrists with institutional footholds outside the asylum and expanding its client base.[80] Still, the reforms never delivered on their promises to transform psychiatry into a medical science. Nor did they resolve psychiatry's basic ignorance. The dream of domesticating madness in the laboratory became more and more elusive. Psychiatrists could not escape the conclusion that "discoveries that threw a flood of new light upon other diseases failed to illuminate the darkness that enshrouded the essential nature of disorders of the mind."[81] In a presidential address before AMPA in 1923, H. W. Mitchell lamented, "It is unfortunate that we cannot direct research into channels that would definitely identify, subject to Koch's law, 'the germ of insanity,' so often mentioned and pictured in Sunday supplements, or in the field of therapeutics, find some simple medical or surgical procedure that would immediately 'cure' the mental disorder."[82] Neurosyphilis proved to be the exception, not the rule. Still, the dream of transforming psychiatry into a medical science never completely died. Mitchell himself maintained hope that while mental diseases "seem to defy solution," psychiatrists could anticipate a "swifter advance" in the coming years.[83] Mitchell's optimism notwithstanding, most psychiatrists came to terms with the fact that ahead of them lay a long, frustrating road.

Beyond Medicine

Reformers' desire to bring psychiatry closer to medicine was tempered by a desire to carve out a distinct identity for psychiatry. They embraced a notion of medical science that was broader than the laboratory and included more than just the physical body. Even the most ardent champions of the laboratory like Lewellys F. Barker recognized that psychiatry required insights beyond those the laboratory could supply. "Psychiatry is preeminently a science of human behavior," declared Barker, "a special discipline that teaches us how to recognize and treat disorders of the powers of adjustment, a branch of knowledge that studies the feelings, the thoughts and the strivings of those who are inadequately responsive to their environment in the hope of helpful therapeutic intervention (diagnostic and curative psychiatry)."[84] Knowledge of anatomy, pathology, and neurology was crucial, but reformers warned that the laboratory should never become "divorced from the personal life of the patient."[85] Psychobiology had to be attuned to the patient in all his or her complexity. Albert M. Barrett, a professor of psychiatry, described the breadth of information relevant to psychiatrists:

> Psychiatry to-day is in a position that makes it possible to bring to the solution of its problems a far wider range of information than ever before. Its interests have been immensely broadened in the general recognition that the problems with which it deals are essentially psycho-biological in their relations. Concisely stated, the problems that interest psychiatry center in the efforts of the personality to adequately adapt itself through its mental functioning to the demands of the social situation in which it must exist. Such a viewpoint brings it in contact with whatever deals with life in its personal and social relationships.[86]

Mental illness was not reducible or analogous to physical disease; it involved more. As such, good psychiatric practice required more. Psychiatrists were "called on to have a more profound knowledge than anyone else."[87]

To widen the psychiatric gaze, reformers cultivated a deep appreciation of the psychological factors of mental illness. Psychobiology's focus on the psychological dimensions was not novel in and of itself. Superintendents themselves had appreciated the psychological dimensions of their patients' insanities. Indeed, the asylum and its mechanism of cure—a calming environment to rejuvenate excited nerves—worked on the psychology of patients. Additionally, folk psychology with psychospiritual and religious dimensions had been part of American culture since the colonial period.[88] What psychobiology added to these efforts was a more deliberate focus on the individual personality through one-on-one psychotherapy.

Once again, Meyer played an instrumental role in promoting psychotherapy. As with everything, his was an eclectic approach. His technique drew from various existing psychological therapies, including hypnotism, therapeutic suggestion, and moral suasion. Influenced by pragmatists, like William James, Meyer maintained that the "backbone of psychotherapy" was "habit training."[89] Viewing mental illness as a by-product of defective habits, the "psychiatrist—user of biography—must help the *person himself* transform the faulty and blundering attempt of nature to restore the balance, an attempt which has resulted in merely undermining the capacity of self-regulation."[90] The goal was to replace bad habits of thinking, ingrained over time, with natural, healthy habits that restore fitness to the personality.

Meyer also dabbled in psychoanalytic thought. Freudian thought was introduced to the United States in the first decades of the twentieth century,[91] and Meyer's early interest lent it some important initial credibility. In psychoanalysis, Meyer saw a set of theoretical ideas that could serve psychiatrists in their quest to understand the complexity of their patients. Yet, Meyer's endorsement of Freud was qualified. Ever sensitive to reduction, he could not countenance what he viewed as Freud's overemphasis on the subconscious and sexual development. Nor could he stomach the dogmatic tendencies of psychoanalysts. For Meyer, psychoanalysis was granted no authoritative status over other therapies; it was part of the psychobiology tool kit to be used when appropriate or expedient.

Meyer never provided much in the way of concrete detail in outlining a distinct psychotherapeutic procedure. As a result, psychiatrists adapted existing practices in ad hoc ways. Therapy reflected a fluid bricolage of existing ideas and basic common sense. More than a specific technique, psychobiology affirmed the relevance of mental and psychological factors for comprehending and treating mental illness. The elevation of mental factors set the stage for the psychoanalytic period to follow (see chapter 3), but for the time being, it amounted to little more than a command to attend to the psychological dimensions of a patient's suffering. Psychiatrists must pursue mental *and* biological facts. These pursuits should be infused with a pragmatic common sense that resisted elaborate theorization. Meyer stated:

> There is much confusion between conflicting schools of psychology, often with unwise dramatization in teaching certain subjects like hysteria, hypnotism, and theories of psycho-analysis by instructors who never have worked with patients and without any opportunity for the student to see the facts first, or ever to see the actual clinical material. For this reason, some of us turn frankly to the sound Huxleyan[92] definition of science as being organized common sense. In a field in which nearly every adult has more practical experience with human nature and human functioning than is set forth in most textbooks of psychology, it seemed wisest not to add too much theory, but to make certain that the worker learns to use all the plain facts.[93]

In short, Meyer endorsed a practical, commonsense approach to psychotherapy, one that drew insights from a variety of circulating theories, both lay and medical, but in the end remained rooted in the facts of the case at hand.

In addition to psychological treatment, psychobiology encouraged social reform efforts. These were pursued under the rubric of mental hygiene, an inclusive program that sought to prevent mental distress through education, early intervention, and public health measures. As psychiatrists' concerns moved beyond the asylum, they turned to issues of mental health in the community and daily problems in living. Taking their cues from public health efforts, psychiatrists hoped through mental hygiene that "mental diseases will decrease just as the infectious fevers have decreased by removal of their causes."[94] E. Stanley Abbot of McLean Hospital elaborated:

> Mental hygiene as a science deals with questions of the environments to which we must adjust ourselves and of our minds by means of which we make our adjustments. It considers what our minds are; how we get them; how they develop; what we are who have them; what we do with them; faulty uses we normals may make of them; various factors, external or internal, that may help or hinder us; ways of promoting the helpful ones; the effects and prevention of harmful factors and compensation for harmful effects.[95]

Meyer nurtured this effort. The evolutionary logic to which he subscribed oriented him toward the significance of an organism's environment. "The emphasis on the living patient became the central characteristic of the American movement destined to reach its culmination in mental hygiene," he promised.[96] By identifying and applying hygienic principles, psychiatrists would take their fight into the community. They would prevent mental illness from emerging in the first place. Thus, Meyer viewed mental hygiene as an enterprise that fused the revolutionizing medical sciences with psychiatry's traditional administrative acumen.

Mental hygiene was institutionalized in the first two decades of the 1900s. In 1908, Clifford Beers, a former mental hospital patient, published a memoir, *A Mind That Found Itself*. The memoir offered a critical account of psychiatric hospital care.[97] Beers approached Meyer for advice on how to help reform psychiatric treatment. Although Beers's memoir focused on institutional care, Meyer steered him toward mental hygiene. In 1909, with Meyer's blessing, Beers founded the National Committee for Mental Hygiene (NCMH). Beers envisioned a cooperative but centralized national movement with a broad mandate, one that would be lay led but dependent on psychiatrists for guidance. Meyer imagined something different: a confederation of local organizations in which psychiatrists took the lead while lay volunteers executed their designs. The two split over these conflicting visions for the organization, and the NCMH adopted Beers's vision.

Among its diverse projects, the NCMH conducted surveys, made reports to influence state policy, published a quarterly journal, disseminated information to the public, supported new hospitals, and worked to create community clinics. However, it was plagued by financial difficulties and never realized its many ambitions. Despite its broad mandate, the NCMH's main contributions were mostly restricted to its surveys on mental health. Nevertheless, as an idea, mental hygiene retained significant cachet among psychiatrists. Like the program of psychobiology of which it was a part, mental hygiene came to mean different things to different people. This flexibility facilitated its wide embrace. Moreover, mental hygiene tallied with psychiatrists' desire to escape the asylum, as it posited a role for psychiatrists outside the crumbling mental hospitals. Finally, mental hygiene presented an opportunity to articulate psychiatry's distinct role in medicine. Whereas other medical specialties homed in on the body, psychiatry's broad expertise was poised to serve as "a liaison science between medicine and social problems."[98] Synthesizing the biological, psychological, and social, psychiatry could teach medicine proper crucial lessons. When laboratory medicine grew in prominence, the "sick man" began to disappear from medical cosmology.[99] By insisting that all doctors receive some training in psychobiology, psychiatry could help medicine rediscover the patient and his or her social milieu. In this way, psychiatry would provide "the synthetic type of mind" that medicine needed to integrate specialized knowledge "into a picture of the individual which is usable therapeutically."[100]

Mental hygiene was not without controversy. As psychiatrists extended their reach, they began to involve more actors in mental hygiene, including new mental health professions like psychologists and psychiatric social workers as well as older competitors like the clergy and law.[101] Mental hygiene came to reflect a diverse array of interests that began to compete over control of its direction. The participation of many interested parties emboldened challengers to psychiatric authority.

The most fraught issue for psychiatrists in mental hygiene, however, was what to do about eugenics. Eugenics arose as a force in the United States between 1900 and 1930. Based on the writings of Francis Galton and Herbert Spencer's notion of "social Darwinism," eugenics had its intellectual origins outside psychiatry, in biology, psychology, and criminal anthropology.[102] More than a science, eugenics was a movement of elites who, wary of the changing demographics of the country, sought to implement reforms to improve the genetic stock of the United States. Eugenicists focused on the role of hereditary factors in the promulgation of social ills. Because individuals with "bad stock" reproduced prodigiously, while those of good stock did not, the evolution of the human race was headed toward general degeneration. Eugenicists conjured policies to reverse these trends. These included "positive" measures to encourage the reproduction of elites and "negative" measures to discourage or prevent the reproduction of the "unfit," via marriage restrictions, immigration control, confinement, and forced sterilization. Eugenicists focused on mental illness and "feeblemindedness" as one of the major problems that accompanied genetic degeneration. The issue of feeblemindedness, a loose diagnosis of mental deficiency believed to be associated with a host of other social ills (crime, poverty, sexual deviancy, etc.), brought eugenicists into close contact with psychiatry.

Psychiatrists were split on whether they should embrace or reject eugenics. On the one hand, eugenics carried a certain allure, especially for psychiatrists in mental hospitals.[103] It offered an explanation for the endless growth in patient population and an excuse for the futility of their treatments. With the stock of the country declining, mental illness increased, swamping the already overrun hospitals. Eugenic ideas could also explain the changing demographics of inpatient populations. New immigrant groups were of lower stock and more prone to mental illness. It was not surprising that mental hospitals were being flooded with patients from immigrant backgrounds. Finally, because eugenics was phrased in scientific terminology and viewed as a legitimate science, it offered yet another means by which psychiatry could assert its scientific bona fides. For this reason, many institutional psychiatrists were sympathetic to eugenics. A 1916 survey conducted by John R. Haynes, physician and leading eugenic reformer in California, revealed that many psychiatrists longed for sterilization programs for "incurables."[104] In 1927, the Supreme Court upheld the constitutionality of sterilization laws in its ruling for *Buck v. Bell*. As these laws spread,[105] some psychiatrists willingly adopted the practice, even arguing that the sterilizations had therapeutic value for female patients. And some advocated for redirecting mental hygiene toward eugenic policies. Since "by far the most important factor with which we have to deal in the consideration of the pathology of the main types of insanity [is] the hereditary influence on insanity," it behooved psychiatrists "to see to it that the mentally superior stocks shall not be supplanted by stocks that are mentally inferior."[106]

On the other hand, eugenics sat in tension with the core tenets of psychobiology. Its narrow focus on hereditary traits violated the spirit of psychobiology's appreciation of the multidimensional nature of mental disorders. While hereditary influences are "powerful etiological factors in the appearance of insanity," APA president Charles Bancroft asserted that they were one factor among many and "too much weight must not be placed upon the so-called stigmata of degeneracy."[107] The uncritical acceptance of hereditary claims ignored the protean nature of mental illness. "The laws of Mendel have not been shown to apply for any single normal human character of simple type, except perhaps eye color," argued Abraham Myerson, then the clinical director at Taunton State Hospital. "To assume then that the vast range of the psychoses (the feeble-minded, the epileptic, character anomaly, criminality, and neuroses) is related to a unit determiner or group of determiners acting as a unit is, to say the least, premature."[108] Others cautioned against adopting such drastic, irreversible measures like forced sterilization on the basis of "insufficient evidence."[109] Diagnostic uncertainty made it difficult "to draw a hard and fast line separating the fit from the unfit."[110] When linked with racist and nativist sentiments, eugenics ideas were dangerous, as they might lead to unjustified sterilization. Finally, the professional benefits of a full-throated embrace of eugenics were not certain. Other than warehousing and sterilizing the unfit, what place did psychiatry have in eugenics? Its role seemed to be restricted to the very institutions many psychiatrists were trying to escape.

On the whole, psychiatry's engagement with eugenics was inconsistent and ambivalent. While leading figures like Thomas Salmon, William White, and Meyer (who sat on an advisory council for the American Eugenics Society) expressed some interest, their correspondence reveals that it was of secondary concern.[111] Eugenics became just another part of psychobiology's sprawling program, never privileged, often disparaged, but retaining a niche nevertheless.

An Elusive Convergence

In 1932, the National Research Council (NRC), the operating arm of the National Academy of Sciences, undertook a study of psychiatry to determine "what the actual state of psychiatric knowledge is and for suggesting certain possible means of advancing our understanding and control of mental disorders."[112] The NRC selected Madison Bentley, professor of psychology at Cornell University, and E. V. Cowdry, professor of cytology at Washington University, to conduct the study. The resulting report, published as *The Problem of Mental Disorder*, was a startling account of a field lacking a center. The bulk of the report was composed of five chapters written by experts representing major points of view within psychiatry—clinical psychiatry, medical psychiatry, neurology, psychobiology, and psychoanalysis. In isolation, each chapter offered a straightforward review of research from a particular perspective. However, when aggregated and set against each other, the chapters highlighted the fragmentation of psychiatry. Psychiatrists disagreed on the most basic aspects of mental disorders. Summarizing their findings, Bentley and Cowdry stressed this disagreement: "The one extreme declares disorder to be not merely mental symptoms and indicators, but a *disease of mind*; the other extreme maintains that disease must imply pathology and that pathology always appears *in bodily tissue*."[113] Moreover, psychiatry had become divided by "partisan emotions."[114] It succumbed to "a confused— many would say in a disordered—state" characterized by the very type of dogmatism against which psychobiological reformers had promised inoculation.[115] If psychiatry was to move forward, it required "a shift in outlook, which would compel men to value facts above doctrines."[116] Although written in dry academic prose, the upshot of the report was unmistakable: as a referendum on the state of psychiatry, it revealed the profession to be an unmitigated mess.

Meyer contributed a chapter on psychobiology to the volume. He positioned psychobiology as "a mode of approach to the study of the organism," one mode among many distinct modes relevant to psychiatry. This positioning spoke volumes as to the declining influence of the paradigm by the 1930s.[117] While Meyer, ever the evangelist, lauded psychobiology, he portrayed it not as the foundation of psychiatry, but as a means to facilitate dialogue across psychiatry's various schools. He emphasized its practical usefulness for organizing clinical practice and psychiatric training rather than its potential to reinvent the psychiatric project. Psychobiology had been reduced from an overarching vision for psychiatry to one school among many jockeying for influence within the fractured profession.

From the start, psychobiological reformers promulgated a broad program to the study and treatment of mental disorders. This was seen as necessary given the depth of psychiatric ignorance coming out of the asylum period. With so little known, reformers encouraged multiple pursuits. The strength of pluralism, as Meyer and other reformers declared, was that amid great uncertainty, it ensured that any research displaying a modicum of promise would be paid its due attention. Wary of closing off possible sources of insight, reformers hedged their bets, encouraging experimentation while refusing to invest all of psychiatry's energy and resources in any one direction. With so little known, the reasoning went, better to cast a wide net than hazard neglecting something crucial. The expectation was that over time, psychobiology's many strands would converge in a comprehensive understanding of mental illness.

The ever-present risk of psychobiology's pluralism was incoherence. With so many moving parts, psychobiology courted confusion, contradiction, and competition. Meyer remained long blind to this problem. Content to rest on his faith in convergence, he failed to explain the relationship between psychobiology's component parts. As a result, psychobiology was always a scraggly beast of a program. It grew over time, by accretion, collecting and discarding appendages, accumulating into a pastiche that defied coherence. Psychobiology not only failed to join the biological, neurological, psychological, and social features of mental illness into a robust conceptualization; it created many different psychiatries, each with distinct assumptions regarding mental illness, how to study it, and how best to treat it. Decades into psychobiology, psychiatry splintered into silos, some promising, others sputtering, but with each "[worshipping] at the different shrines of psychiatry, each one of us in our own way."[118]

Most psychiatrists specialized, focusing their individual attentions on specific corners of psychobiology. Some maintained their existing commitments to mental hospitals. Others aspired to a medical identity that tried to apply the latest medical theories and laboratory techniques to the study of mental illness. Others turned to psychology, combining psychoanalytic ideas with other, more commonsense psychotherapeutic notions to treat the mind through its thoughts. And still others sought to cultivate a more expansive notion of medicine, one that integrated the social and the biological and was attuned to prevention and mental hygiene. Psychiatrists of different schools entered into fierce competition with each other for resources, prominence, and prestige, working to discredit one another in the quest to claim the mantle of the one true psychiatry. The grand synthesis that psychobiological reformers promised receded as a goal. Indeed, it had come to be seen as hopelessly naïve.

Fragmentation jeopardized psychiatry's professional credibility. Efforts aimed at solidifying psychiatry's medical credibility sputtered. New institutions—the research institute and the urban mental hospital—intended to be the embodiments of psychiatry's commitment to laboratory science and serve as the next foundation of psychiatric power failed to achieve reformers' expectations. Having been misled by the promise of the asylum, state legislatures were reticent to invest more resources into mental health. This hampered the growth of novel organizations. Psychiatric research institutes never caught on nationally; only a few states followed the lead of the New York Pathological Institute in establishing them. Those that were created were plagued by financial insecurity and suspicion from psychiatrists in existing mental hospitals. The effort to create urban mental hospitals for acute cases fared a little better. These institutions brought psychiatry in from the rural countryside and expanded its reach into less serious cases of mental disorders. Yet, like the research institutes, the new mental hospitals never achieved their promise. The scientific advances were scarce, their therapeutic innovations problematic, and their funds consistently in short supply. In practice, the urban mental hospitals became appendages of the existing mental hospital system; they provided short-term care while shipping difficult cases to be warehoused in traditional asylums in the country.

The new institutions not only failed to meet reformers' expectations; they created new problems. Psychiatric practice bifurcated into two distinct sectors: traditional long-term hospital care and shorter, inpatient care in urban centers. This development reified the distinction between chronic (read: helpless) cases in custodial care and less severe (read: treatable) cases treated in short-term facilities or outpatient settings. This distinction would shape professional identities, institutional rationales, and patients' fates for decades. In creating and segregating a population of chronic hopeless cases, the new institutional division of labor encouraged reckless experimentation. Psychiatrists' overzealous embrace of new treatments has burned the profession over and over. Psychosurgery, then various shock therapies, and eventually lobotomies were all adopted to great fanfare, only to be abused, exposed as fraudulent and even cruel, and thus transformed into symbols of the profession's corruption. Even so, institutional psychiatrists never learned caution; they continued to experiment on patients for decades. The allure of a treatment that would place psychiatric treatment on par with their medical peers proved too strong to resist, especially when coupled with hospital psychiatrists' desperation to do something for the intractable cases under their care. Under the guise of treatment, psychiatrists developed innovative ways to torture their patients.

Psychiatrists fell further behind their medical peers. Medicine proper had consolidated its authority, vanquished alternative challengers, and possessed boast-worthy discoveries. Psychiatry could make no such claims. Any conceit that psychiatry, through psychobiology, would instruct other medical specialties in a fuller, more robust approach to care was abandoned. Worse, it struck many as delusional. Grand ambitions gave way to deep insecurity. Psychiatrists judged themselves harshly. "There is a current feeling among medical men that there is comparatively little scientific research being done in psychiatry," observed Dr. Jacob Kasanin of the Boston Psychopathic Hospital. "It may seem to us as psychiatrists that a great deal of work is done in our field, yet when one compares the total amount of research in psychiatry with other branches of medicine, one can see the difference very readily."[119] Under psychobiology, psychiatrists had lost more ground to their medical brethren.

Psychiatry's expeditions into the community also had mixed professional consequences. Mental hygiene promoted awareness of mental health, revealing the extent of its prevalence and its less severe manifestations. This broadened understanding of mental illness helped facilitate some psychiatrists' move out of the asylum and set the stage for the subsequent psychoanalytic revolution in psychiatry. Still, psychiatrists were never able to assert their control over mental hygiene, nor were they able to effectively articulate the specific expertise they brought to these endeavors. Worse, mental hygiene encouraged the rise of competing mental health professions, who over time would come to challenge psychiatry's authority. As such, psychobiology's ventures into psychological and sociological territories never amounted to more than an unfocused gesture. The gesture was significant rhetorically, but like so much during this eclectic period, its execution was fumbled.

Most damning, psychobiology produced little insight of note. It was unclear what psychiatry was, much less what it knew. Decades into this period of experimentation, of diverse research operating under the pretenses of a medical science, psychiatry's ignorance seemed as intractable as ever. In 1933, psychiatrists J. C. Whitehorn and Gregory Zilboorg described the state of psychiatric research in disconcerting terms:

> It is generally recognized that psychiatry is in great need of scientific research. Many are urging it, others agree to it, none deny its importance. However, there is no unanimity of opinion as to what to search for, nor when and where and how. Thus, one may observe one group of investigators spending a great deal of painstaking and expensive labor in the search for specific causes of a mental disease, called schizophrenia, while others would deny its existence, as a disease, and yet others may be heard proclaiming with greater or lesser caution the discovery of its cure.[120]

Just as August Hoch had noted, in 1900, that psychiatry lacked basic agreement as to what variables were relevant, Whitehorn and Zilboorg observed that thirty years later, psychiatrists were still struggling with the basic questions "as to what to search for, nor when and where and how." What was a good idea? What was a bad one? How could psychiatrists tell the difference? Psychiatry was "not lacking in theories," but it lacked the shared epistemological assumptions necessary to adjudicate between theories.[121] Decades of pluralism had left it unclear how best to proceed. Psychobiology's central tenet—that mental illness was complex and multifaceted—exacerbated this problem. It was one thing to recognize the multiple dimensions of mental disorder; it was quite another to figure out how they fit together. In this sense, the protean character of psychiatry's object was both the point and the problem of psychobiology. Unable to figure this out, psychiatry remained "in a maze" with little clear direction emanating from decades of experimentation.[122]

Still, it would be wrong to view psychobiology as an unmitigated disaster for the professional aspirations of psychiatry. Its most marked success was neutralizing the threat from neurologists. The Guiteau trial had been an embarrassment to both psychiatrists and neurologists. But in its aftermath, overt antagonism gave way to greater integration. Psychobiology deserves much of the credit for this rapprochement, as it offered a bridge between psychiatric and neurological camps. It constructed an eclectic space under which both neurology and psychiatry could operate through a division of labor but as part of the same overarching program. As psychiatric reformers pivoted away from the asylum and embraced European medical science, they found themselves having more in common with neurologists than their superintendent forbearers. This intellectual compatibility was strengthened by more regular interaction. The divide between neurologists and superintendents had long had a geographical, urban/rural component. The new institutions created by psychobiological reformers brought psychiatrists back to urban centers and into closer proximity with neurologists. For their part, neurologists, working in private practice, viewed the new psychiatric institutions as a means to support their practices and as a potential source of employment.[123]

While psychobiology encouraged cooperation between neurologists and psychiatrists, in the end the two were drawn together by a common foe. As nonmedical professionals, encouraged by mental hygiene, began to stake claim to mental illness and offer treatment, neurologists and psychiatrists joined forces to thwart these incursions into their jurisdictions. Taking their cues from medicine proper, which had deployed licensing and examinations to eliminate alternative medical sects, the APA began working with the American Medical Association (AMA) and the American Neurological Association (ANA) to develop educational standards and erect legal safeguards. In 1934, the American Board of Psychiatry and Neurology was organized. Although separate certifications were granted for psychiatry and neurology, they were conferred by the same board. Through this cooperation, the distinction between the two professions, though never fully eroding, carried fewer professional stakes. Increasingly, they were viewed as complementary endeavors. Neurology handled structural problems pertaining to the brain, while psychiatry, as the broader specialty of the two, dealt with the more prevalent and amorphous problems classified as mental illness.

The resolution with neurology notwithstanding, by 1940 psychiatry found itself once again in a precarious position, its dilemmas manifold. The profession had been pulled apart by centrifugal forces. It had achieved important licensing and certification protections, but it was unclear what distinct expertise these certifications signaled. Even as psychiatrists attempted to move away from inpatient mental hospitals (née asylums), psychiatric power remained dependent upon them, for it was the only place where psychiatrists' authority went unchallenged. The problem was that this role conferred little prestige and little interesting work. As the profession split in different directions, psychiatrists were presented with fundamental problems of choice that they had long deferred. Where should it focus its attention? Dedicate its resources? Invest its energy? Psychobiology bet that a coordinated, multipronged attack on its ignorance would, over time, lead to a synthesis. This bet did not pay off. It would be up to the next generation to figure out the way forward.

Conclusion

What are we to make of the psychobiological period in psychiatry? How are we to assess the pivot from a profession of asylum superintendents to something broader, more diverse, less cohesive? Should we dismiss it as misbegotten? Should we deride psychobiology as "derationalizing"?[124] As a nice but empty slogan? Or does it deserve more credit?

For their part, historians have not been kind to psychobiology, either ignoring the period or dismissing it as intellectually vacuous.[125] They have been just as dismissive of Meyer, the figure who came to embody psychobiology's contradictions. His critics disparage him as a "psychiatric anarchist,"[126] while his supporters trip over themselves to note his flaws.[127] Psychobiology lacks the tragic arc of the asylum era, the perceived arrogance and ultimate comeuppance of the psychoanalytic period, or the persistent zombie promise of contemporary biomedical psychiatry, in which efficacy appears tantalizingly close to psychiatrists' grasp. But more than anything, it lacks cohesion, revealing the disarray of a profession in search of an identity and a solution to its ignorance.

However, when taking a longer trajectory, the psychobiological era emerges as a critical inflection point in psychiatry's history of ignorance. Psychobiology did not resolve psychiatric ignorance, but through its experimentation, reformers hit upon the means by which subsequent generations of psychiatrists would attempt to manage its fallout. In this, it left an enduring legacy. This legacy has three dimensions: intellectual, habitual, and tactical. First, many of the ideas, concepts, and theories developed and legitimated during this period of experimentation would come to exert significant influence over subsequent reformers. During certain periods and reinventions, these ideas might be de-emphasized, but they rarely disappeared altogether. Instead, they sat dormant, incubated in isolated places, ready and available to be taken up and promoted by the next generation of reformers. Psychoanalytic reformers of the mid-twentieth century who would steer psychiatry toward the psychological would build on psychobiology's crude forays into psychotherapy. The community mental health movement in the 1960s and 1970s would try to reclaim mental hygiene to broaden the reach of the profession. And throughout psychiatry's existence, however complicated and fraught the relationship might become, psychiatric reformers have appealed to medicine as a model to imitate. In this sense, the psychobiological period, despite all its conflicts and contradictions, handed subsequent generations of psychiatrists a suite of ideas that came to shape the intellectual history of psychiatry.

Second, this period also witnessed the emergence of distinct tactics that would become central to the management of ignorance moving forward. The first was rhetorical in nature. To explain the persistence of ignorance, psychobiological reformers located its source in the character of mental illness itself. When assessing its lack of progress vis-à-vis general medicine, psychiatrists attributed their difficulties to the fact that mental illnesses were more resistant to the type of simple, monocausal explanations afforded by germ theory. This rhetorical move ennobled psychiatric ignorance, portraying psychiatrists as courageous in their willingness to take on such a difficult task. Second, psychobiological reformers engaged in the production of promise, couching their appeals in a future axiom, projecting a time when ignorance would be overcome. Meyer's insistent promotion of psychobiology's convergence exemplified this tactic. The damaging effects of *current* ignorance were minimized by an appeal to *future* expectations in which such ignorance was resolved. Mental illness was unknown and difficult to know, but not unknowable. This tactic bought reformers time and allowed psychiatrists to acknowledge ignorance without undermining their professional aspirations. Indeed, with promised resolution in hand, ignorance could be even construed as a positive, a call to arms that spurred innovation. Third, in their attempt to derive authority from an association with the laboratory revolution sweeping medicine, psychobiological reformers engaged in *bandwagoning*, or the attempt to link psychiatry to external research programs perceived to have widespread credibility. Neurosyphilis became a symbol that forged a link between psychiatry and medicine. In addition to its cultural and symbolic dimensions, bandwagoning also encompasses institutional and organizational elements, like the establishment of new allies and new organizations. This was evident in the creation of psychiatric research institutes and new urban mental hospitals intended to mirror similar reforms within medicine proper. Commonsense notions of ignorance view it as a property of thought and thus assume that its resolution entails the construction of sounder arguments or the discovery of new ideas; these organizational tactics reveal that the war of ideas is waged not just through words alone.

Finally, and most importantly, this period established reinvention as the overarching means by which reformers met ignorance and the crises it caused. During this time, reinvention became *the* template for subsequent reactions to professional crisis, the habit to which reformers would return again and again. Faced with an exposure of its ignorance, psychobiological reformers did not seek to tweak or build upon the existing asylum system, but rather tried to reinvent the profession altogether. They sought to shed the burdens of the past by reformulating the epistemological, ontological, and institutional bases of psychiatry. Reformers dispensed with an expertise rooted in administrative management. In its place, they sought to articulate a distinct medical identity, aspiring to a revolution on par with medicine proper, committed to the laboratory sciences but retaining the pluralistic appreciation of nonbiological factors in the treatment of mental illness. In the process, the ontological understanding of mental illness itself changed. Earlier understandings of mental illness as nervous exhaustion gave way to an appreciation of the protean character of mental illness. From the one-size-fits-all treatment of the asylum era, reformers spawned a new agenda broad and diverse in its character, reflecting and respecting the character of mental illness itself. In future periods, the details of reformers' reinventions would change (e.g., their intellectual arguments, institutional bases, the understanding of mental distress, etc.), but the pursuit of a dramatic reinvention persisted. To domesticate ignorance, reformers would seek to reboot the profession, and in the process, wipe the slate clean. Consequently, despite its contradictions and failings, the psychobiological period established the habit of reinvention that subsequent reformers would return to again and again. More than anything, this was its most important legacy.

Yet, when resorting to reinvention, subsequent reformers would draw an important lesson from psychobiology's failure. There was a fatal flaw in Meyer's approach to ignorance. Research programs require constraints lest they devolve into a state of unboundedness. Born of a reasonable—and, some might argue, noble—recognition of the depth of psychiatric ignorance, Meyer encouraged open-endedness in the psychiatric project. His great latitude and his cultivation of diverse programs sent the psychiatric project sprawling in all directions. Beyond an appreciation of the multidimensional character of mental illness and its embrace of an ethos of pluralism, psychobiology provided little guidance to psychiatrists. It placed almost no restrictions on the range of possibilities. As a result, psychiatrists succumbed to a type of professional anomie, a state of normlessness that bred confusion.[128] Rather than tame psychiatric ignorance, psychobiology multiplied it, birthing new questions in ever-increasing corners without supplying the requisite structure to answer them. In the future, then, reformers would choose a course that Meyer rejected; they would pursue focused reinventions.

THREE

Ignorance Repressed

Few events in the history of American psychiatry have taken on such mythical proportions as Sigmund Freud's one and only visit to the United States in 1909. Invited by G. Stanley Hall, president of Clark University, Freud was asked to give a series of lectures on psychoanalysis in celebration of the university's twentieth anniversary. This visit is often portrayed as *the* key moment in which Freud introduced his radical new ideas about the mind to the country that would become, improbably, his staunchest defender.

The record, however, rebuts the more hagiographic takes on Freud's US trip. The invitation was never intended to be a grand introduction of Freud. It was an academic conference, one with an impressive roster of speakers, but a conference nonetheless. Freud was not feted as conquering intellectual hero. He was not even the main draw, as many of the other twenty-nine speakers had reputations far outdistancing his. The honorary degree Freud received did not reflect an endorsement of psychoanalysis; this honor was granted to all who spoke on topics related to psychology and education. Freud was not the sole representative voice of psychoanalysis; also invited were two of his acolytes, Sandor Ferenczi and Carl Jung, the latter of whom was more popular in the United States than Freud.[1] Perhaps for these reasons, Freud himself initially balked at the invitation, agreeing to participate only after Hall increased his stipend. Even then, Freud treated the task with some disregard, procrastinating in finalizing his remarks until the morning he was scheduled to speak.

Freud's half-heartedness sprang from his unfavorable opinion of the United States. Throughout his life, he was quick to dismiss the United States, voicing misgivings that exceeded the typical arrogant dismissals of European elites. He saw Americans as prudish, sexual hypocrites. He mocked their democratic strivings and corresponding broadmindedness as indicating a lack of taste and cultured judgment.[2] For Freud, Americans were purveyors of anti-intellectualism and shallow materialism. And they were unlikely converts. The conference would be a chore.

Yet, despite his initial reservations, Freud seems to have enjoyed the experience.[3] At the time of the invitation, Freud was a little-known Viennese neurologist, his fledgling psychoanalytic movement striving for legitimacy. The conference provided an opportunity to preach psychoanalytic thought to an impressive audience, a veritable who's who of early twentieth-century American thought that included Franz Boas, Emma Goldman, William James, Adolf Meyer, and Edward Bradford Titchener. Each morning between September 7 and 11, Freud gave his lectures in German. His plan for the lectures, however belatedly conceived, was to synthesize the field of psychoanalysis "condensed almost to the point of caricature" for "practical Americans."[4] In this way, Freud served as his own popularizer. And by all accounts, he received a sympathetic hearing. While some in the audience audibly gasped at his ideas regarding childhood sexuality, coverage of his lectures was, on the whole, favorable.[5] Luminaries like Hall, James, and Meyer offered their encouragement. Moreover, the trip gave Freud time to cultivate closer relationships to those, like Abraham A. Brill and James Jackson Putnam, who would become the most vocal American advocates of psychoanalysis. Therefore, while the conference did not cement Freud's place in the United States, it did lay the foundation for psychoanalysis to make unanticipated inroads there. Before the trip, psychoanalysis was viewed as just one of many competing mental health cures in the United States; afterward, it became the topic du jour in psychiatry.

Still, although the visit was a pleasant surprise, Freud never shed his mistrust of the United States. Upon returning to Europe, he reportedly remarked to his English colleague Ernst Jones that "America is a mistake, admittedly a gigantic mistake, but a mistake nevertheless."[6] He would never return.

The irony, of course, is that this giant mistake became the place where Freud's ideas achieved their greatest influence and firmest professional endorsement. It would take a couple decades and much modification for it to happen, but by the end of World War II, American psychiatry was transformed into a bastion of psychoanalysis. During the middle decades of the twentieth century, psychiatry reinvented itself once again, this time in the image of Freud. Writing in 1961, George C. Ham, psychiatrist and chairman of the Department of Psychiatry at the University of North Carolina, observed:

> Psychoanalysis as a theory, as a method of investigation, and as a technique of treatment has in a few short years been strikingly, if unevenly, integrated into medical education, research and practice. This represents a radical change

from two decades ago. During these 20 years, the chairmanship of several departments of psychiatry have been awarded to men who were fully trained psychoanalysts; many others to men well acquainted with the principles and concepts of psychoanalysis. The majority of other medical school departments of psychiatry have included as fundamental principles many of the discoveries and basic concepts of psychoanalysis.[7]

As psychoanalysts captured the leadership of the profession, American psychiatry became almost synonymous with psychoanalysis. According to Iago Galdston, a prominent New York psychiatrist, it had become "difficult to conceive" of a psychiatry without Freud.[8] To be a psychiatrist meant being an interpreter of the mind's irrepressible subconscious forces.

This chapter examines the psychoanalytic period from roughly 1930 to 1970, situating it within the longer history of psychiatric ignorance discussed thus far. As psychobiology unraveled, the profession descended once again into crisis. Psychobiology's sprawling, unwieldy agenda fractured the profession. Psychiatrists lacked consensus on the nature of mental distress and no clear articulation of the distinct contribution of psychiatry to sorting it out. Harry Stack Sullivan, one of the most influential psychiatrists of the interwar period, groused that psychiatry "is not science nor art but confusion."[9] Its very purpose was unclear, its object as mysterious as ever. To move forward, psychiatrists Henry Elkind and Carl Doering insisted that psychiatrists needed to establish "the phenomenon we are talking about to be a really existing thing" to contribute something "beyond the meagre observation that some people are insane, a fact which is pointed out by the laity and of itself seldom needs any confirmation by the psychiatrist with the help of his numerous and intricate theories."[10] Psychobiology had yielded little in the way of insight beyond common sense.

By 1930, psychiatrists were back to square one, forced to again confront their stubborn ignorance. In response, psychiatry split into two distinct wings, which, despite some overlap, practiced in parallel universes. On the one side were psychiatrists who worked in the public mental hospital system. Burdened with hopeless cases and relegated to a custodial role, institutional psychiatrists embraced a somatic view of mental illness and experimented with harsh medical treatments that had harmful, often tragic, effects on their patients. This wing will be discussed in the next chapter. In this chapter, I examine the more aspirational wing of psychiatry, reformers who adopted psychoanalysis as a means to shore up the credibility of psychiatry. These reformers took up Freud's ideas, modified them into a distinct ego psychology, and used them to transform psychiatry.

Existing historical scholarship on the psychoanalytic period is contentious, fluctuating in response to the intellectual currents of the day. Freud
has long been a lightning rod for controversy and, to this day, he inspires
intense polemics. During the height of psychoanalysis, supporters like
psychiatrist-historian Gregory Zilboorg depicted the psychoanalytic reforms
as a triumph of humanism that elevated the mind to its deserved prominence.[11] However, as psychiatry shifted to a biomedical model in the 1980s,
psychoanalysis has suffered in historical esteem. The "Freud Wars"[12] of the
1980s and 1990s were won by Freud's critics, and today the psychoanalytic
period is depicted as a hiatus, a disruptive detour in psychiatry's quest to
become a medical science.[13] "Depending on the interpreter or historian,"
notes writer Lisa Appignanesi, "[Freud] is the heroic conquistador of the secrets of the unconscious, the great innovator whose talking cure definitively
altered the treatment of madness, or the manipulative fraudster who
launched a movement out of a mixture of fabrication and speculation."[14]
Susceptible to hagiography on one side and condemnation on the other, the
historical assessments of the psychoanalytic period are rife with caricature
and ax-grinding. But I am not interested in relitigating the "Freud Wars."
Nor do I intend to synthesize internecine controversies and byzantine elab-
orations of psychoanalytic thought.[15] Rather, I focus on the reception of
psychoanalysis in the United States and its relationship to the professional
politics of American psychiatry. Freud's thinking had a greater impact in
the United States than anywhere else in the world. Psychoanalysis became
dominant after World War II, only to suffer a rapid decline in the 1970s. I
examine this rise and fall as unfolding not to some unique logic particular
to psychoanalysis, but rather according to deeper, more enduring dynamics
involving psychiatry's struggle with ignorance. The psychoanalytic period was
not as anomalous as it is often portrayed; its unfolding repeated the profession's now habitual cycle of managing ignorance through reinvention.

Psychoanalysis furnished American psychiatric reformers with a new theoretical edifice to make sense of the bewildering data that had overwhelmed
psychobiology. It also provided a vehicle for the reassertion of psychiatrists
as *the* indispensable authorities on matters related to mental health. But
most importantly, psychoanalysis offered psychiatrists a new way to manage
their ignorance. It did so through mystification, or the process of making
expertise inaccessible to external judgment. As articulated and practiced,
psychoanalysis, with its theoretical complexity and hermeneutic interpretation, was largely immune to public scrutiny and outside meddling. Its
production of knowledge—and, in turn, its eruptions of ignorance—were
kept behind closed doors, cloistered in the impenetrable interaction of the

analyst and analysand. This mystification was given an ontological gloss, as psychiatrists reframed mental distress as neuroses emanating from dark recesses of the unconscious. Neuroses could only be revealed by a trained analyst, who possessed the interpretive skill necessary to decode superficial symptoms and unearth the suppressed meanings of madness. Thus, psychiatric expertise became the restricted province of adepts.

The obfuscation at the heart of the psychoanalytic reinvention allowed psychiatrists to recapture what historian John Harley Warner calls "professional mystery."[16] When combined with institutional developments emanating from World War II and favorable cultural currents of the postwar period, psychoanalysis did not just stabilize the legitimacy of psychiatry for the three decades between 1940 and 1970. It enabled psychiatrists to reach levels of prestige unmatched both before and after. However, as sure-footed as the profession seemed, psychoanalysis was always in tension with psychiatry's claim to a medical identity. Changing scientific norms within medicine during the 1970s, especially those related to standards of evidence and methods of assessment, brought this tension to a head. In an environment that demanded greater accountability, the mystification of psychoanalysis became untenable. Under such conditions, psychiatry's ignorance could no longer be repressed.

Translating Freud

Contrary to what many may think, psychotherapy in the United States did not originate with the importation of Freud and psychoanalysis. At the time of Freud's visit, a handful of versions of psychotherapy were already circulating throughout the country. These domestic psychotherapies had been developed by nonmedical, often religious, mind-cure movements and faith healers, like Christian Science, the New Thought Movement, and the Emmanuel Movement.[17] Most psychiatrists maintained a healthy skepticism toward these psychotherapies, viewing their practitioners as charlatans and content to keep them at arm's length. The promise was that the psychotherapy promoted by psychobiology did little to distinguish psychiatrists from these other mind-cure therapies. Psychobiology offered an eclectic mixture of ideas that amounted to little more than commonsense treatments focused on habits. As with most things, psychobiology insisted that attention be paid to psychological factors but offered little guidance of how to translate this into concrete practice. A distinctly psychiatric approach to psychotherapy, one with broad appeal, remained elusive. For this, reformers would turn to Freud, transforming psychoanalysis into something distinctly American.

A host of cultural changes contributed to the eventual ascendency of psychoanalysis within American psychiatry. First, many of Freud's core ideas resonated with the domestic psychotherapies that had captured some of the cultural zeitgeist during the first decade of the twentieth century. For example, like psychoanalysis, early spiritual therapeutics focused on character development and maintained an appreciation of unconscious forces.[18] Psychoanalytic reformers tapped into this wave of interest, co-opting the growing obsession with the individual fostered by mind-cure movements.[19] They also rode other cultural changes that dovetailed with Freudian ideas. During this time, argues historian Nathan G. Hale, American culture experienced something of a crisis in sexual mores, as a subset of the population began to chafe at the traditional puritanical strictures and Victorian sensibilities.[20] With its emphasis on psychosexual development, psychoanalysis appealed to the avant-garde challenging the sexual status quo: a "psychotherapeutic culture," infused with psychoanalytic ideas and speaking the language of personal reflection, caught on among writers, intellectuals, and urban elites.[21] These cultural changes combined to create a crucial opening for psychoanalysis in psychiatry.

While these cultural trends were important, it was war, more than anything, that elevated psychoanalysis. World War I accelerated the changes in sexual mores that made Freud more palatable, and its barbarous violence seemed to confirm psychoanalysis's bleaker insights.[22] The brutality of trenches and the seeming senselessness of the war demanded some sort of explanation. As a "philosopher of the irrational and the brutal in human nature," Freud was positioned to provide one.[23] Indeed, in response to the war, Freud revised his already pessimistic view of humanity into a downright tragic one. Stressing the darker forces of the human psyche, he elaborated his notion of the "death instinct" and the irreconcilable tension between the individual and civilization.[24] In addition to highlighting the irrational forces at work in human behavior, other elements of World War I appeared to corroborate psychoanalytic theory. The prevalence of "shell shock," for example, supported Freud's insights regarding the importance of dreams and origins of neuroses in trauma.

For many American psychiatric reformers, World War I lent credibility to psychoanalytic ideas. And insofar as psychiatrists could be transformed into adepts in this tradition, psychoanalysis presented an opportunity to legitimate their profession. The sheer mental anguish the war produced underscored the need for their service. "The Great War, responsible for so many tragedies, was not wholly devoid of benefits," observed Lewellys F. Barker, "and among these must be counted the awakening of the medical profession, of the military authorities and of the public to the extraordinary and unsuspected prevalence of mental defects and of disorders of the emotions and among the young men who were drafted."[25] By the end of World War I, the United States boasted the most psychoanalysts in the world,[26] but psychoanalysis's dominance over American psychiatry was only just beginning.

If World War I lent credence to Freud's ideas, World War II was pivotal for the consolidation of American psychiatry around them. First, the influx of European Jewish analysts fleeing Nazism invigorated the American psychoanalytic movement, conferring upon it a degree of intellectual heft. By 1943, 149 exiled psychoanalysts and psychiatrists had been relocated to the United States.[27] Second, psychiatrists' participation in the war effort afforded new institutional opportunities that drew it closer to medicine. At the time of US entry into World War II, the US Army had just thirty-five psychiatrists on staff; by the end, this number had ballooned to nearly a thousand.[28] The surgeon general created a medical division of psychiatry (to accompany its two other divisions, medicine and surgery) and placed it under the control of William Menninger, an advocate of psychodynamic psychiatry who established the influential Menninger Foundation along with his brother, Karl. Under Menninger's guidance, psychiatrists' influence over military operations grew. Menninger insisted that every military physician receive basic training in the principles of psychoanalysis.[29] Psychiatric services were set up near combat areas, and two psychiatric hospitals were created stateside to meet the growing needs of soldiers returning home. Psychiatrists, notably Harry Stack Sullivan, also created a screening system for recruits. This screening was no rubber stamp; psychiatrists exercised their authority to the tune of rejecting nearly two million recruits.[30]

World War II was American psychiatry's coming-out party, "a capstone for the trend toward making psychoanalysis 'practicable.'"[31] As William Menninger recalled fondly, during the war, "psychiatry struggled from the rear seat in the third balcony to finally arrive in the front row at the show."[32] The war gave psychiatry a renewed sense of purpose and confidence, and by its end, the profession had been transformed. Psychiatrists now possessed an explanatory framework to combat their ignorance. But more importantly, in psychoanalytic psychotherapy, they now possessed a marketable skill that could distinguish them from competitors and that they could sell to a new clientele of urban, cosmopolitan elites during the postwar economic boom.

Ego Psychology

American psychiatrists did not merely adopt Freud's ideas. They modified them to fit their needs. In the process, they transformed psychoanalysis into something less overtly sexual, more optimistic, and more medical in character. Incidentally, this transformation did not have Freud's blessing. He balked at these changes, deriding American psychoanalysis as "a kind of hodge podge" that lacked rigor.[33] Freud continued to rebuke his American colleagues for what he saw as their indiscriminate ways until his death in 1939. Nevertheless, despite Freud's objections, it was American psychiatrists who became most avowedly Freudian.

A neurologist by training, Freud became frustrated with the search for the somatic basis of neurosis and, early in his career, turned to its psychological dimensions. As a therapeutic technique and a method of investigation, psychoanalysis grew out of Freud's evolving metapsychology of the mind. His initial topographical model of the mind focused on the distinction between the mind's conscious and unconscious elements, the latter vaster than the former. Freud held that mental distress arises from a conflict between the unconscious—a repository for repressed feelings, desires, instincts, and conflicts—and the conscious mental life of the individual of which he or she is aware. The origins of these conflicts can be traced to early childhood and psychosexual development, namely, the inability of the child to reconcile his or her sexual drives with normative expectations (most famously articulated in the idea of the Oedipus complex). Later, Freud amended his conceptualization of the mind, overlaying his topographical model with a structural model, consisting of the id, ego, and superego. The id, or unorganized part of the personality structure that contains basic instinctual drives, conflicts with the superego, or societal strictures conveyed via socialization primarily by the family. The ego must reconcile the competing demands of the id and the superego to allow unconscious desires to be expressed or satisfied in ways appropriate to the external demands of the world. Absent this resolution, an individual is susceptible to neuroses.

Freud's articulation of neurosis was broad; the difference between the sane and insane, the normal and the pathological, was a matter of degree. Every individual was susceptible to unresolved tensions between the unconscious drives and the constraints civilization placed upon their realization. For Freud, we are all a bit neurotic. Thus, psychoanalysts were less interested in delineating different types of mental illness and more focused on attending to the specific manifestations of neuroses among their patients, however minor or major.

Psychoanalysis, Freud argued, distinguishes itself from other mind cures because it is the only therapy to move past manifest symptoms to penetrate the mind at a depth necessary to address the fundamental conflicts of a patient. Psychoanalysis taps into a patient's unconscious to undercover the suppressed, unmet desires that manifest as neurotic symptoms. Because the unconscious is perceived as largely inaccessible, psychoanalysis is often described in archaeological tropes. Analysts must *unearth* the unconscious through processes like dream analysis, free association, and transference. The manifestations of the unconscious are subtle, rarely straightforward or obvious. Given this elusiveness, psychoanalysts maintain constant vigilance in observing patients. Nothing is immaterial; the most irrelevant-seeming detail of a dream or a slip of the tongue is fodder for insight in the hands of a skillful psychoanalyst.

In the process of appropriating psychoanalysis, American psychiatric reformers modified Freud's vision. Retaining some of the eclecticism of psychobiology, they selectively adapted psychoanalysis to create a more practical, less dogmatic approach.[34] Finding Freudian thought overladen with technical jargon, too obsessed with sex, and too pessimistic, Americans embraced a more fluid version, which they deemed "ego psychology." Based on Freud's structural model, ego psychology focuses on the unconscious defense mechanisms of the ego. These mechanisms—reaction formation, denial, projection, isolation of affect, and so on—are established in childhood, replayed in adulthood, and become the organizing principles of one's personality. Thus, ego psychology de-emphasizes unconscious desires of the id to emphasize the patient's personality and ego defenses. The American psychoanalyst Rudolph Loewenstein described this reorientation as one from "instinctual aspects of pathogenic conflicts" to "analyzing the patient's resistances."[35] The focus on ego defenses, however, presented a practical problem. Whereas the id has "motivation" to reveal itself in analysis, wishing the recognition and realization of its unconscious desires, psychoanalytic treatment is "a menace to the embattled ego and its unconscious, characterological defenses," which work so efficiently because they are invisible.[36] Analytic techniques like free association that reveal the id by suppressing ego defenses are inadequate to illuminating those very defenses (e.g., repression, rejection, projection, reaction formation, etc.). As a result, ego psychology demands more cooperation from the patient to identify the ego's defense mechanisms. Over time, defenses can arise in the context of the analytic encounter as they play out in the talk-and-talk-back of the therapeutic encounter, often through the dynamics of transference.

Ego psychology evolved in the United States under the guidance of Heinz Hartmann, who was instrumental in shifting the emphasis and aims of psychoanalysis.[37] Drawing inspiration from Darwinian evolution, and echoing similar ideas within psychobiology, Hartmann introduced adaptation as central to ego development. Just as organisms evolve in relation to their environment, so too does the mind evolve in relationship to early family dynamics and society more generally. Under the rubric of adaptation, ego psychology attends to disruptions in developmental processes that result in the structure of the psyche itself. Maladjustments lead to neurosis. To treat neurosis, ego psychology tries to neutralize problematic defenses and adaptations so as to assist a patient's "process of coming to terms with the environment."[38] American psychoanalysts, therefore, traded Freud's emphasis on early sexual development for an analytic encounter that incorporated the entirety of the patient's life so as to identify problematic patterns in the ways in which the ego responds to his or her environment.[39] They dealt with more concrete objects like interpersonal conflicts, tracing current conflicts back to problematic defense mechanisms that emerged in reaction to, say, family dynamics.

Consequently, in American hands, psychoanalysis became something more moralistic, practical, and conservative.[40] Freud always maintained modest goals for treatment, famously remarking that the goal was to turn "hysterical misery into common unhappiness."[41] American psychoanalysts offered an optimistic twist. More so than their European counterparts, American psychoanalysts pursued outcomes like sublimation, encouraging their patients to transform socially unacceptable desires into more acceptable outlets, and neutralization, by which the ego stripped drives of their aggressive and sexual qualities. In the process, psychoanalysis became something both more *and* less radical. American psychoanalysts sought ambitious treatment outcomes. They promised patients a more profound change than the alleviation of neurotic symptoms; they pledged "a character-changing therapy" that resonated with American ideals of self-reliance.[42] But this was often done in the name of conformity, as they sought to help a patient achieve what Hartmann termed "social compliance."[43] American psychoanalysts jettisoned Freud's more provocative and revolutionary ambitions to readjust the individual to societal demands.[44]

Thus transformed, ego psychology provided American psychiatric reformers with a framework to bring coherence to the psychiatric project in the wake of the confusions left by psychobiology. Whereas Meyer provided little direction on how to navigate all the factors pertinent to a particular case, Freud provided psychotherapy with a "theoretical superstructure" that could be brought to bear on idiosyncratic cases.[45] Armed with sensitizing concepts and trained ears, psychoanalysts could identify the specific origins of their patients' psychological distress. "Since the advent of psychoanalysis," argued APA president and influential psychoanalyst William A. White, "we [psychiatrists] for the first time have our vision directed to where the real trouble has taken place, and our interest centered upon the actual mechanisms that are producing the symptoms."[46] Psychoanalysis replaced the "hit and miss type of psychotherapy, which lacked any sound theoretical foundation," with a sophisticated system.[47] The secrets of the mind thus revealed, psychiatric ignorance would be overcome.

In practice, most American psychiatrists did not become dyed-in-the-wool adepts of psychoanalytic theory. Instead, they remained heterodox, selecting elements of psychoanalysis that fit their particular needs.[48] Indeed, most psychiatrists identified as "psychodynamic,"[49] rather than "psychoanalytic." Karl Menninger's book *The Human Mind* provides an excellent distillation of this American brand of psychoanalysis. One of Menninger's many attempts to popularize psychoanalysis, *The Human Mind* argues that while psychiatrists had long been "clustered within the forbidding walls of mysterious castles on the out-skirts of a few villages," they had come to recognize the mind as something more than "the brain's little bag of tricks."[50] Freud was instrumental in this, having discovered "a method for learning systemically about these hidden things in people's minds."[51] His "greatness" (which "is impossible to overestimate") was that he provided "a theory about the way in which instinct acts to motivate human conduct."[52] Inspired by this, Menninger, like his psychodynamic peers, articulated a psychiatry that attended to the personality of the patient in order to facilitate "readjustment by an attack on some sort of conscious and unconscious conflicts that produce the distress."[53] Rather than a rigid doctrine, American psychodynamic psychiatry constituted an orientation attuned to the dynamics between the subconscious, the ego's defense mechanisms, and the patient's environment, particularly his or her interpersonal conflicts.

Whether American psychiatrists embraced orthodox Freudianism, ego psychology, or the more fluid psychodynamic psychiatry, psychiatry during the middle of the twentieth century was reimagined through Freud. Psychiatrists had transformed themselves into interpreters of the unconscious forces, healers of minds, and menders of personalities.

Mystifying Knowledge

In a 1956 article in the *American Journal of Psychiatry* (*APJ*), Maxwell Gitelson, an influential member of the Chicago Institute for Psychoanalysis, observed that psychoanalysis was wrapped in a certain "mystique."[54] This mystique was neither negative nor unusual; it was no different "from the mystery which attaches to all outposts of science, whether in mathematical physics or on the frontiers of biology."[55] Indeed, mystique was crucial to science, as it supplied the necessary awe that garners public support and insulates it from premature criticism. To move forward as a science, psychoanalysis, Gitelson argued, should not aim for more transparency, but should harness its mystique.

Upon this air of mystery, psychiatrists solidified their professional authority. Psychoanalysis provided psychiatrists a new stance vis-à-vis their ignorance, one that thwarted criticism by rendering their knowledge opaque to outsiders. In psychoanalysis, Freud introduced a distinct epistemology and understanding of the nature of psychiatric knowledge. This epistemology was oriented around depth interpretation secured in the intimacy of the psychoanalytic encounter. Couched in often obtuse jargon, Freud's theoretical edifice brought a measure of coherence to the psychiatric encounter. But psychoanalytic theory was no cookbook for therapeutic practice. Instead, it provided sensitizing concepts that induced a way of thinking about a case, and techniques by which to read the latent meaning in manifest signs. The real work of psychoanalytic knowledge production was an emergent property of the dynamics of the psychoanalytic encounter. Treatment was tethered to the specificity of the patient and the skill of the particular psychoanalyst. For this reason, psychoanalysis as a therapeutic practice defied codification.

The psychoanalytic style of reasoning was laid out in in-depth case studies. Early in psychoanalysis's founding, the long case history was the central "genre for reporting psychoanalytic results" and became "the vehicle for representing the theory and methods of psychoanalysis."[56] In Freud's writing, the trials of Anna O., Rat Man, and Wolf Man provided concrete instantiations of psychoanalytic reasoning. By studying these cases, psychoanalytic initiates gained familiarity with a particular way of thinking about their patients' distress. Accumulated, taught, and endlessly debated, these cases supplied a "lexicon of narrative patterns" that psychiatrists adapted, via analogical reasoning, to make sense of the individual cases before them.[57] Cases disciplined the eye and ear of the psychiatrist so that psychoanalysis could become, in the words of American analyst Trigant Burrow, a "microscope of the mind."[58]

The epistemology of psychoanalysis rested on a cultivation of depth interpretation and case-based reasoning. Historians of science Carlo Ginzburg and Anna Davin argue that, distinct from positivistic sciences, psychoanalysis embraces conjectural knowledge, an "interpretive method based on taking marginal and irrelevant details as revealing clues."[59] This reasoning shares affinities with detective work. It involves piecing together disparate, often ambiguous data to achieve a coherent account. And indeed, the imagery of detective work appeared in psychiatric discourse of the period.

When discussing the challenges of learning psychoanalysis, Adolf Meyer pointed out, "Not everybody is born a detective. Not everybody can venture upon the ground of rather delicate constructions and interpretations."[60] Karl Menninger insisted that because "the human mind is a complex mass of motives and mechanisms apt to go awry," it "requires expert technical sleuthing" to discover why.[61] No clue is too insignificant to ignore; A. A. Brill, a leading American psychoanalyst, asserted, "The main base of Freud's psychology is that there is nothing accidental or arbitrary in the psychic life, that everything has reason and meaning."[62] To unlock the unconscious, psychoanalysts had to heed slips of tongues or attend to dream imagery to overcome the mind's defense mechanisms. This thorough forensic investigation could not be rushed, nor short-circuited. It demanded persistence and an abundance of time.[63]

This dogged pursuit of clues is necessary given psychoanalysts' understanding of mental distress. Mental distress, or neurosis, results from subterranean conflicts, long repressed and hidden from view. In the standard American textbook on psychoanalysis of the time, the *Problems of Psychoanalytic Technique*, Otto Fenichel stated, "Neurosis is a complicated phenomenon. One can get one's bearings in a complicated subject only if one adopts, as a basis, a definite system of orientation with definite coordinates to which to refer all phenomena."[64] For Fenichel, psychoanalysis enabled the psychiatrist to penetrate the surface symptoms, which were "a *substitute* for something repressed," and "make the unconscious accessible to the ego, that is to help the ego to understand that something it has passively experienced is really actively brought about by a part of itself."[65] The roundabout techniques analysts deployed (dream analysis, free association, etc.) aimed at "subsurface exploration," lulling the patient's conscious mind into a state of compromised vigilance, so as to allow the unconscious to come through.[66] Impervious to easy observation, neurosis was difficult to divine even for the most practiced analysts. This framing of mental distress had an added benefit vis-à-vis the politics of ignorance. Expanding on an argument made by psychobiological reformers, psychoanalysts attributed at least some psychiatric ignorance to the character of mental distress itself. Neurosis was, by its nature, hard to understand. But here psychoanalysts went further than their predecessors. For them, mental distress was buried deep in the inaccessible recesses of the mind. No wonder it resisted easy elucidation.

For reformers, all this amounted to a notion of psychiatric expertise that was inaccessible to anyone not trained in psychoanalysis. Psychoanalysts' main knowledge claims—the insights they produced—were rigorous *interpretations* specific to the patient. Diagnostic labels were not enough. More than just facile, they were misleading and dangerous. Psychoanalytic theory might articulate broadly what *kinds* of conflicts might produce neurotic symptoms, but the individual analyst's mandate was to work closely with the patient to understand the specific roots of his or her distress. At the end of the day, the causes of neurosis were specific to the individual, arising from his or her own psychosocial development and interpersonal relationships. They would only be revealed "by inquiring most intimately into the psychic life of the individual" to "delve in the deeper mainsprings of his character."[67] Thus articulated, analytic expertise became manifest in "a clairvoyant understanding of a stranger's personal problems."[68] American psychoanalytic reformers, in articulating a distinct ego psychology, may have downplayed the more baroque hermeneutic gymnastics of Freud. Nevertheless, they maintained a view of expertise based on an almost indescribable, acquired feel, one that was restricted to psychiatrists.

Reinvented as such, what psychiatry purported to offer were depth interpretations. In an article, "The Problem of Interpretation," Rudolph Loewenstein described the seemingly ineffable process of coming to an interpretation as it was understood by American psychoanalysts of the period.[69] Loewenstein defined interpretation as explanations by which psychoanalysts lead patients to greater knowledge of themselves. The process of forming interpretations was delicate. Before even considering interpretation, analysts must create an environment that loosens "the barrier or censorship existing normally between conscious and preconscious process" and be trained on "the inner experiences of the patient."[70] Once a proper milieu conducive to interpretation was created, the patient and psychoanalyst could get down to the hard labor of interpreting the patient's neurotic symptoms, to "move from the surface to the so-called depths."[71] Interpretation was "drawn by the analyst from elements contained and expressed in the patient's own thoughts, feelings, words and behaviors."[72] The psychoanalyst allowed the patient to speak unencumbered. Over time, the psychoanalyst tactfully steered the patient toward the observation that his or her behaviors display certain characteristic patterns. Once the patterns of behavior and the character of the ego defenses were accepted by the patient, they then worked together to identify the origins of neuroses in critical events in the patient's life. But in Loewenstein's formulation, the process of coming to and conveying an interpretation was a long, fraught, and fragile endeavor. The patient did not receive the interpretation willingly, but resisted as his or her ego defenses asserted themselves. The patient and analyst must work through complex mechanisms like transference, in which the patient redirects his or her feelings onto the analyst and thus erects obstacles to therapy. Interpretation had to be pitched at the proper time, in the proper sequence, in the appropriate words, and at the proper level of comprehension for the particular patient. As such, psychoanalysts had to possess an indefinable skill, which Loewenstein called "analytical tact," or an "intuitive evaluation of the patient's problems which leads the analyst to choose, among many possible interventions or interpretations, the one which is right at a given moment."[73] Only through careful, pains-taking persistence did the patient accept the interpretation and achieve "dynamic changes."[74]

When done correctly, psychoanalytic treatment produced a particular kind of knowledge. At its core, it was knowledge that dealt "with the individual experiences of a human being."[75] It aimed "at widening the conscious knowledge of the individual about himself."[76] But it would be incorrect to suggest that psychoanalytic knowledge was pitched solely at the individual level. Rather, psychoanalysts reached their interpretations by applying theoretical concepts to idiosyncratic cases. Here, a balance in abstraction had to be struck.[77] A psychoanalyst had to help the patient obtain "insight at a more generalized level than the insight he might gain from pure introspection, but much less abstract than are scientific formulations."[78] Psychoanalytic knowledge ascended above the individual case to reveal patterns of thoughts and behaviors that psychoanalytic theory had developed. But once such patterns were identified, the interpretive practice pivoted back to the specificities of the case in order to secure individual self-knowledge. Ultimately, the purpose of interpretation was not to elaborate theory—although this might happen as a result—but rather to facilitate personal insight for the patient. Or, as Loewenstein described it, the interpretive act aimed not at uncovering the Oedipus complex, but the "specific individual experiences which constitute the manifestations of the Oedipus complex of the person."[79]

Psychoanalytic knowledge, therefore, was characterized by insularity. It emerged behind closed doors in the subtleties of the psychoanalytic encounter. It could only be assessed by those involved in that encounter. The Hungarian-American analyst Franz Alexander stated:

> Psychoanalysis is the most individual type of treatment which medical science has ever produced. Each case is a unique problem. What the therapist is primarily interested in is not the nosological classification of a person, not in what way he is similar to others but in what way he differs from them. Every person has his own potential formula of adjustment.[80]

The purpose of interpretation was not to impose a wholescale rereading of the patient's biography or personality, but rather to illuminate "what is already in the preconscious—and just a *little bit more*—which thereby become capable of entering consciousness."[81] Or, in the words of Loewenstein, it was to "add to their [patients'] knowledge about themselves" so as "to produce those dynamic changes that we call insight."[82] The goal sought was adjustment, to help a patient "to remain an individual in a complex society and to express his individual inclinations on a realistic and socially constructive level by becoming a dynamic actor in the social process, by creative participation in it."[83] As such, psychoanalysts sought to produce useful, case-specific insights. Whether an interpretation was correct or not was determined, not according to some sort of external standard, but by whether it helped relieve the patient's suffering.

This kind of knowledge was resistant to outside, independent corroboration. The context of discovery and the context of justification, the generation of the hypothesis/interpretation and the assessment of it, were all contained within the psychoanalytic encounter. In effect, this made external assessment as to the accuracy and efficacy of psychoanalytic knowledge nearly impossible. This is not to suggest that analysts adopted an anything goes approach to their interpretations or rejected generalization altogether. The theoretical apparatus and the exemplary cases organized psychoanalytic practice and established a basis of shared assumptions against which analysts might assess each other's work. But still, the final word on an interpretation came from within the psychoanalytic encounter, not from without.

The opacity of American psychoanalysis was reinforced by other features of its practice and training. First, it was achieved in part by the spatial arrangement of the analytic encounter. To accomplish this delicate investigative operation, psychoanalysts stressed the importance of the creation of an analytical space. Traditionally, the couch has been the symbolic center of this space, and in turn, central to production of psychoanalytic knowledge.[84] Lying supine with the analyst out of view, the patient could speak his or her mind unencumbered. This created both a safe space and a sense of "placelessness," a setting that removed the patient from the vicissitudes of his or her life.[85] Only in such a space could the relevant clues erupt from the subconscious and circumvent the ego's defense. Second, the resulting interpretation was understood as an emergent property of the dynamic relationship between the psychoanalyst and analysand.[86] It was hard to glean from outside this context. Indeed, attempts to subject the dynamic to outside scrutiny did violence to it. For this reason, analysts rejected formulaic approaches to therapy. Sensitive to the emergent, dynamic quality of each analytic encounter, they underscored the uniqueness of each encounter; Fenichel argues that "the infinite multiplicity of situations arising in analysis does not permit the formulation of general rules about how the analyst should act in every situation, because each situation is essentially unique."[87] Finally, the mystification of psychiatric knowledge was reinforced by the strictures imposed on analytic training. The only way to learn psychoanalysis was through extensive apprenticeship with another analyst, which was coordinated by independent psychoanalytic institutes. The psychoanalytic mind-set was learned interpersonally and experientially. Freud's recommendation that all analysts must themselves be analyzed became dogma in the United States, "an inflexible and central fact of analytic education."[88] Trainees had to undergo psychoanalysis in order to understand and learn psychoanalysis.

All this served to render psychoanalytic knowledge inaccessible to outsiders. By definition, outsiders could not adequately assess psychoanalytic claims. Edward Strecker, an influential midcentury psychiatrist, observed that once it was determined "that the psychoanalytic doctrine cannot be understood without the experience of a successful personal analysis," criticism of its fundamental tenets by outsiders was excluded as illegitimate.[89] Abraham Myerson, an early critic of psychoanalysis, complained that this stricture was a "very ingenious subterfuge for escaping criticism": "So long as you have not been psychoanalyzed," he observes, "you cannot judge the results of psychoanalysis. But I am not a surgeon and yet I can judge the results of surgery."[90] By positioning themselves as the sole arbiters of what were nontransparent knowledge claims, American psychoanalysts protected themselves from outside criticism.

The epistemology of psychoanalysis therefore held great appeal to psychiatric reformers wanting to combat perceptions of ignorance. Reformers reoriented psychiatric thought toward the individual, narrowing the scope of its claims to individual patients and insulating these claims from criticism. If each patient's neurosis arose in response to his or her own psychosexual development or interpersonal conflicts, any demand that psychiatry provide a generalized explanation of neurosis was circumspect. Moreover, psychoanalytic knowledge was produced in what sociologist Michael P. Farrell calls "collaborative circles," a group of peers who share similar goals and who, through long periods of dialogue and collaboration, negotiate a common vision.[91] The insularity of these circles protects certain intellectual commitments and assumptions from interrogation. Within their circles,

American psychoanalysts might challenge each other's interpretations or question their fealty to certain theoretical ideas, but this questioning never touched the central tenets of psychoanalysis.

Through psychoanalysis, therefore, psychiatric expertise was cordoned off, restricted to like-minded, similarly trained thinkers. Psychoanalysts were able to draw firm boundaries between themselves as knowers and others as non-knowers. This gave psychiatry an air of mystery and went a long way in hiding their ignorance.

A Psychoanalytic Science

Mystification only works when accompanied by authority. People are willing to extend trust and the benefit of the doubt to those whom they perceive as possessing legitimate authority. The dilemma facing psychoanalytic reformers was how to secure such authority amid the public failures of psychiatry. For this, they once again turned to medicine, seeing in it both a source of prestige as well as a template for institutionalizing professional power.

Much of the original appeal of psychoanalysis to psychiatric reformers was that it promised to offer a *medical* approach to psychotherapy distinct from the popular lay, religious therapies that threatened psychiatry's jurisdiction. Freud, as American psychiatrists repeatedly pointed out, was himself a doctor, as were the overwhelming majority of his early followers.[92] His ideas grew out of neurology, and although they would later be seen as offering a psychological alternative, Freud conceived of psychoanalysis as an extension of medicine. The problem for American psychiatrists trying to frame psychoanalysis as medical was that Freud himself was adamant that its practice need not be restricted to physicians. Physicians, Freud insisted, "have no historical claim to the sole possession of analysis."[93] Furthermore, medical training often contradicted the spirit of psychoanalysis; it was "more or less the opposite of what he [the analyst] would need as a preparation for psycho-analysis," in that it ignores "the mental side of vital phenomena."[94] For these reasons, Freud maintained that psychoanalysis should not be "swallowed up by medicine" or turned "into a mere housemaid of Psychiatry."[95]

The issue of lay analysis became a proxy debate for the medical status of psychoanalysis and opened a major rift between American psychoanalysts and their European counterparts. European psychoanalytic institutes remained open to lay analysts, despite the predominance of physicians within their ranks. In the United States, however, the adoption of psychoanalysis was caught in the whirlwind of professional politics. Reeling from the ruin of public mental hospitals, mired in the confusion fostered by psychobiology and threatened by its ignorance, American psychiatrists were determined that psychoanalysis remain restricted to doctors. Safeguarding this restriction became a paramount concern for reformers. If reformers were to ride the psychoanalytic reinvention to professional power, lay analysis could not be countenanced. In the 1920s, American psychoanalysts limited the right to practice psychoanalysis to individuals trained at accredited medical schools, a decision Freud himself derided as "more or less equivalent to an attempt at repression."[96] In 1938, the American Psychoanalytic Association (APsaA) limited its membership to physicians. This increased tensions between American and European psychoanalysts, and by the 1930s, American psychoanalysts were isolated from the international community. Isolation, however, did not inoculate Americans from this controversy. Disputes over lay analysis erupted with the influx of analysts to the United States during World War II, many of whom were barred from practicing psychoanalysis and excluded from membership in American analytic institutes. In response, the profession began to enforce these restrictions with "a new zeal."[97] In 1951, the AMA, APA, and APsaA reasserted their position, releasing a joint statement condemning lay analysis.

Even with the prohibitions on lay psychoanalysts, reformers still had to convince their domestic medical peers that psychoanalysis was, "first of all, a medical procedure."[98] In this, they were not starting from scratch. Some of the groundwork had been laid by psychobiology, which had started to legitimate the relevance of mental factors in medicine writ large. And despite the laboratory revolution, case studies were still accepted as important forms of medical knowledge. Psychoanalytic knowledge would not have been seen as that beyond the medical mainstream. Still, the affinities were tenuous. Reformers had much to do to transform psychoanalysis's hermeneutic, interpretative tendencies into something that could be reasonably seen as a medical practice.

To this end, American psychoanalytic reformers went out of their way to stress the scientific character of psychoanalysis. In his 1938 presidential address to APsaA, Alexander laid out the vision of a scientific psychoanalysis. Alexander argued that as psychoanalysis "shifted its center from Europe to this country," it was transformed.[99] The days of psychoanalysis as a "movement" that debated "philosophical issues regarding human nature" were in the past.[100] In the "tolerant and critical atmosphere" of the United States, reformers were able to transform psychoanalysis into an "unemotional" science; American psychoanalysts were not "disseminators of a gospel" but "self-critical scientists."[101] The embrace of ego psychology reflected a conscious attempt to make psychoanalysis more empirically grounded. Literary imagery and metapsychological musings gave way to a more straightforward concentration on patient behavior and ego defenses. By these means, psychoanalysis became something less obviously hermeneutic, less jargoned, while retaining the emphasis on interpretation. American psychoanalysis still required expert interpretation to identify a patient's ego defenses, link them to the patient's biography, and ultimately to his or her neurotic behaviors. Defenses were more concrete and observable, but not *too* concrete. The interpretative leaps might be shorter, but psychotherapy still demanded the clairvoyant skill of the trained analyst.

By stressing its empirical basis, reformers tethered psychoanalysis to medicine. Still, the fit was not seamless. Mental illness, reconceptualized as neurosis, could not be described "in terms analogous to those which describe a physical illness," as "neither the location nor the causative agent nor the pathology can be simply stated."[102] Zilboorg said:

> We may not overlook the fact that psychiatry was born out of medicine and matured by medicine. By the same token we may not overlook the fact that the psychiatrist, dealing more directly with the inner life of man than the doctor representing any other medical specialty, has always had to draw upon certain special prejudices concerning the human mind, or upon various philosophies prevailing at a given time, in order to create for himself a medicopsychological frame of reference usually not found in autopsy material or purely physiological observations or speculations.[103]

Psychoanalysts brought something extra, beyond medical expertise, to their practice, but the fit with medicine was still awkward.

Reformers attempted to flip psychoanalysis's differences with medicine to their advantage. They pitched psychoanalysis as a means to reform medicine proper and overcome its long-standing oversights. According to this argument, psychoanalysis presented an opportunity to expand the boundaries of medicine and introduce more complexity into mainstream medical thought. APA president Leo H. Bartemeier argued, "The great technological advances that have taken place in medicine within the last three-quarter century raise this threat—the loss of the personal relationship with the patient."[104] Psychoanalysis could counteract this trend by imbuing medicine with an appreciation of the role of personality in illness and the importance of the doctor/patient relationship in the healing process. For this reason, American psychoanalysts promoted psychosomatic medicine, seeing it as a vehicle to introduce psychoanalytic principles into mainstream medical practice and, in the process, assert a place for psychiatry in medicine.[105] Incorporating psychoanalytic elements could yield a more effective, more humane medicine. However inelegant the attempt to frame psychoanalysis in a medical vein, it was sufficient enough to secure a place on medicine's bandwagon (provided, that is, that psychiatrists accepted a somewhat marginalized position within medicine and stayed in their lane). This association with medicine conferred a degree of legitimacy upon psychiatry. And after World War II, psychiatry entered a period of influence unwitnessed since the early asylum period. Having acquitted themselves admirably in the war effort, the federal government rewarded psychiatrists by passing the National Mental Health Act in 1946 that established the National Institute of Mental Health (NIMH). The NIMH's broad mandate included funding mental health research, supporting training programs for mental health workers, and providing state grants for clinics and treatment centers. While the relative amount given by NIMH to psychoanalysis was small in comparison to that given to non-analytic competitors, psychiatrists in general benefited from the training programs.[106] Their ranks swelled.[107] Seventy percent of NIMH's initial budget went to subsidizing training, and the number of psychiatrists in the United States increased from 4,700 to 27,000 between 1968 and 1976.[108] Psychiatrists also benefited from the federal expansion of the Veterans Administration (VA), which provided new employment opportunities. With state legislatures now resistant to investing in psychiatry after being burned, the federal government replaced them as the patron of psychiatry. And it proved to be a generous benefactor.

If the shifting fortunes of psychiatry in general were dramatic, they were even more so for psychoanalysts within psychiatry. By the 1960s, psychoanalysis had become hegemonic in psychiatry. The transformation of psychoanalysis into ego psychology allowed for the widespread embrace of psychoanalytic ideas within American psychiatry, however eclectic and selective it might be.[109] Membership in the APsaA grew from ninety-two members in 1932 to 1,300 in 1968.[110] Psychoanalysts established twenty US training institutes as well as twenty-nine local societies. With the election of William A. White to APA president in 1925, they ascended to the leadership of the APA and would dominate these positions well into the 1970s.[111] Psychoanalysts also held chairs of most prestigious psychiatry departments nationwide. Increasingly, the very identity of being a psychiatrist rested on "a full knowledge of the principles of psychoanalysis."[112]

Reconstituted under psychoanalysis, psychiatrists displayed a high level of confidence, some might say arrogance. "Psychoanalysis," proclaimed APA president Kenneth Appel, "has brought the greatest contribution in the history of psychiatry; it brought light where there was darkness, order where there was chaos, and understanding where there was only description."[113] Psychiatric discourse brimmed with excitement and hope for "a new era of progress."[114] The future was bright, expectations high. "Perhaps no other discipline," argued Charles Ernest Goshen, director of the APA's General Practitioner Education Project, "is presented with such unique opportunities as is psychiatry in bringing about a comprehensive understanding of man from a knowledge of both man's biology and his humanity."[115]

Psychoanalysis had an additional benefit. It facilitated psychiatry's move out of the deteriorating public mental hospital system, a move initiated during psychobiology but still incomplete. "Psychoanalysis made it possible to treat respected and upper-class members of the community, thereby enhancing the prestige of psychiatric practice," observes sociologist Rose Laub Coser. "At the same time, it fostered the opportunity for treatment in a private doctor's office, the symbol of a physician's devotion and service to patients."[116] By 1958, only 16% of psychiatrists worked in traditional state hospitals.[117] The popular image of the psychiatrist became identified with private, office-based psychotherapy. Even the maligned archetype of this image reflected this shift. Satirists mocked "the bearded man of short stature, either bald or with a luxuriant crop of matted hair, hypnotic eyes and Germanic accent, who sits behind his subject and listens for exactly fifty minutes to the outpourings of the troubled soul."[118] The image of psychiatric patients changed as well; the institutionalized and chronically insane gave way to the well-heeled urban neurotic. Via psychoanalysis, psychiatry had been reinvented.

Return of the Repressed

Psychiatric expertise under psychoanalysis was built on mystification. Psychoanalysis supplied not just a new way of thinking about mental distress, but also a way of thinking that was insulated from outside criticism. The very idea that its benefits could be externally judged ran anathema to its spirit. The efficacy of psychoanalytic treatment could not be assessed according to some *general* criteria when its claims were *specific* to the needs of the patient as they emerged in the psychoanalytic encounter. By treating this encounter as sacrosanct, psychoanalysts protected their practice from prying eyes.

Charges of ignorance can arise from diverse sources. The asylum era was undermined by the exposure of cure rates; the fraudulent numbers supplied critics with evidence of inadequate knowledge. During the psychobiological period, charges of ignorance arose from the perception that things were spinning out of control. In the psychoanalytic period, a feeling of staleness with the prevailing paradigm was at play, but the clamoring for change arose mostly from outside sources who began to demand greater accountability in psychiatric treatment. The mystification of psychiatric expertise, which yielded professional gains in the 1950s and 1960s, became a liability in the 1970s, as forces conspired to insist on transparency from psychiatrists. Changing epistemic norms in medicine coupled with new ways of paying for health care rendered the retreat to the analytic encounter unacceptable. As newer, cheaper, and seemingly more effective drug therapies were developed, the burden was placed on psychiatry to justify the time, money, and intensive labor involved in psychoanalytic treatment. Unable and/or unwilling to provide the demanded evidence, psychiatrists exhausted the goodwill they had accrued. The public was less willing to countenance psychiatrists' obscurantism. This left psychoanalysts vulnerable to criticisms that they were hiding their ignorance behind their appeals to the individual and complicated theories that could not be tested; in other words, that they were unscientific.

The dominance of psychoanalysis had coincided with the "golden age" of American medicine, in which physicians were accorded tremendous and unquestioned authority on medical matters.[119] Insofar as psychiatry maintained its association with medicine, however marginalized, it basked in medicine's glow. However, a series of medical controversies—like the thalidomide controversy in the early 1960s and the revelation of the Tuskegee syphilis experiments in 1972—eroded public trust in medicine. In response, the federal government changed how it regulated medical experimentation and treatment.[120] The FDA rewrote its drug approval protocols, promoting randomized controlled trials (RCTs) as the gold standard of evidence. Specific therapies had to be shown to work on specific conditions. Case studies were downgraded under the new evidentiary regimes; in the face of demands for quantification and replication, they were dismissed as anecdotal and abandoned as legitimate evidence.[121] The rise of managed care and health maintenance organizations (HMOs) in the 1970s drew attention to the increasing costs of health care. Insurance companies began to assert more control over treatment. Taking some of the decision making out of physicians' hands, they would only cover cost-effective, demonstrably efficacious therapies. Of psychiatrists, they demanded shorter therapeutic procedures.[122] Insurance companies also created a paperwork infrastructure to monitor treatment, requiring formal diagnoses and measured outcomes. As a result of these developments, the period of deference to doctors was being replaced by a focus on evidence. And this new environment was hostile toward the kind of opaque claims to expertise on which psychoanalysts had long depended. Although "evidence-based medicine" would not gain full steam in the United States until the 1990s, its precepts and logic were beginning to be imposed on medical practice to the professional detriment of psychiatry.

Demand for standardized, empirical evidence spelled trouble for psychoanalysis. Although psychiatrists claimed the mantle of science for psychoanalysis, these claims were always fragile. They were dependent on *how* one defined science. Psychoanalysts maintained a broad view of science as an ethos. To be scientific was to approach questions deliberately and to pursue explanations of sufficient depth, using theory to guide explorations. But the changing norms articulated a view of medical science grounded in proper techniques, or the careful application of transparent and replicable research methodologies. This put psychoanalysis at a great disadvantage. A science attuned to repressed, inner subjective states, especially unconscious ones, faced what historian George Makari calls "daunting epistemological problems" when it came to the demands of scientific objectivity.[123] During psychoanalysis's heyday, psychiatrists too often eschewed research, deferring to "nonpsychiatrists" to conduct it, all the while remaining "too satisfied within the present framework of knowledge, hypotheses, and theories."[124] Attempts to clarify its theoretical claims went unfulfilled, lending credence to criticisms that psychoanalysis contained "still too much gobbledygook and too much excess ideological baggage."[125] When demand for standardized research increased during the 1970s, it raised questions that were difficult for psychoanalysts to answer. Could there be general criteria applied to assessing psychoanalytic interpretation when insight was understood as an emergent property of the psychoanalytic interaction? Could one create a standard measure of recovery, when treatment was premised on the capabilities and needs of the particular patient? Could one accommodate the strictures of RCTs to study psychoanalysis when so much depended on the idiosyncratic relationship between the analyst and analysand? Was psychoanalysis fundamentally untestable?

Many critics answered these questions negatively. For some, psychoanalysis was not amenable to scientific investigation, because it was simply not a science. Philosopher Karl Popper famously argued that psychoanalysis, like Marxism, proffered untestable hypotheses that could not be falsified.[126] As such, it failed to meet the standard of a scientific theory in principle. Armed with this Popperian critique, some critics argued, for example, that one could not prove that a child did *not* have an Oedipal conflict.

Philosopher Adolf Grünbaum took a different tack.[127] Rejecting Popper, Grünbaum argued that psychoanalysis *was* falsifiable. Psychoanalysis rested on what he termed the "Tally Argument"; an interpretation was "accurate" to the extent that it "tallied" or resonated with the patient and led to an improvement in his or her condition. In this way, psychoanalysis placed "clinical confirmation on an epistemic throne" and could be assessed accordingly.[128] Drawing on existing research, Grünbaum concluded that psychoanalysis failed to meet its own criteria of success; it was shown in "at least well over 125" studies to have no therapeutic benefit over competing psychotherapies.[129] Observing the long-standing resistance among psychoanalysts to test efficacy, Grünbaum argued that "when Freudian theories are subjected to experimental or observational tests, the results do not support them; they fail the test."[130]

Psychoanalysts reacted to these criticisms in two ways. Some refused to countenance such arguments on epistemological grounds. The idea of testing and comparing the results of psychoanalytic encounters was logically inconsistent with psychoanalysis itself. The emergent, dynamic, and particularistic character of the psychoanalysis precluded the kind of standardization and codification that the new evidentiary commitments required. "Psychoanalysis," argued Trigant Burrow, "is a process which is strictly individual and must be so because unconscious mechanisms cannot be investigated in the presence of a third person."[131] Any attempt to assess psychoanalysis by someone outside this interaction, or according to some external standard, did violence to it. Thus falling back on mystification, these proponents declared their opposition to the new evidentiary norms. They refused to "follow blindly where the results of the double-blind study lead us!"[132] In taking this stand, the psychoanalysts courted a schism with medicine, desiring to escape, once and for all, the irony that "psychiatry rests its claims for professional status on a profession that is hostile toward it."[133]

Other psychoanalysts tried to accommodate the new demands. They sought to develop analytic-friendly evaluations. But these efforts were beset with problems. For example, in 1947, the APA, upon the insistence of psychoanalysts like Lawrence Kubie, appointed a committee to evaluate the results of psychoanalysis. From the start, the committee was plagued by basic issues of categorization, operationalization, and measurement. Could psychoanalysts agree on interpretations and common diagnostic assessments? On appropriate standards of treatment? On general measures of recovery and cure? The study limped on for years. It was not published until twenty years later, and even then, it drew muddled conclusions. On measures of symptom relief, it discovered that psychoanalysis was not very effective, but the authors noted that for most psychoanalysts, symptom relief was not the intended target. The deeper, more "structural" personality changes were harder to pin down. The clearest finding of the report was that the qualities of the psychoanalyst mattered a great deal, thereby throwing a wrench in any research, like RCTs, that tried to control for this factor.

As medicine proper adopted the new evidentiary norms, the difficulties of molding psychoanalysis to fit them presented professional problems. The association with medicine had been crucial to shoring up the legitimacy of psychoanalysis. With this under threat, the always tenuous association fractured into a "vexing" relationship between psychiatry and "the rest of medicine."[134] As Freud's promotion of lay analysis suggested, there was nothing inherent to psychoanalytic treatment that required medical expertise. American psychoanalysts adopted this requirement for professional reasons. But they never resolved the otherness of psychiatry within medicine. Psychiatrists themselves had long acknowledged this ill fit. "No other specialty of medicine has had a history so strange, nor a relation to human thought so intimate as psychiatry," insisted Alan Gregg, an officer at the Rockefeller Foundation. "No other specialty of medicine deals with diseases whose initial signs can be so easily confused with moral lapse."[135]

Medicine had been revolutionized and professionalized under the rubric of disease specificity, that diseases should be thought of as entities existing outside the unique manifestations of illness in particular patients.[136] Psychoanalysts, on the other hand, took the personality as its object of intervention. Even if they used the term "disease," they understood it in a fundamentally different way, as "the logical outgrowth of the particular personality in its efforts to solve a particular problem (or perhaps several problems)," a part of the patient, not as "an intruder or an invasion from without."[137] As new norms of empirical testing took hold, psychoanalysts found it difficult to gloss over this long-standing tension with prevailing medical conceptions of illness.

Tensions came to a head over the issue of diagnosis. Diagnosis was central to this new regime of evidence, for without reliable diagnoses, researchers cannot create the comparable groups of patients that RCTs require. But psychoanalysts had long held "an aversion to diagnosis," arguing "that it is not the label but the problem that concerns the therapist."[138] Affixing a label to a patient's unique problem was reductionistic and antithetical to the psychoanalytic mode of reasoning. In addition, psychoanalysts did not conceive of mental distress as discrete entities, instead maintaining a view of neuroses existing on a spectrum, with every individual more or less neurotic. The line between the sick and the well could not be easily drawn. This clashed with the push to standardized psychiatric knowledge. Vague, generic diagnoses of "neurosis" no longer sufficed. Roy Grinker Sr. warned his fellow psychiatrists:

> In a sense many contemporary psychiatrists have been working upstream against the forces opposing concepts of syndromes and accurate diagnostic criteria. The unpopularity of diagnosis and knowledge of the life history of describable entities is a reaction against the "disease" concept in psychiatry and the overemphasis on individual dynamic processes. Yet the pendulum has swung too far away in the direction of concern only with "the problem" of a specific patient (or client).[139]

Research funders, government agencies, and insurance companies, in demanding firm diagnoses, had swung the pendulum away from core psychoanalytic assumptions.

On the issue of diagnostic reliability and validity, psychiatry was found wanting. Particularly damning was the infamous research conducted by David L. Rosenhan, an American psychologist. As described in his article "On Being Sane in Insane Places," published in *Science*, Rosenhan sent eight healthy pseudo-patients to twelve mental hospitals to try to gain admittance.[140] All were admitted, despite reporting the vaguest of symptoms (pseudo-patients were instructed to claim that they were hearing unclear voices saying mundane things like "empty," "hollow," and "thud").[141] As if these admittances were not damaging enough, Rosenhan's subjects reported that the only individuals who questioned their mentally ill status were the patients themselves. When one hospital administrator objected to Rosenhan's methods, he agreed to send more pseudo-patients to give the hospital the opportunity to screen potential admittances more thoroughly. When the hospital announced that they had identified over forty pseudo-patients, Rosenhan informed them that he had never sent any. Drawn in devastating plainness, Rosenhan concluded, "It is clear that we cannot distinguish the sane from the insane in psychiatric hospitals."[142] Psychiatrists were unable to achieve this most basic of tasks.

Diagnostic uncertainty was a reflection of bigger issues. Psychiatric ignorance, repressed under psychoanalysis, aggressively reasserted itself in psychiatric discourse during the 1960s and 1970s. Psychiatrists began to lose faith in psychoanalysis and question whether it was ever all that it was cracked up to be. The "practical accomplishments" under psychoanalysis "have been few and the progress disappointingly slow."[143] The promised "revolution or what we call a 'breakthrough' has not appeared," as "the etiologies of most disorders are unknown."[144] Once again, the threat of professional fragmentation reared its head. Psychiatrists had become bogged down in irrelevant internecine theoretical conflicts. In turn, psychiatry's boundaries became "shifting and diffuse, and where etiological uncertainties and competing theories are more the rule than exception."[145] In his 1975 presidential address to the APA, John Spiegel lamented, "Every profession must endure controversy, but the current disagreements within the profession of psychiatry boggle the mind."[146] Once seen as innovative and avant-garde, psychoanalysis now appeared retrograde to many psychiatrists. It was "showing its age" and had "suffered a marked loss of momentum," admitted psychoanalyst Joseph G. Kepecs.[147] "Psychoanalysis, once a revolutionary movement," he continued, "has now become relatively conservative."[148]

As it had in the past (and would again in the future), psychiatry under psychoanalysis had fallen prey to the enticements of the latest new thing. In its quest for prestige, argued psychiatrists Ames Fischer and Morton Weinstein, psychiatry had "no rival among medical specialties in its susceptibility to fads and its readiness to board the newest bandwagon" and no equal in their tendency "to be overenthusiastic in their acceptance of currently 'stylish' methods and techniques."[149] The expectations for psychoanalysis, like the "stylish" reinventions before it, went unfulfilled. Psychoanalysis had become, in Grinker's words, "a crumbling stockade of proprietary dogmatisms" that "maintain[ed] itself aloof from the progress of behavioral science and look[ed] askance at conceptions of rigor."[150] Psychoanalytic psychiatrists found themselves facing emboldened critics, many of them their professional peers, "who argue[d] that psychoanalysis is passé, that its theoretical constructs are outmoded, that it is a dubious therapeutic technique at best, and that its costliness in both time and money can no longer be justified in the face of newer and more effective techniques for symptom amelioration."[151] Psychiatry was relegated to the status of a second-rate medical profession, as arbiters of conditions unwanted by other fields. These unwanted conditions brought professional instability, as they risked being confiscated by other branches of medicine. Psychologist George W. Albee observed that "when a real organic cause is discovered to be the significant underlying factor in the production of disturbed behavior . . . the treatment of these conditions is removed from the psychiatric field."[152] Psychiatry's jurisdiction began to crumble, circumscribed as it was to contested ailments poorly understood from within a dominant psychiatric paradigm that was showing its age.

Conclusion

The patient paced, ten, twelve, fourteen hours a day. In the seven months since Dr. Raphael Osheroff had been admitted to Chestnut Lodge, his anxiety and depression had worsened, and with it, the pacing. The raspy footfalls of his slippered feet echoed the halls. His feet swelled, blistered, and blackened, his heels bruised. Bursitis shot waves of pain through his hips. He shed forty pounds. Osheroff's mood grew increasingly agitated, and his relationship to the psychoanalytic staff soured. They dismissed his ceaseless pacing as non-compliance. Little did the staff know that the endless shuffling they observed day in and day out would become an indictment of their entire mode of treatment, a symbol of a psychiatric era in decline. Little did they anticipate that the pacing patient would file a lawsuit that would throw into question the very legitimacy of psychoanalysis.

Osheroff, a nephrologist from Maryland, had committed himself voluntarily to Chestnut Lodge in January 1979. He was suffering from depressive symptoms that arose after a business failure and his second divorce. In selecting Chestnut Lodge, Osheroff placed his care in the hands of an august hospital with a well-deserved reputation as a bastion for psychoanalytic/psychodynamic treatment.[153] Three decades earlier, psychiatrist Alfred H. Stanton and sociologist Morris S. Schwartz had been invited by the Lodge to conduct a study of its wards.[154] They noted that the care at the Lodge—which they deemed quite good—was suffused with an unusually strong commitment to psychoanalysis, a commitment that verged on ideological dogma:

> There was a general consensus among practically all personnel at the hospital about the nature of mental illness and its proper treatment. Most articulate patients and substantially all the staff took it for granted that mental disorder was the result of interpersonal difficulty, and that the effective treatment of it was in interpersonal terms. "Psychotherapy" and "treatment" were synonyms in this hospital, in contrast to certain other hospitals where insulin or some other therapy is "treatment."[155]

In its firm opposition to somatic treatments, the Lodge operated "as an almost inexorable propaganda machine" for psychoanalytic principles.[156] Indeed, the Lodge was a major proponent of treating schizophrenia via psychotherapy, a controversial approach that many psychoanalysts themselves objected to. Decades later, when Osheroff arrived at the Rockville, Maryland, facility, the Lodge maintained its reputation as a center for psychoanalytic treatment.

The staff diagnosed Osheroff with an affective disorder (manic-depressive illness, depressive type) and a personality disorder (narcissistic personality disorder). In their treatment program, they focused on the latter. The plan was to restructure Osheroff's personality through "safe regression." Applying a combination of milieu therapy and "confrontative psychotherapy," doctors hoped to break down Osheroff's defenses. This, they believed, would help him overcome his tendency to blame his struggles on external factors and get him to take responsibility for the events in his life.[157] Only then could his depressive symptoms be addressed. Osheroff's doctors anticipated that the treatment would require three years of inpatient care and another decade or so of outpatient treatment.

Initially cooperative, Osheroff started to resist his treatment and resent his doctors. Feeling demeaned and punished, he decompensated. In an unpublished memoir, Osheroff described a "journey deeper and deeper into the depths of an inferno that Dante himself could never conceive of in his most tortured or creative moments."[158] He began to pace.

After seven months, Osheroff's parents removed him from the Lodge. They checked him into Silver Hill, a private hospital in Connecticut, where he was immediately put on lithium. Within weeks, his condition improved. After three months, he was discharged. But Osheroff returned to a life in shambles. During his months of institutionalization, he had lost his medical license, become embroiled in a conflict with his ex-business partner, and lost custody of two of his children. Seeking redress, Osheroff filed a civil lawsuit against Chestnut Lodge for negligence and medical malpractice. In the suit, he claimed that the Lodge had misdiagnosed his condition. By prioritizing his personality disorder, they neglected to treat his depressive symptoms, which should have been "very easily treatable" with available medications.[159] In their "doctrinaire refusal to recognize and utilize state-of-the-art somatic therapies," Lodge doctors never even considered somatic treatment an option, nor did they disclose "alternative therapeutic modalities" to Osheroff.[160] Because of their philosophical blinders, the staff failed "to recognize that some mental incapacities are physiological in origin."[161]

In response to the charges, the Lodge appealed to long-standing psychoanalytic principles to justify their focus on Osheroff's underlying personality disorder. Reflecting their psychoanalytic commitments, they viewed his depressive symptoms as epiphenomenal to the true problem, which resided in Osheroff's personality. Until his personality disorder was resolved, nothing could be done for the depression. In addition, the Lodge blamed Osheroff himself for the treatment's failure. He was resistant to treatment, unwilling to address his own ego defenses. His subsequent improvement at Silver Hill, retorted the Lodge, was explained away as the result of his willingness to cooperate with the staff there, not the curative power of the drugs themselves.

The lawsuit was settled out of court by the State of Maryland Health Claims Arbitration Board. Siding with Osheroff, they awarded him $250,000 in damages. After numerous appeals, the suit was settled for an undisclosed amount.

Osheroff v. Chestnut Lodge established no legal precedent and garnered almost no media attention. Nevertheless, within psychiatry, it set off a maelstrom. The case became symbolic of the beleaguered standing of psychoanalysis and portended its coming replacement. It highlighted the growing rift between proponents of the long-dominant psychoanalytic perspective and a new generation of reformers brandishing a biomedical view of mental illness.

Although the case received scant coverage in the mainstream press, it was discussed in every academic department and arbitrated on the pages of professional journals. The most prominent discussion of *Osheroff* was an exchange between two Harvard psychiatrists, Gerald Klerman and Alan Stone, featured in the *American Journal of Psychiatry*. The central issue at stake in their exchange was the legal notion of "respectable minority rule." This rule protects physicians against claims of malpractice and negligence if (1) the treatment involves medical issues in which there are divergent schools of medical thought; and (2) their conduct is in line with a respectable position within this dispute, even if that position is in the minority.[162] Coming to Osheroff's defense, Klerman denied that this rule was applicable; the case was not about "psychotherapy versus biological therapy, but, rather, opinion versus evidence."[163] As Klerman saw it, on one side, there were proven drug treatments; on the other, psychoanalytic ideology. Psychoanalysis was not substantiated by an adequate evidentiary research base and was therefore not a respectable position. The Lodge had acted irresponsibly, and if the profession, beholden to psychoanalytic interests, was unwilling to set appropriate treatment guidelines, it was "understandable" that patients would seek out the courts to do so.

Defending the Lodge, Stone stressed the lawsuit's dangerous implications for the profession.[164] Arguing that Klerman was overstating the evidence in support for psychopharmaceutical drugs, Stone contended that Klerman's real agenda was "to promulgate more uniform scientific standards of treatment in psychiatry, based on his own opinions about science and clinical practice."[165] Although establishing no formal legal precedent, Klerman worried that *Osheroff* was already becoming a means to establish a de facto therapeutic precedent. Biological psychiatrists critical of psychoanalysis were trying to use the courts to impose a monolithic vision for psychiatry. This was dangerous politics. Stone demanded that "the legal standard of care should reflect the 'collective sense of the profession,' not the partisan opinions of one particular group and certainly not the latest unreplicated and evolving scientific evidence."[166] Asking the legal system to adjudicate legitimate professional disagreements courted disaster, as it might prematurely establish an inappropriate standard and undermine psychiatrists' autonomy.

Both Klerman and Stone appealed to psychiatric ignorance in marshaling their arguments. For Klerman, recognition of ignorance served to warn against the dogmatism he saw among psychoanalytic psychiatrists: "In the current situation in psychiatric practice, where there are large areas of ignorance, it behooves individual practitioners and institutions to avoid relying on single treatment approaches or theoretical paradigms."[167] Like psychobiologists before him, he cautioned against premature closure and called for open-mindedness in the face of ignorance. But this openness had to have limits, and for Klerman, the appropriate standards for assessing claims were imported from biomedical science, particularly RCTs. Stone likewise acknowledged the gaps in psychiatry's knowledge base, but followed its logic to a different conclusion. Under conditions of uncertainty, the respectable minority rule is indispensable. It protects "the diversity of reasonably prudent professional opinion and different approaches to the practice of the healing arts against the rigid orthodoxy."[168] With so much unknown, it was wrong to circumscribe research to theories and treatments that were amenable to the shifting evidentiary whims of medicine. Consequently, while both sides acknowledged psychiatric ignorance and agreed that it demanded openness, they diverged in how they perceived psychoanalysis's potential to overcome this ignorance.

The debate raged on, but *Osheroff* had a chilling effect on psychoanalytic treatment. Forever after it, psychoanalysts had to consider the threat of legal sanction when formulating a treatment program that accorded with their cherished psychoanalytic principles.

In the late 1970s, psychiatry yet again descended into turmoil, of which *Osheroff* was but one example. The psychoanalytic reinvention had unfolded according to an all-too-familiar pattern. Reformers promulgated the expectation that psychoanalysis would correct the misguided errors of the psychobiological era. By bringing a measure of coherence and a clear direction to psychiatry, psychoanalysis promised insight into, and resolution of, the most basic questions pertaining to mental distress. Like the reforms before it, reality never caught up to the hype. The psychoanalytic dream proved to be a chimera. Ignorance persisted. It was hidden and obscured, but enduring. As outside actors began to demand greater accountability, it was once again exposed. Psychiatry, claimed APA president Perry Talkington, became a "profession under attack" besieged by internal and external critics.[169] Crisis ensued. As "a feeling of nihilism" took hold, psychiatrists were forced to grapple with "the unsettling and bewildering feeling that what they have been doing has been largely worthless and that the premises on which they have based their professional lives were partly fraudulent."[170]

However, even as the psychoanalytic period repeated the well-worn pattern of crisis–reinvention–crisis, it developed new wrinkles in the management of ignorance. The first was a conscious effort to secure new sources of patronage. One strategy available to collective actors when suffering setbacks is to switch arenas of conflict, to relocate the struggle to spaces in which they may have a better advantage.[171] For nearly a century, psychiatry had been dependent upon state legislatures to support the mental hospitals that formed the institutional bulwark of its authority. Over time, however, psychiatry had exhausted the legislatures' goodwill and patience. Given psychiatry's checkered and tense relationship with state legislatures, legislators were unlikely to accept the claims of psychoanalytic reformers on trust. This trust was essential for an expertise so dependent on mystification. World War II, however, offered psychoanalytic reformers an opportunity to court the federal government and reduce psychiatry's dependence on state legislatures. Claiming success during the war effort, reformers shifted their arena of focus to the federal government, securing funding through the NIMH and jobs in the VA system. These resources were harnessed to not only grow the profession, but build and fund an organizational infrastructure for psychoanalytic psychiatry beyond that of the system of mental hospitals.

More crucially, psychoanalytic reformers mitigated psychiatric ignorance through mystification (at least for a while). Professional power and expert authority is rooted in the control over knowledge, achieved through a set of mechanisms that control the supply of and demand for professional work. Central to this power is the issue of transparency, or lack thereof. Professions are granted authority on the basis that they possess specialized knowledge that is inaccessible to others.[172] This demands that professional knowledge possess the quality of "cognitive indetermination"; it cannot be too transparent lest it become accessible to those outside the profession, thereby negating the need for special professional privileges.[173] To some extent, then, professional expertise is always shrouded in mystery. Psychoanalysts, however, took obfuscation to an extreme. Psychoanalytic knowledge emerged behind closed doors in an inaccessible space and trafficked in theories and interpretations that could only be judged by those trained in its tradition. The psychoanalytic encounter, and to a lesser extent its psychodynamic spin-offs, was transformed into an "occult object," something mysterious to those on the outside looking in.[174] By this means, psychiatrists recaptured some of their "professional mystery."[175]

Just as important as rendering psychiatric knowledge opaque, psychoanalysis obscured psychiatric ignorance. It enclosed ignorance in the psychoanalytic encounter, while articulating a scope of expertise resistant to criticisms of *general* ignorance. Psychoanalytic reformers recentered

psychiatric expertise as pertaining to the specificities of the individual patient. The knowledge it produced was less generalized knowledge on the
nature of mental illness and more in-depth insight into the particular manifestations of neuroses they saw in their patients. Expectations focused on
individual-level outcomes; the proof of psychoanalysis's pudding lay in the
self-understanding it lent to the patient. Thus, while psychoanalytic psychiatrists hid their ignorance under elaborate theories and a posture of certainty,
the true power of the psychoanalytic paradigm derived from its obscurantism and relative imperviousness to outsiders. As long as patrons and authorities more or less accepted psychoanalytic premises, mystification remained
an effective means to manage the potential fallout from ignorance.

The mystifying nature of psychanalytic knowledge and the influx of new
support from federal sources enabled psychiatry to achieve a degree of authority it had never known. Changing evidentiary norms, however, ruptured
the trust propping up psychoanalytic mystification. The federal government
as well as new actors, like insurance companies, began to demand an accounting. These actors insisted that psychiatry bend to the new standards
of evidence in medicine, to submit itself to external validation. The way to
assess the efficacy of treatment was recalibrated. No longer could assessment be restricted to the subjective judgment of the patient; psychiatrists
now had to demonstrate objective, quantifiable evidence of efficacy. In such
an environment, the opacity of psychoanalysis became a liability. Unable
and unwilling to succumb to this accounting, psychoanalysis came under
intense criticism and rapidly lost authority. Its ignorance was once again
laid bare, and the legitimacy of psychiatry, in turn, suffered.

New calls for reform echoed across the profession. But what would replace the psychoanalytic paradigm? By the 1980s, biomedical reformers
were poised to take over. But the story of their emergence will have to wait.
For while the aspirational wing of psychiatry was embracing psychoanalysis, the institutional wing was languishing in public hospitals, trying desperately to escape the decaying situations in which they found themselves.
The shift in orientation toward private practice facilitated by psychoanalysis
went some of the way toward facilitating the profession's escape. But in the
1960s, another possible direction appeared. Community psychiatry made
its bid for reinventing psychiatry. Stressing social, environmental, and even
political factors, community psychiatrists pursued an ambitious program to
prevent mental distress, with psychiatrists at the helm as social engineers.

FOUR

It Takes a Community to Raise a Profession

For Walter Jackson Freeman II, the chief threat to psychiatry was not over-zealousness, but dithering inaction. With little patience for psychotherapy, Freeman believed that the secrets to mental illness lay in the brain, and from the beginning of his career in 1924, he doggedly pursued promising somatic treatments. In the 1930s, he came across the work of a Portuguese neurologist, Egas Moniz, who was performing "leucotomies" on his mental patients, a surgical procedure that cut nerve fibers in the brain. Inspired, Freeman and his colleague, James Winston Watts, a neurosurgeon at George Washington University, performed their first neurosurgical operation in 1936. They dubbed their procedure a "lobotomy."

The rationale for prefrontal lobotomy drew on an amalgam of ideas that had been circulating since the psychobiological era. The frontal lobes were thought to be the seat of psychic activity in which ideas are stored. For the mentally ill, maladaptive thought processes had become habitual and entrenched in the frontal lobes. Severing the connections between the prefrontal cortex and the anterior frontal lobes would relieve the "the emotional response to the pathologic ideas," or so the thinking went.[1] Upon this specious rationale, Freeman and Watts justified the drastic surgery. And families, desperate for treatments, found their way to the two enterprising doctors, most notably the Kennedy family, who had the surgery performed on Rosemary Kennedy.[2]

Early lobotomies were complicated and cumbersome. Drilling holes into the skull required the skill of a well-trained neurosurgeon, like Watts, and all the staging of modern medical surgery. This limited their appeal.

Convinced of the revolutionary treatment on his hands, Freeman began to tinker with the procedure. In 1946, he introduced the transorbital lobotomy to American psychiatry. Freeman described the new procedure in technical language that belied its horrors:

When the patient is unconscious, I pinch the upper eyelid between the thumb and finger and bring it well away from the eyeball. I then insert the point of the transorbital leucotome into the conjunctival sac, taking care not to touch the skin or lashes, and move the point around until it settles against the vault of the orbit. I then drop to one knee, beside the table, in order to aim the instrument parallel with the bony ridge of the nose, and slightly toward the midline. When the 5 cm. mark is reached, I pull the handle of the instrument as far laterally as the rim of the orbit will permit in order to sever fibers at the base of the frontal lobe. I then return the instrument half way to its previous position and drive it further to a depth of 7 cm. from the margin of the upper eyelid.[3]

A transorbital lobotomy involved driving a trocar into the brain through the eye orbit. Once inserted, Freeman pivoted the trocar back and forth to sever the white fibrous matter connecting the cortical tissue of the prefrontal cortex to the thalamus. The procedure took mere minutes—and little surgical skill—to perform. (The story, perhaps apocryphal, is that Freeman refined his technique by practicing with an ice pick and a grapefruit.) Freeman's "innovation" primed lobotomy for widespread dissemination. It could now be performed by psychiatrists in mental institutions or even their own offices. There was no need for neurosurgeons or surgical operating rooms. Freeman's lobotomy promised a cure that psychiatrists could wield on their own.

Dismayed by Freeman's wanton experimenting, Watts split with him, refusing to endorse lobotomy as an "office procedure" performed by untrained psychiatrists. Unchecked by Watts's tempering influence, Freeman embarked on his career work, promoting transorbital lobotomy to any psychiatrist who would listen. This he pursued with a combination of missionary zeal and the tricks of a seasoned salesman. To support his claim that lobotomy was "an effective means of treating all but the most severe and chronic cases of schizophrenia," Freeman published misleading statistics of its efficacy alongside dramatic case studies of miraculous recoveries of former patients.[4]

In 1948, Freeman began traveling to mental hospitals throughout the country, performing lobotomies on patients and training staffs in the technique. During the summer of 1951, he embarked on a kind of macabre road trip, traveling to seventeen states plus Canada, Puerto Rico, and Curaçao. At one point, Freeman drove 11,000 miles in a five-week stint, and at his peak, he drove his trocar into as many as 225 patients in just twelve days.[5]

Save for his doggedness and willingness to travel, Freeman was no anomaly. Such an overzealous character has been found all too often throughout the history of psychiatry. But if the 3,500 lobotomies performed by Freeman himself might be explained away by his almost religious conviction in the procedure—he was a "maverick" and true believer, according to a biographer[6]—the other 17,000 lobotomies performed in the United States between 1936 and 1951 are not as easily accounted for. They cannot be reduced to the work of a single zealot maiming patients under the false pretense of science. The fact of the matter was that lobotomy was seen as a respectable tool in the armamentarium of hospital psychiatry. It won endorsement from esteemed figures like Adolf Meyer and the preeminent neurophysiologist John F. Fulton. In 1949, Moniz was awarded the Nobel Prize in medicine for developing the technique.

Today, because lobotomy has become *the* symbol of psychiatric abuse in the popular imagination, it is hard to comprehend how the barbaric-seeming practice caught on. To attribute its popularity to Freeman's sales acumen alone is too simplistic. Instead, lobotomy's appeal attested to the extent to which the psychiatric mental hospital system had deteriorated by the 1940s and 1950s. Despite the rebranding, mental hospitals had never recovered from the failed asylum period. The day-to-day experiences of institutional psychiatrists offered an unrelenting reminder of their ignorance and impotence. The choices presented to institutional psychiatrists were stark: either embrace a custodial role and focus on containing their patients' madness or experiment with new treatments out of a sense that things could not possibly get worse. Under these conditions, transorbital lobotomy had its allure. It held up the promise that mental hospitals could become "active treatment centers," that psychiatrists could shed their custodial role to become doctors with cures.[7] It also projected a future in which the locus of psychiatric practice would be removed from the mental hospital. In Freeman's formulation, lobotomy offered a distinct *psychiatric* treatment that validated psychiatrists' distinct expertise. Even if it was reserved as a "last resort, the end of the line," a significant number of patients fell into this category.[8] Compelled to do *something*, hospital psychiatrists cut.

Like ECT, metrazol therapy, and surgical bacteriology before it, lobotomy never became the cure-all it promised to be. Its efficacy a mirage, it did little to improve the station of hospital psychiatrists. Lobotomy fell into disfavor and ignominy, leaving in its wake only the blank stares of its victims.

While lobotomy did not provide the escape from the mental hospital, psychiatrists never gave up the dream. In the second half of the twentieth century, institutional psychiatrists found an alternative route out, not via the trocar but via the program of community psychiatry. This chapter examines the brief but significant attempt to reinvent psychiatry along the lines of community psychiatry in the 1960s and 1970s. Turning attention away from the more aspirational psychoanalytic wing of psychiatry, it addresses the long-languishing institutional wing, which had developed its distinct reforming impulses, most of which were focused on breaking free of the stultifying mental hospital. Psychiatry owed its existence to the mental hospital. It originated there. Whatever the profession's other difficulties, the mental hospital provided a stronghold of uncompromised authority, a place where psychiatrists' power went unchecked. Whereas psychiatrists encountered resistance when they tried to extend their jurisdiction to patients with less serious forms of mental illness, they faced little opposition when it came to the chronically mentally ill. As long as there was a need for long-term inpatient care, there was a need for psychiatrists, however unglamorous the work.

Like their psychoanalytic peers, institutional psychiatrists grappled with ignorance. Psychiatry dealt "with the most complex of all phenomena which we know in the universe, the highest organization of anything we know, viz. the nervous system, and its product the human mind."[9] And while psychiatrists might speak "glibly of 'discoveries' and 'new insights,'" these amounted to little more than "restatements in modern idiom of truths about the human mind which have been known to the wise men throughout the ages."[10] In their failure to alleviate the suffering under their charge, institutional psychiatrists confronted psychiatric ignorance, not in the abstract, but daily in their concrete dealings with their patients. Reduced to a custodial role, they were overwhelmed by patients they could not help and critics they could not shake.

In response to these difficulties, a group of reformers envisioned a world in which mental hospitals were not needed. Embracing an activist orientation, they hoped to move psychiatry into the community, where care would be provided outside the walls of the hospitals in a network of community-based services. As coordinators of a diverse, comprehensive network of services, psychiatrists would increase the scale of their influence, becoming consultants on a wide array of societal ills. Such was the expectation of this new reinvention. And it started with a bang. Under the banner of "community psychiatry," psychiatrists helped dismantle the system of mental hospitals in the 1960s. Reformers petitioned the federal government to replace these hospitals with more flexible and dynamic community-based care. With the passage of the Community Mental Health Act in 1963, psychiatrists claimed victory for deinstitutionalization.

The celebrations, however, were short-lived. A mere decade into the community reform effort, it faltered. Community psychiatry was built more on slogans than actual research. Rather than offer a positive program of community care, it amounted to little more than a negative critique of mental hospitals and a naïve commitment to deinstitutionalization. Community psychiatrists never "fully appreciate[d] how little they know concerning the factors that contribute to or militate against the development of neuroses and psychoses."[11] Mental hospitals were shuttered, but the comprehensive network of community-based services never materialized, hampered by a lack of funding, a lack of purpose, and eventually a lack of psychiatric interest. Clear that the expectations of community psychiatry would not be met, psychiatrists walked away from it in the 1970s.

In terms of the politics of ignorance, community psychiatrists did not propose new ideas or even promise much in the way of future insight. They drew on long-standing ideas within psychiatry, now reframed in psychodynamic terms, that pointed to environmental factors in propagating mental illness. Reformers merely assumed that psychiatrists possessed expertise relevant to engage with the social world. To withhold this expertise was to abdicate their social responsibility. Consequently, the community psychiatry reinvention tried to manage ignorance by diluting it, spreading it far afield so as to obscure its depth. Whereas psychoanalytic reformers narrowed their focus, framing psychiatric expertise as penetrating knowledge of the individual psyche, community psychiatrists sought to broaden psychiatry's reach into social and cultural factors related to mental health. And yet, despite their differences in scale and scope, both reinventions succumbed to the same fate, a dramatic rise and a meteoric fall.

The fall for community psychiatry would be far more damaging in its impact. In their embrace of community psychiatry, psychiatrists rejected its institutional origins. However problematic and ineffective these institutions were, they had long been the stronghold of psychiatric power to which the profession retreated when challenged. When dismantled, psychiatry found itself homeless, faced with intense competition and having renounced its responsibility to its original clientele, patients with serious mental illness. Furthermore, their ignorance assumed a more visible form; these patients, once sequestered out of sight, could now be seen on the streets of every major American city. In a history of failures, deinstitutionalization would be psychiatry's most damaging professionally.

Snake Pits, 1945–1960

From their inception, mental hospitals, née asylums, formed the institutional backbone of American psychiatry. Although their luster dulled after the asylum period, they remained a significant part of psychiatry's identity, even as reformers, first with psychobiology and then psychoanalysis, sought to reconfigure psychiatry outside their walls. While the elite aspirational wing filled the pages of psychiatric journals and articulated the profession's aspirations, institutional psychiatrists continued to toil away in mental hospitals, marginalized to the periphery of professional politics but plugging along nonetheless. Indeed, up through World War II, the bulk of psychiatric practice remained institutional. On the eve of World War II, the public mental hospital system employed more than two-thirds of APA members.[12] In 1945, state hospitals had a resident population of about 430,000, of which approximately 88,000 were first-time admissions.[13] Patients with chronic mental illness in long-term inpatient care comprised the bulk of psychiatry's clientele.

Still, psychiatrists had developed a deep ambivalence toward mental hospitals. On the one hand, the hospitals embodied the profession's origins and justification for its emergence. Psychiatry was founded on the promise that it could cure mental illness and mitigate the social problems it caused. State legislatures accepted this pitch and funded asylums. In doing so, they endorsed psychiatrists' jurisdictional claim over chronic mental illness. Psychiatrists held this claim unchallenged, even *after* the asylum's promises were exposed as empty. The control over this clientele—a control exercised through mental hospitals—afforded a degree of professional security, a hard floor for psychiatry's authority. And significantly, it was in the mental hospitals that psychiatric practice and philosophy hewed closest to medicine. Here, psychiatrists deployed treatments that at least looked like medicine. Here, psychiatrists maintained a more somatic view of mental illness than their psychoanalytic peers, who, having turned their attention to the psychological dimensions of mental illness, strained to maintain their link to medicine.

On the other hand, conditions in the mental hospitals had degraded to such a degree that many psychiatrists reached the conclusion that they were unsalvageable. This decline was driven by the related problems of overcrowding and underfunding. As discussed in chapter 1, all other factors aside, mental hospitals faced a simple numbers problem, a "silting up" stemming from the accumulation of chronic cases. As long as demand remained consistent, a fatalistic logic took hold and created an irresolvable problem for mental hospitals. They could not discharge patients at a rate commensurate to those they were asked to take in. Because public mental hospitals were required to accept everyone, there was little that psychiatrists could do to stem the tide. As a result, institutions constructed to hold 250 patients reached populations of up to 10,000 by the 1940s. Overcrowding was compounded by decreased funding from state legislatures. Between 1930 and 1945, legislatures preoccupied with first the Great Depression and later World War II ignored mental hospitals.[14] The result, noted APA president Kenneth E. Appel, was a mental hospital system in which "treatment can scarcely be said to exist for the majority. It is mostly care and custody. Mass methods, herding and regimentation, are the rule."[15] All mental hospitals faced these challenges, although well-heeled, private mental hospitals were able to soften some of their effects.[16]

Institutional psychiatrists tried to maintain a modicum of control amid this untenable situation. "Living in remote areas" made it hard; the isolation from their peers robbed them "of interchange of ideas and stimulating normal human relationships."[17] Nevertheless, this isolation did not dissuade institutional psychiatrists from experimenting with new treatments, albeit with typically terrible results. The treatments followed a trajectory of hype and disappointment similar to that of lobotomy. They would be introduced as revolutionary, accompanied by exaggerated claims of efficacy. Desperate to do something for their patients, institutional psychiatrists adopted them with enthusiasm. Anything that held hope was tried. Treatments like ECT and various shock therapies spread faster than their empirical support. Thin anecdotal reports were enough to convince institutional psychiatrists to give them a whirl. However, as psychiatrists came to witness firsthand their inadequate effects, they abandoned hope in the treatments as cures. Yet, despite this waning enthusiasm, most treatments lingered as a part of institutional psychiatrists' tool kit, to be trudged out in a desperate attempt to do something about the most intractable patients, often less for therapeutic reasons than as a means of controlling patients.[18]

The one innovation that avoided this fate was chlorpromazine. Developed in France in 1954, chlorpromazine, or Thorazine, as it was marketed in the United States, was used to treat a host of conditions, including schizophrenia, mania, psychomotor excitement, and other psychotic disorders. At the time, Thorazine was seen as a significant breakthrough by many institutional psychiatrists. It was "found to be of unusual value in the symptomatic control of neuropsychiatric disturbances."[19] The broad adoption of the drug became a big reason that lobotomy fell out of favor. Still, the implications of Thorazine, and the host of psychopharmaceutical treatments that followed, took a while for psychiatry to sort out. Psychoanalysts, in particular, viewed drug treatments with skepticism; they worried that the medications might inhibit the patient from achieving insight. Others saw the drugs "as an adjunct treatment, either as a last resort, when the patient is found not to be responding to psychotherapy, or as an 'opening gambit' early in therapy, sometimes on the first visit and often in response to a request from the patient."[20] And while demonstrating better efficacy than previous somatic treatments, Thorazine was not without significant negative side effects, most notably tardive dyskinesia, or involuntary repetitive body movements. Therefore, while Thorazine injected some much-needed optimism into institutional care—inducing "a wave of enthusiasm for a pharmacodynamic approach"[21]—its effect on psychiatry's professional identity and authority was more ambiguous.

Because of their isolation, many of the developments within mental hospitals occurred outside the public purview. Occasionally, intrepid journalists like Nellie Bly or ex-patients like Clifford Beers would draw public scrutiny, but after a brief period, interest would subside. However, in the postwar period, events conspired to shine a glaring spotlight on mental hospitals. During World War II, conscientious objectors, many of whom were Quakers, were sometimes sent to work in mental hospitals as an alternative to military service. When the war ended, some of these objectors wrote exposés of the conditions they observed. For example, journalist Albert Q. Maisel published a provocative article, "Bedlam, 1946," in *Life* magazine based on reports from conscientious objectors. Accompanied by graphic photographs, the article likened conditions in mental hospitals to Nazi concentration camps.[22] Maisel reported on the horrors of state mental hospitals, which through "public neglect and legislative penny-pinching" had degenerated "into little more than concentration camps on the Belsen pattern."[23] Patients endured regular beatings, which were "covered up by a tacit conspiracy of mutually protective silence and a code that ostracizes employees who 'sing too loud.'"[24] Understaffed by poorly trained workers, the hospitals did not treat most patients. Instead, they subjected them to violent control:

> Thousands spend their days—often for weeks at a stretch—locked in devices euphemistically called "restraints": thick leather handcuffs, great canvas camisoles, "muffs," "mitts," wristlets, locks and straps and restraining sheets. Hundreds are confined in "lodges"—bare, bed-less rooms reeking with filth and feces—by day lit only through half-inch holes in steel-plated windows, by night merely black tombs in which the cries of the insane echo unheard from the peeling plaster of the walls.[25]

The vivid analogy Maisel drew between Nazi concentration camps and American mental hospitals was echoed by others. In an article entitled "An American Death Camp," Harold Orlansky, anthropologist and author, asserted that the "American asylum manifests, in embryo, some of the same social mechanisms which in Germany matured into death camps."[26] Other accounts reinforced this bleak picture even if they did not resort to the Holocaust analogy. These included *Out of Sight, Out of Mind*, a book by Frank Leon Wright that drew on over 2,000 firsthand reports, as well as the popular novel *The Snake Pit*, by Mary Jane Ward, which was made into a major motion picture.[27]

In 1948, journalist Albert Deutsch published *The Shame of the States*, perhaps the most scathing rebuke of institutionalized psychiatry. Deutsch was an established authority on psychiatry, having written a history of the profession in 1937. In the 1940s, he turned his investigative eye toward mental hospitals. Observing that no mental hospital met the APA's own standards, he hoped that publicizing the conditions of mental hospitals would spur reform, an "all-out effort to cure every curable patient and to bring all the others up to their maximum point of improvement."[28] Deutsch visited mental hospitals throughout the country, and in each he discovered overcrowding, the cruel use of restraints, aloof and inaccessible doctors, and a climate of suspicion and brutality. While noting the presence of violence and physical brutality, Deutsch focused on the subtler indignities visited upon patients. "One of the most poignant scenes in a mental hospital—one witnessed on every visit—is that of patients timidly pulling at a doctor's arm or coat as he rushes through the wards on rounds," he recounted.[29] Some of the hospitals spent less than $0.65 a day per patient, all but prohibiting treatment and leading to what Deutsch deemed "euthanasia through neglect."[30]

The outcry caused by these exposés stimulated social scientific investigations into mental hospitals. Among the numerous academic studies, none is more famous and enduring than Erving Goffman's *Asylums*.[31] Goffman worked as an assistant athletic director at the National Institute of Mental Health in Bethesda, Maryland, and culled his observations from this experience.[32] He conceptualized the mental hospital as a type of "total institution," a place of residence and work where a large number of like-situated individuals were cut off from the wider society and led enclosed, formally administered lives.[33] Goffman focused on the constant pressures the mental hospital applied to the patient personality. Commitment to an institution, he argued, results from contingency and personal betrayal. Once committed, a patient's behavior is filtered through the lens of mental illness and interpreted as indicative of his or her insanity. Over time, a patient's former identity diminishes as he or she is socialized into the institution. Eventually each patient is transformed into someone docile and dull, whose every act, and indeed manner of being, serves to confirm his or her status as mentally ill. The resulting behaviors reflect not the symptoms of a pathology, but "deliberate self-defensive moves used by victims of an all-engulfing total institution."[34] In short, Goffman argued that rather than treating mental illness, mental hospitals produced it through the degrading process of institutionalization. The mental hospital was not a treatment center, but a "hopeless storage dump trimmed in psychiatric paper."[35] Written in sharp, clear prose, Asylums offered a damning critique of mental hospitals that would be incorporated into the antipsychiatry movement and criticisms of psychiatric labeling and social control.

While the deterioration of mental hospitals and the harsh conditions therein had multiple causes, psychiatrists were held primarily responsible. "The story of this unconscionable isolation forms a sorry chapter in the history of American medicine," wrote mental health activist Mike Gorman, "and I, for one, am not possessed of enough blessed charity to exculpate the many practitioners of the medical arts who knew better but turned their backs on their sick brethren."[36] Targeted, many psychiatrists tried to deflect responsibility. Some of the "blame-it-on-the-war school," as Deutsch referred to them,[37] pointed to the effects of wartime rationing and inadequate government support. Others deflected critiques by pointing to the complicated nature of mental illness.

For many institutional psychiatrists, however, the exposés underscored the difficulties of their trade and highlighted the need for reforms for which they had long been clamoring. While unhappy about the unwanted attention and concerned about fallout, they shared many of the same concerns regarding what mental hospitals had become. In 1946, the APA broke with tradition and urged psychiatrists to speak out about the problems of the mental hospital.[38] And by 1960, Matthew Ross, medical director of the APA, spoke to the growing resignation many psychiatrists felt toward mental hospitals: "To be sure we are still fighting the battle of the mental hospitals . . . Now, however, we are no longer so sanguine about the potential of the large public hospital as a treatment center. We are arming ourselves with a new set of slogans, virtually all of which focus on alternatives to the large mental hospital or modifications thereof and virtually all of which entail a dispersion of psychiatry into the community."[39] Fatigued by degraded mental hospitals, reformers turned a wistful eye to the community.

Into the Community

Psychiatric reformers had been trying to escape the mental hospital since the end of the nineteenth century; in the 1960s, they finally did. In 1963, President John F. Kennedy signed the Community Mental Health Act, which provided federal funding for the creation of community mental health centers (CMHCs) throughout the United States. Many psychiatrists supported deinstitutionalization, a label affixed to projects oriented around two broad goals: to decrease the institutional mental health population, on the one hand, and to develop alternative community-based services for the mentally ill, on the other. During the psychoanalytic period, the profession's energy and aspirations had shifted toward private practice. As the APA leadership began to acknowledge the failures of mental hospitals, community reform efforts gained steam in the 1950s and 1960s, when a group of psychiatric reformers articulated a new vision for the treatment of chronic mental illness. The mental hospital had become an embarrassing albatross, and many psychiatrists were quick to embrace the promises of community mental health. As the embodiment of this vision, the Community Mental Health Act dealt the final blow to the public mental hospital system, in effect completing the long process of deinstitutionalization, which had begun in the 1950s.[40]

The inspiration for community psychiatry had deep roots in psychiatry, dating back to its origins. During the asylum period, superintendents emphasized the environmental causes of mental distress and adopted a version of what would later be called "milieu therapy," the manipulation of the asylum environment to effect a cure. Because its environment was *the* treatment, superintendent exerted tremendous energy on designing the asylum milieu. When asylums began to buckle under the weight of overcrowding, some superintendents endorsed an alternate model, one that continued to stress the importance of the environment but sought to transform the asylum from a centralized institution into a decentralized system of detached housing or cottages. These efforts drew inspiration from a small town in Belgium, Geel (or "Gheel," as most Americans called it), which has been a symbol of a decentralized community care for the mentally ill for centuries.[41] According to legend, Geel's patron saint, Saint Dymphna, preached tolerance and charity toward those with mental illness. Her local gravesite became associated with miraculous cures of mental illness, and Geel became a pilgrimage destination for the mentally ill. From the thirteenth century on, residents of Geel embraced their role of providing support for these mentally ill pilgrims, establishing a long tradition of foster care that afforded patients freedom of movement. Geel's more dispersed community-based care captured the imagination of early American psychiatrists,[42] especially those who supported a cottage system. A few institutions, like Eastern State Hospital in Virginia, even adopted this decentralized model.[43] While community psychiatrists in the 1960s rarely appealed directly to Geel, they shared many of its tenets.[44]

Advocates of community psychiatry, however, did draw direct links to the early mental hygiene movement. Formally institutionalized in 1909 with the founding of the National Committee for Mental Hygiene, the NCMH was hampered by squabbling between psychiatrists and lay leaders over who would command its efforts (see chapter 2). Nevertheless, the mental hygiene movement introduced a public health emphasis into psychiatry. It drew attention to "broad social factors which psychiatry takes into account in its study of mental processes—processes influenced by the circumstances of family life, municipal conditions, environmental influences, not to speak of the acquired habits and tendencies represented in the constitutional reaction of the individual patient."[45] Although never amounting to a coherent program, the mental hygiene movement created space within psychiatry for the consideration of preventive efforts. Later community psychiatry reformers mined this for inspiration.

The momentum behind community approaches to mental health care grew after World War II. During the war, the "battalions of Psychiatry" not only helped defeat the Axis powers, but also learned critical lessons that would inspire community psychiatry.[46] In the opinions of the psychiatrists involved, the war demonstrated the efficacy of treating patients in non-institutional settings. Treating soldiers closer to the front in temporary settings seemed to facilitate a more rapid return to the front.[47] Extraction and removal of the mentally ill from their situations—the foundation of institutional care—was, by contrast, counterproductive. Soldiers improved quicker if they received short-term, *in situ* care. In addition, World War II seemed to validate the efficacy of therapeutic communities, or team-based approaches to mental health care that humanized care by limiting confinement and encouraging communal interaction.[48] According to William Menninger, this lesson presented psychiatrists with a stark choice in the postwar period:

> One road leads to a continuation of its preoccupation with the end results of mental disease, i.e. concern about patients committed to state hospitals. The other road, however, invites psychiatry to discover how it can contribute to the problems of the average man and to the large issues in which he is involved. Which road will psychiatry follow?[49]

In the decades after the war, many psychiatrists would pursue the community road less traveled.

The war also gave birth to a more activist, political wing of psychiatry. Frustrated by constraints on psychiatric practice during the war and what they perceived to be the APA's weak response to their complaints, a group of fifteen "Young Turks," led by William and Karl Menninger, formed the Group for the Advancement of Psychiatry (GAP) in 1946.[50] Committed to social activism and attuned to the environmental causes of mental distress, GAP sought to push psychiatry, and the APA specifically, into a more active engagement with political and social issues.[51] GAP activists expanded psychodynamic ideas regarding the significance of interpersonal relations outward to the furthest reaches of the social and political sphere.

Although small in number—at its height it had approximately 150 members—GAP became an influential force within the APA during the 1950s, as its members captured a disproportionate share of the APA leadership positions. GAP organized committees to study a wide swath of issues that included Cooperation with Governmental (Federal) Agencies, Cooperation with Lay Groups, Public Education, Racial and Economic Problems (later changed to Social Issues), and Preventive Psychiatry. The committees produced three to four reports a year, on everything from traditional psychiatric topics like lobotomy and mental hospitals, to less conventional ones like racial desegregation, foreign diplomacy, and nuclear energy. The reports reflected a willingness to look beyond the traditional confines of psychiatry. And while their recommendations carried no formal authority, they circulated widely and possessed significant weight among many psychiatrists.

In their reports, GAP members laid out a new vision for psychiatry. They admonished the "Old Guard" institutional psychiatrists as reactionary conservatives, preoccupied with harmful somatic treatments. Instead of a profession fettered to an institution, they favored a dramatic increase in the scope of psychiatric concerns, promoting "the application of psychiatric principles to all those problems which have to do with family, welfare, child rearing, child and adult education, social and economic factors which influence the community status of individuals and families, inter-group tensions, civil rights and personal liberty."[52] In 1950, the GAP Committee on Social Issues published a report, entitled "The Social Responsibility of Psychiatry, A Statement of Orientation," which offered a "set of tentative principles" for a more politically engaged psychiatry.[53] The report endorsed a broad understanding of mental distress, "a more elastic view of illness as a qualitative and quantitative deviation from a hypothetical norm of bio-social adaptation."[54] It made six recommendations. Psychiatrists should redefine the concept of mental illness to emphasize "the dynamic principles which pertain to the person's interaction with society"; examine "the social factors which contribute to the causation of mental illness"; consider more fully "the dynamic process of intra- and intergroup relations"; attend to specific "group psychological phenomena" related to community mental health; identify criteria for healthy social organization; and develop "criteria for social action, relevant to the promotion of individual and communal mental health."[55] Thus, in addition to psychiatrists' traditional role of treating mentally illness, GAP would have them become consultants par excellence, advising leaders and policymakers on a host of society's ills. Anything less than full engagement, and psychiatrists "would surely be guilty of dereliction of duty did we not make a conscientious effort to apply whatever partial knowledge we now possess in the interests of counteracting social danger and promoting healthier being, both for individuals and groups."[56] While GAP never achieved the expansive vision it laid out, it pushed psychiatry further away from institutional care by drawing attention to social issues.

Finally, community psychiatry was encouraged by the increased involvement of the federal government in mental health care. The Mental Health Act of 1946 established the NIMH and granted the institute a wide mandate to fund research and training programs in mental health broadly construed (see chapter 3). Under the directorship of Robert Felix, the NIMH emphasized community-based endeavors. A founding member of GAP, Felix became the first NIMH director in 1949 and held the position for fifteen years. During his tenure, he stamped the institute with his public health approach to mental illness.[57] Felix framed the history of psychiatry as part of "man's growing awareness of his environment and of his responsibilities as a social animal."[58] In order to understand the fundamentally social character of man's problems, psychiatry needed to comprehend how the social environment contributed to mental distress, how "the community can be nurturing and helpful or it can be toxic and hostile."[59] While the other national institutes of health were preoccupied with basic biomedical research, the NIMH's funding portfolio under Felix reflected the public health background of its leadership as well as an aversion to traditional hospital care. It supported epidemiological research in order to gauge the prevalence of mental illness in the community and funded research, not just in medicine, but also in the social and behavioral sciences. As the NIMH came to dominate mental health research—its budget skyrocketed from $8.7 million in 1950 to over $100 million in 1960[60]—the most innovative research it funded was focused on issues outside the public mental hospitals. Insofar as the federal government received its cues and guidance from the NIMH, its agenda would come to inform federal mental health policy. The promise underwriting this policy was that community-based approaches "can lighten immeasurably, and for all time, the great burden the mental illnesses have in the past placed upon mankind."[61]

The Great Escape

As inheritors of these traditions, community psychiatry reformers wanted to "go and fight mental illness on the highways and byways."[62] Committed to values of personal freedom and communal responsibility, they called for a "community revolution."[63] In doing so, they stretched the concept of mental distress and, in turn, psychiatrists' scope of potential influence. This "more elastic view" of mental illness drew on ideas already floating in the psychiatric ether.[64] It carried echoes of psychobiology, which rejected the false dichotomy between the biological and social, as well as the psychoanalytic/psychodynamic ideas regarding the fluid boundary between sanity and insanity, common misery and neurotic suffering.[65] By blurring the distinction between mental health and illness, community reformers captured a greater number of problems under psychiatry's purview. They also appreciated a larger universe of potentially relevant causes for mental distress. Taking ego psychology's focus on interpersonal relationships, they expanded it from a focus on the family to incorporate larger historical, social, and political forces into their concerns.[66] The end result was a view of mental illness more capacious than even that of psychobiology, one that demanded a psychiatry with interests far beyond mental hospitals and individual psychotherapy. A 1973 APA position paper summarized this shift in emphasis: "The concept of mental illness has been broadened from one in which psychiatry was concerned almost exclusively with psychotic patients (who represented a small percent of the population) to one in which the emphasis has become the commitment of the community's total mental health resources to serving and maintaining the mental health needs of the entire population."[67]

How exactly psychiatrists were to serve the "mental health needs of the entire population" remained vague. Community psychiatry offered more of an orienting framework than a concrete program of reforms. Portia Bell Hume, a pioneer in mental health, defined community psychiatry "as the embodiment of principles and practices derived from clinical psychiatry (psychobiology), public health, social welfare practice, and from scientific research. Its methods and techniques are drawn from the evaluation, treatment, and control of psychiatric disorders in a variety of public programs and administrative settings, as well as from the professional practice of the psychiatric and parapsychiatric professions."[68] Many community psychiatrists were content to leave it at that, to assert that it was psychiatry's responsibility to intervene broadly while providing few specific details as to how. Everyone could agree that social and environmental factors were crucial to the mental health equation, and that psychiatrists, as experts in mental illness, should play a role in addressing these factors. Beyond this, psychiatrists would just need the "courage to proceed with half-knowledge," as one psychiatric textbook put it.[69] Proceeding with "half-knowledge" meant that psychiatrists had to be willing to embrace a more activist mentality, a willingness to intervene in the prevailing social and political issues of the moment, even despite its knowledge gaps. A stated commitment "to situate the origins of mental illness in the interplay between the self and societal forces" led to repeated calls for wide-ranging interventions in psychiatric discourse throughout the 1960s and into the 1970s.[70] In turn, psychiatrists were drawn into controversies that dovetailed with antiwar, civil rights, feminist, and countercultural movements, and many were more than willing to take explicit positions on these topics.[71]

Psychiatric reformers, however, faced challenges when trying to convince their colleagues to follow them into the community. To do so, they had to encourage their more skeptical peers to reconfigure their professional identities, either as institutional psychiatrists or as psychoanalytic/psychodynamic talk therapists. To get psychiatrists outside the traditional places of work, either in mental hospitals or analyst offices, they needed to convince them that psychiatry thus reformed would encompass "a variety of roles, each with a multiplicity of functions, each employing a number of procedures and techniques."[72] Community psychiatry certainly had *a* place for the more traditional psychiatric roles, but these efforts were to be part of a broader social program. In essence, they needed to persuade the average American psychiatrist to "turn his [sic] eyes away from the individual patient toward the community."[73]

Many of their peers were not persuaded. Opponents to community psychiatry raised numerous objections. They worried that efforts "to expand and press into all cracks and crevices of man's dissatisfaction" would lead to a psychiatry that was "unhappily schizophrenic."[74] Of utmost concern was psychiatrists' status as physicians. Every insistence that psychiatry was not just a branch of medicine but also "a branch or application of psychology, sociology, of ethnology, of philosophy," was met by retorts that psychiatrists had to "first be good physicians."[75] "I am concerned about maintaining our integrity as physicians," expressed Matthew Ross, psychiatrist and former medical director of the APA. "I am concerned with the clarity of our image of ourselves as physicians."[76] In raising these concerns, critics anticipated a professional risk. The further psychiatry moved away from medicine, the more it left itself vulnerable to competition from nonmedical mental health workers. Psychiatry's medical bona fides had long distinguished them from these competitors, and to risk compromising it was professionally foolish.

Additionally, critics of the reforms argued that community psychiatry was built more on slogans than rigorous research. Once again, Ross quipped, "If a historian a hundred years from now had no source materials to work with other than slogans, I suspect he could reconstruct a fairly accurate intellectual history in the period 1948–1960."[77] Henry Warren Dunham, a sociologist known for his epidemiological research, dismissed community psychiatry as the latest "therapeutic bandwagon," a fad that elided the problems in psychiatry's knowledge base.[78] "Why do psychiatrists think that it is possible to treat the 'collectivity' when there still exists a marked uncertainty with respect to the treatment and cure of the individual case?" he asked. "How are we going to take the first preventive actions if we are still uncertain about the causes of mental disorders?"[79] It was one thing to proclaim that social and environmental factors mattered; it was quite another to figure out how to stem their effects with tangible policies.

Finally, opponents cautioned that an explicit political turn was dangerous to the profession's cohesion and might undermine its ethical norms. An issue that first arose with GAP, critics of community psychiatry worried that psychiatrists in positions of authority would impose their political views on others. This was anathema to science. After all, the common denominator for APA membership was "not one of political persuasion but of professional pursuit."[80] Psychiatry risked its neutral and objective authority as an observer of the human condition if it got too political.

Given this internal resistance, how did community psychiatry reformers achieve significant legislative and policy reforms? Much of the answer lay in the fact that critics also shared reformers' distress about the state of psychiatric mental hospitals. Not only had conditions in the hospital deteriorated; they had been exposed. With each new withering exposé, the profession's prestige took a hit. Pressure for reform mounted. Insofar as community psychiatry positioned itself as *the* alternative to mental hospitals, there was a professional logic to supporting some of its ambitions, if not embracing it as a wholesale reinvention. Nearly all psychiatrists recognized the professional disaster they were courting if psychiatry continued to be equated with institutional care in the public eye.

In CMHCs We Trust

In 1964, Roy Grinker Sr. expressed what many psychiatrists were feeling about their profession:

The professional view held by psychiatrists is today mixed and confused. Psychoanalysis, for which many have sacrificed so much, has not become the therapeutic answer; it seems to be mired in a theoretical rut vigilantly guarded by the orthodox and except for relatively few examples, prevented from comingling with science. The great breakthrough promised by the modern psychosomatic approach, with its concepts of specificity of psychological etiology of degenerative diseases, has succumbed to the hard facts of multiple causation and critical phases of development.[81]

For those dissatisfied with the elitist, individual-level focus of psychoanalysis and somatic treatments in state mental hospitals, an alternative emerged. Community mental health centers (CMHCs) promised an expanded role for psychiatry, a program of total treatment that penetrated all facets of society. Rather than congregating and segregating the chronically mentally ill or restricting therapeutic care to the cosmopolitan wealthy, CMHCs would achieve comprehensive care for all, no matter a patient's station or level of mental distress. Inpatient treatment would remain a last resort, but the locus of mental health treatment would be shifted to the community. Rather than remaining "isolated from the rest of the community," CMHCs would become the means by which psychiatry would be transformed.[82] Under the watchful guidance of psychiatrists, these "truly interdisciplinary collaborative" ventures would become the hubs for coordinating all facets of mental health care.[83] And as directors of CMHCs, psychiatrists would be in command.

Community reforms received an unlikely boost from institutional psychiatry itself. Prior to deinstitutiosnalization, a handful of institutional psychiatrists experimented with reorganizing their mental hospitals. These efforts focused on patient autonomy, freedom of movement, and greater opportunity for patient self-governance. They also began to favor team-based approaches to care, in which psychiatrists worked with other mental health professionals, medical professionals, and social scientists to develop comprehensive treatment programs. In the psychiatric vision of team care, psychiatrists were to maintain ultimate authority, but there was a growing consensus that treating the mentally ill was a collective endeavor that demanded multiple kinds of expertise. Most significantly, the new psychopharmaceutical treatments suggested that with proper management, many mental patients could live fuller lives outside institutions. In this regard, Thorazine helped reshape psychiatrists' calculus of what was possible for their patients.[84] The antipsychotic drug altered both the actual practice of treating serious mental illness—drug therapies supplanted psychosurgery—and the prognosis of patients with these conditions. For the first time, the efficacy of a treatment seemed to meet its hype; psychiatry appeared to have discovered the long-sought-after magic bullet.[85] The development of additional psychopharmaceutical treatments like lithium and imipramine was perceived as a signal of a new era in psychiatric treatment. Drugs went from being "adjunct" treatments to the means by which it would become "possible to care for more patients outside the hospital."[86] For this reason, President John F. Kennedy pointed to these developments as a justification for federal community-based programs in a message to Congress: "These breakthroughs have rendered obsolete the traditional methods of treatment which imposed upon the mentally ill a social quarantine, a prolonged or permanent confinement in huge, unhappy mental hospitals where they were out of sight and forgotten."[87]

The shift to community-based care, policy-wise, was driven by developments external to psychiatry as well. Community psychiatry resonated with a more general shift in welfare policy. During the Depression and the New Deal, and then later in Kennedy's New Frontier and Johnson's Great Society programs, American welfare policy had moved from an "indoor" institutional focus, mostly overseen by state legislatures, to "outdoor" non-institutional policies, like Medicare and Social Security insurance, that were federal grant-in-aid programs.[88] Second, the social sciences had been invigorated in the postwar period, facilitated by the GI Bill and new federal funding streams. Social scientists produced a slew of epidemiological research indicating the seemingly high prevalence of mental illness in the community.[89] Such research revealed an unmet demand for community-based services that could be developed and maintained via the funding apparatus of federal welfare programs.

Riding these developments both within and outside psychiatry, community-based reforms gained political momentum. In 1955, the APA Executive Committee and the AMA Council on Mental Health met to plan a comprehensive study on mental health treatment. That same year, Congress passed the Mental Health Study Act, which provided $1.25 million in funding for three years for the study. The Joint Commission on Mental Health and Illness was formed, and in 1961, it published its report. The report inventoried the difficulties facing psychiatry. According to it, the search for effective treatments of mental illness was undercut by two factors—"the absence of knowledge about specific causes and specific cures in the diagnosis and treatment of the psychoses" and the apathy of the public toward mental illness, which "tends to disturb and repel others rather than evoke their sympathy and desire to help."[90] Noting the limited effects that regular exposés and the public scandal had on reform, the Commission argued that more than moral indignation was needed to effect real change. While the Commission "did not presume to present wholly definitive conclusions or universally approved recommendations," it did express unqualified support for CMHCs and community-based initiatives.[91] Puzzled with "the continued existence of these 'hospitals' that seem to have no defenders, but endure despite all attacks," it called for the integration of mental hospitals with the surrounding communities and recommended that "a national mental health program should set as an objective one fully staffed, full-time mental health clinic available to each 50,000 of the population."[92] Immediately, the NIMH, still under Felix, released a position paper supporting the report and echoing the claim that CMHCs were the most appropriate means to tackle the problems identified in the report. Felix reasoned:

> General public acceptance of this philosophy—and it cannot come too soon for the good of the mentally ill—will be tantamount to a national decision to eliminate so far as we can the prolonged hospitalization and institutionalization of the mentally ill. Communities will do what they long since should have done, namely, provide the facilities and services that will forestall hospitalization whenever possible and give the convalescent mentally ill every chance to achieve maximum psychological and social recovery.[93]

The winds of federal mental health policy were blowing in the community's direction.

In October 1963, in a bold new approach to mental health treatment, Kennedy signed the Community Mental Health Act of 1963 into law. The act provided federal grants to states to create local mental health centers. While deinstitutionalization was already underway, the new law accelerated it by making community-based care a national priority. Felix, like many of his community psychiatry peers, was bullish: "I believe that the effect of the Centers Act will be revolutionary, for it will make it possible, as the years roll on, for hundreds of communities to develop true community mental health centers within which—or from which—a network·of services may develop."[94] Psychiatry, now oriented toward the community, would admit "no separation of prevention, treatment, and rehabilitation," but rather would work to create a network of interdependent services that would allow the mentally ill to receive the treatment they needed without having to be institutionalized.[95]

Promises Unfulfilled

The push for community psychiatry had taken on the character of a social reform movement. Driven by utopian impulses, psychiatrists spoke grandly of the reforms, exclaiming promises "of ending forever the neglect and isolation which has been the lot of the mentally ill, both in and out of hospitals, since the dawn of time."[96]

It was not to be. Within a decade, it was clear that community psychiatry was nowhere near accomplishing its ambitious promises. The swiftness of its collapse was remarkable, especially when compared to past psychiatric reform efforts.

By the mid-fifties, CMHCs had become yet another example of psychiatry's malfeasance. In 1974, a group associated with consumer advocate Ralph Nader published a report on them.[97] Their findings were damning. While "good intention" may have driven the establishment of CMHCs, the report observed that "their current disarray is painfully obvious."[98] Most centers failed to provide even a modicum of the diverse services they promised (i.e., diagnostic services, rehabilitative services, precare and aftercare services, training, research and evaluation, etc.). At best, "the centers represent a Band-Aid approach to a number of social sores that will continue to fester regardless of the amount of first aid"; at worst, they exacerbated inequality in care, systematically ignoring "the program's directives to serve the poor."[99] CMHCs lacked focus, having extended "the definition of mental illness to include a kaleidoscope of disorders from organic and functional psychoses to neurotic disorders, alcoholism, drug addiction, school learning difficulties, juvenile delinquency, employment and marital problems, and even political dissent."[100] Community psychiatrists had taken on so broad an agenda that it defied rational planning. Without proper federal oversight, a clear mandate, or adequate funding, CMHCs failed their constituents. By 1977, CMHCs served just two million people.[101] The admittedly problematic system of mental hospitals had been dismantled for a non-system. The chronically mentally ill were left to their own devices.[102]

The Nader report lay much of the blame at the feet of psychiatrists, who by insisting that mental health efforts be directed by medical professionals "brought to their newest realm their business acumen, upper-middle-class bias, and professional hubris to burden this massive federal subsidy."[103] Some psychiatrists treated the centers as personal fiefdoms and financial windfalls, abusing the public's trust. They became more focused on preserving their organizations' existence than providing care. With the situation out of hand, the report concluded that the best way to save the centers would be to remove them from psychiatric and medical control. Indeed, the CMHCs seemed to have fallen into "the familiar pattern of past mental health reforms that were initiated amid great moral fervor, raised false hopes of imminent solutions, and wound up only recapitulating the problems they were to solve."[104]

Deinstitutionalization had two interrelated goals—to decrease the inpatient psychiatric care and to relocate services to the community. These broad goals, however, never coalesced around a coherent program but rather unfolded in an expedient and disjointed way. Unfortunately, while reformers accomplished the first goal of deinstitutionalization, they failed to create an adequate replacement, much to the detriment of psychiatry and its most vulnerable patients. Reformers dismantled the mental hospital system. In 1955, the population of mental patients in state and county mental hospitals numbered 559,000. In 1970, this number had decreased to 338,000, and by 1988, it was down to a meager 107,000, an 80% decrease in thirty years.[105] California adopted the most aggressive approach, decreasing its institutionalized population from a peak of 37,490 in 1959 to 5,715 in 1977.[106] Such rapid and wholesale discharge was also encouraged by the availability of federal funds under Medicaid, Medicare, SSI, and SSDI.[107]

While reformers were successful in depopulating mental hospitals, they never completed the second task of replacing the state mental hospital system with a robust community-based one. State legislatures saw deinstitutionalization as a means to divest from mental health care and the burden of caring for the chronically mentally ill. And federal legislation never laid out a realistic plan of what to do with the newly discharged patients. Mental hospitals were shuttered without adequately thinking through, establishing, or funding viable alternatives. Less than half of the proposed CMHCs were built nationwide. Those that were established faced manifold problems. A 1977 Government Accounting Office report noted that among the sundry difficulties, the implementation of CMHCs suffered from poor leadership, failure to plan, lax administrative and monitoring procedures, and uncoordinated service-delivery operations.[108] They also faced constant funding shortages, as legislation repeatedly underestimated their costs. Federal funding slowed during the Nixon administration, but the death knell for many of the embattled CMHCs came with the election of Ronald Reagan, who abandoned funding for the programs almost altogether.[109] Aside from a handful of local success stories, the community psychiatry reforms were an unmitigated disaster, what historian Edward Shorter calls "one of the greatest social debacles of our time."[110]

This rapid failure stemmed from the ill-conceived manner in which the community-based reforms were pursued. In their haste to move on from the mental hospital, reformers accepted the purported benefits of community-based interventions at face value. Reformers wanted desperately to believe in the reforms. One striking feature of these efforts was the absence of empirical support or even calls for research into community-based measures.[111] Supporters took for granted that community care would be more effective. Repeating these claims in a mantra-like fashion gave them the veneer of truth, despite almost no empirical support. CMHC directors seemed allergic to research. Those who acknowledged the dearth of evidential support deflected concerns by arguing that eventually the centers themselves would provide it: "Unfortunately, at our present state of knowledge, primary prevention of mental illness or disorder is possible in only a few instances; but the centers will provide us with data for epidemiological studies which can lead to further development of preventive techniques."[112] But even then, directors avoided program evaluations, lest they cast negative light on their efforts. The lack of critical interrogation of community psychiatry's expectations stemmed, in part, from the abject deterioration of state mental hospitals and the public relations problems they presented. In comparison, *any* change seemed better. And because the influence of the social milieu in shaping mental health seemed so obvious, CMHCs fell prey to the all-too-common "arrogance of preventive medicine";[113] reformers remained utterly confident in their interventions despite the inherent challenges they presented.

The lack of a carefully conceived program and the expedient, uneven way in which it was implemented resulted in confusion. Basic questions went unanswered. What was "the community"? Should it be described "in geographical or functional terms"?[114] Did the delineated "catchment areas" that CMHCs were supposed to serve have a tangible existence? Or were they mere statistical artifacts created via policy prescriptions? Was the belief that an "open warmth of community concern" would lead community members to "do what they long since should have done" based on reality?[115] Or did it represent a misplaced faith in a mythical ideal of community? And who should CMHCs primarily serve? Was their main purpose to coordinate care for the chronically mentally ill so they could avoid institutionalization? Or was their mandate to promote mental health generally? In addition to these dangling questions, reformers subscribed to problematic assumptions that led their efforts astray. Community-based care assumed that patients had access to resources like housing and supportive networks, that they could obtain and hold jobs, that they could advocate for themselves, and that communities in fact wanted to help. In holding such assumptions, community psychiatrists were "sociologically naïve," according to anthropologist Sue Estroff.[116] By the time these assumptions were recognized as incorrect, it was too late to change course.

Community psychiatrists had fallen victim to their own hype. They accepted rose-colored slogans in place of a plan. But realities on the ground quickly disabused their romantic notions of community. Local politics, it turns out, could get quite messy. Psychiatrists found their efforts consumed in its "territorial disputes," as they were forced to negotiate "jurisdictional politics" and "vested interests."[117] Disillusioned, many psychiatrists concluded that the political engagement of community psychiatry was better in theory than in practice. As many psychiatric reformers before them, they dove headlong into a new reform in an effort to set the profession on a more enlightened course. And, like many of these predecessors, the initial expectations proved to be naïve and exaggerated.

Psychiatrists critical of community psychiatry were all too happy to point out how reformers had been seduced. From the start, they cautioned their peers that they were "arming ourselves with a new set of slogans," not a coherent plan.[118] The rapid failure and retreat from CMHCs confirmed their suspicions. Avrohm Jacobson, psychoanalyst and professor of psychiatry, insisted:

> We are too much taken with such appealing slogans as "treat the whole man," "treat the man in his setting," "conduct war upon mankind's ills." Individuals still need to be treated despite those who would stamp out disease with statistics, social action projects, and organized factories for research. When we are primarily concerned with the individual, we constructively serve the community. But if primarily we serve the community, we run the risk of assuming that all individuals can be treated without our knowing their history, birth, development, emotional responsiveness, attachments, areas of fear and of hope, and moments and ways of strength.[119]

For these critics, the community mental health movement "glorified the concept of community without adequately understanding it," and "in retrospect, its rhetoric is a considerable embarrassment."[120] Psychiatrists had succumbed to a "typical American attitude: 'Don't stand there mumbling; do something!'" wrote psychologist Norman W. Bell and psychiatrist John P. Spiegel. "Even if we don't know what to do, there is the national assumption that some action is better than none at all."[121] Community psychiatry came to represent all that was wrong with psychiatric reforms—the embrace of style over substance, the reckless rush to adopt the newest thing, and the inevitable disappointment when none of the rosy projections came to fruition.

Within a decade of their establishment, psychiatrists withdrew from CMHCs. But they could not avoid the professional fallout of their failures.

CMHCs were conceived as collaborative interdisciplinary endeavors that emphasized a team-based approach to care. In supporting them, psychiatrists created opportunities for their professional competitors.[122] Because psychiatrists could not handle the labor demands of its ambitious program themselves, they had to lean on other mental health professionals. This gave psychiatrists' competitors a platform to promote their own professional agendas. As a result, psychiatrists found themselves "under heavy assault from clinical psychologists, psychiatric nurses, social workers, and psychiatric technicians, who are clamoring for equal authority, equal status, and equal recompense."[123] They tried to reassert their authority by appealing to their medical expertise, but the very logic of community psychiatry undermined the power of such claims. In the daily activities of the CMHCs, medicine proper was but a small portion of the actual work. "Severely questioned by his [sic] fellow workers," it was becoming less evident what the community psychiatrist brought to the table, aside from medication management.[124] And why did the right to prescribe justify control over community care and its broadened notion of mental health? Community psychiatry, which began as a way to increase the professional authority of psychiatry, became a liability. "Mental health is in the saddle and riding psychiatry," warned Ross;[125] by 1970, most psychiatrists agreed with this diagnosis and jumped off the bandwagon.

Of particular concern was the rise of clinical psychology. For most of its history, psychology had been an academic discipline more attuned to laboratory research than treating patients.[126] Insofar as they intervened clinically, their role was circumscribed to the administration of psychometric instruments. In 1940, there were essentially no clinical psychologists. But, like psychiatry, psychology received a boost from World War II.[127] Gaining treatment experience during the war, psychologists began to make incursions into clinical practice. They too benefited from increased federal funding, increased demand for mental health services, and increased institutional ties to schools, the military, the court system, and the VA.[128] In 1949, at a meeting in Boulder, Colorado, psychologists established standards for clinical training, thus formalizing an applied wing to complement their research wing. Between 1949 and 1959, the percentage of members in the American Psychological Association who had a private therapeutic practice grew from 2.3% to 17%.[129] Competing with psychoanalysts, clinical psychologists developed therapeutic techniques, like cognitive behavioral therapy (CBT), that were less time intensive, more cost effective, and more amenable to randomized controlled trials. And, despite continued efforts on the part of the APA, AMA, and APsaA to form a united front and declare psychotherapy a medical treatment, clinical psychology continued to grow unchecked. Psychiatrists' dominance over psychotherapy was already weakening in the late 1950s and early 1960s. The shift toward the community exacerbated this trend. Psychiatrists had moved into a terrain that, in many ways, was more favorable to psychology given psychologists' long-standing ties to community institutions (e.g., schools).

While the community reforms fomented professional competition, their more lasting professional legacy was the dismantling of psychiatry's traditional institutional base. Psychiatric authority had long been justified by its control over mental hospitals and, in turn, the jurisdiction over patients with serious mental illness. It was from this foundation that psychiatrists launched their incursions into private practice and less serious forms of mental distress. By supporting deinstitutionalization, psychiatrists broke up the very system upon which its existence had long depended. In the process, they abandoned the chronically and severely mentally ill, who now fell through the newly created chasms in the mental health system. Thus, at the very moment that professional competition was intensifying, psychiatric reformers had destroyed much of what made them distinct from other mental health professionals as well as the very institutions to which they had always retreated in times of crisis.

Conclusion

By the 1970s, both community psychiatry and psychoanalysis were in disarray. Around the same time, a global antipsychiatry movement burst onto the scene to mount an existential challenge to psychiatry. Rather than a cohesive entity, the antipsychiatry movement was a rather elastic and amorphous conglomeration of interests, encompassing an array of agendas that fed off each other. Some critics were legatees of the tradition of mental hospital exposés; others were civil rights advocates who challenged the commitment laws. Some directed their ire at psychoanalysis, others toward new drug treatments. Some focused on the most overt examples of psychiatric abuse, others on the subtler processes of stigma and labeling.[130] Some trafficked in academic circles; others reached wide audiences (most famously Ken Kesey's 1962 novel, later made into an Oscar-winning movie, *One Flew over the Cuckoo's Nest*). Yet, while the criticisms were diverse, they merged into a damning critique of psychiatry, one rooted in the idea that psychiatrists were agents of social control.[131] To antipsychiatry activists, the horrors of psychiatric treatment and the profession's failed incursions into everyday life reflected an arrogant overreach and callous meanness. Moreover, underlying this overreach was a profound ignorance that antipsychiatry activists were all too happy to point out.

No one played the role of irritant better than Thomas Szasz, the "enfant terrible" or "bête noire" of psychiatry.[132] A psychiatrist himself, Szasz spent the majority of his career at the State University of New York. A committed libertarian, Szasz penned scathing critiques of his peers, unfurling vicious attacks on their pretensions to medicine. "Psychiatry is conventionally defined as a medical specialty concerned with the diagnosis and treatment of mental diseases," states Szasz. "I submit that this definition, which is still widely accepted, places psychiatry in the company of alchemy and astrology and commits it to the category of pseudoscience. The reason for this is that there is no such thing as 'mental illness.'"[133] To Szasz, psychiatrists abused the medical metaphor in order to transform "problems of living" into seeming pathological diseases.[134] Unlike medicine, however, these "counterfeit" mental "diseases" lacked a physical or biological basis.[135] They were not discovered or proved, but invented and proclaimed. All this "fakery and pretense" allowed psychiatrists to "share in the prestige and power of the physician" and, in turn, cloak their oppressive practices in the guise of medical science.[136] With its false diseases and bad faith analogies, psychiatry, to Szasz, was engaged in a modern form of witch hunt.[137]

Szasz took an inflexible stance on the profession's ignorance. It was not temporary, nor resolvable. Instead, mental illness was unknown, because as a myth, it did not exist. Its biological cause would never be discovered because it had no biological nature; it was just a vacuous metaphor put in the service of legitimizing a profession whose true task was social control.[138] Even so, Szasz was not willing to give up on psychiatry altogether. He proposed a psychiatry of ethics based on a theory of personal conduct, one that focused on helping patients deal with their problems of living. In this, he hoped to "effect a much-needed and long-overdue rapprochement between psychiatry on the one hand, and ethics and philosophy on the other."[139] At a time when the prestige of psychoanalysis was waning, Szasz's vision offered little appeal to psychiatrists concerned about their professional standing. Without staking a claim to medicine, how would psychiatrists distinguish themselves from other mental health professionals?

Aghast, most psychiatrists responded Szasz with vehement objections. Wounded that one of their own would make such "exaggerated, biased, alarmist, impractical, and even erroneous" claims—"the kind of harangue which would be expected from a demagogue rather than a responsible scientist"[140]—psychiatrists roundly denounced him. In a talk entitled "The New War on Psychiatry," Henry Davidson took Szasz to task for his irresponsible comments, especially his "most spectacular impeachment," the "comparison of psychiatric examinations with witch hunting."[141] By misleading "the less sophisticated elements of the public," primed by decades of bad press, Szasz was encouraging the perception that psychiatrists "are a menace to our patients."[142]

However, an undercurrent of anxiety and insecurity colored psychiatrists' retorts to the antipsychiatry movement. Psychiatrists could swat away the more exaggerated and hyperbolic criticisms, but their core concerns could not be as easily dismissed. Indeed, many psychiatrists were beginning to hold similar concerns themselves.

Psychiatry's embrace of community psychiatry unwittingly provided fuel for their opponents. And the failure of this reform left their professional status seriously compromised. In 1967, APA president Harvey Tompkins asked his peers, "How can we deny that there is rampant in our society an element of distrust of our intentions and practices as physicians, reflective of many images that must discomfit us if for no other reason than that they are so widespread?"[143] Eight years later, then APA president John P. Spiegel chronicled the uncertainty plaguing all branches of psychiatry:

> Is "action for mental health" anything but a slogan? Is community mental health based on solid empirical evidence of its efficacy? Can psychoanalysis and other long-term psychotherapies be justified on the basis of either credible theory or tested results? Are the psychotropic drugs curing patients or merely watering down their symptoms? Is not the whole enterprise more of an illusion—a successful public relations effort, perhaps, but certainly not the practical and effective application of a body of scientifically certifiable findings or theories?[144]

Paranoia and gloom pervaded psychiatry. In his presidential address before the APA, Perry C. Talkington declared the beleaguered profession to be "under attack, both internally and externally."[145] Talkington went on to chronicle the many forces impinging on psychiatric authority—lawyers challenging commitment laws, the FDA demanding proof of efficacy, insurance companies usurping the control over treatment, mental health competitors encroaching on their jurisdiction, and antipsychiatry activists maligning their hard work. Psychiatrists sounded stern warnings that the profession had to grapple with "a sense of contempt toward the mental health enterprise, radiating vaguely from a variety of quarters."[146] Absent a forceful response, psychiatry risked death by a million cuts.

With psychiatry's ignorance as exposed as ever, calls for patience to uphold the status quo were not only naïve; they were dangerous. Psychiatrist E. Fuller Torrey, who himself would come to assume the role of psychiatric gadfly later in his career, assessed the situation in stark terms. Despite treating more patients than ever, "psychiatry is dying," and, likening it to a platypus, he asserted that the profession was "an evolutionary dead end, unable to defend itself and headed toward extinction."[147] Would it survive?

As a failed reform effort, community psychiatry unfolded according to psychiatry's familiar script. Hype for community psychiatry begat unreal expectations. Yet, hype gave way to disappointment, as the professional benefits accrued from the move to the community were outweighed by the problems it created. With psychiatric ignorance persistent, the reinvention was abandoned. But despite the similar script, the underlying logic driving community psychiatry differed from previous reinventions in important ways. The previous generation of psychoanalytic reformers had turned inward, narrowing psychiatric expertise until it could be captured, veiled, and mystified in the psychoanalytic encounter. Community psychiatry reformers, on the other hand, expanded psychiatry outward, increasing its purview and broadening what fell under its jurisdiction. They tried to insert psychiatry into all facets of social life. In doing so, they sought to alter the focus of psychiatric concern, to reorient the profession away from the individual to the community. The broadening gesture of the community psychiatry reinvention also departed from that of psychobiology. Psychobiological reformers had proposed a diffuse, widespread program so as to avoid premature closure of potentially fruitful venues for research. It dispersed in multiple directions to pursue insights wherever they might be. But psychobiological reformers maintained their focus on the individual patient. Community psychiatrists' shift in object and change in scale was driven less by a research agenda—witness their uncritical sloganeering—and more by a desire to alter the institutional base of the profession. In turn, community psychiatry as a reform acted on ignorance differently. Changing the scale of psychiatric concern, it tried to mitigate psychiatric ignorance by diluting it. Rather than beginning with an appreciation of psychiatric ignorance, community psychiatrists assumed they already possessed the relevant expertise to speak on community problems. In claiming that psychiatry had something to say about everything, perhaps few would notice it had little to say about anything.

Community psychiatry also differed from previous reinventions in the speed with which it unfolded. The hype/disappointment dynamics were compressed, unfolding over a single decade rather than multiple ones. Community psychiatry failed quicker. In its quick failure, however, the ephemeral community psychiatry reinvention left two significant legacies that shaped the politics of ignorance going forward. It was an impactful reinvention, despite never really getting off the ground. Deinstitutionalization, undertaken with the support of many psychiatrists, dismantled the mental hospital system for all intents and purposes. In 1955, there were 340 beds in psychiatric hospitals for every 100,000 Americans; by 2010, that number would drop to fourteen beds per 100,000.[148] Psychiatrists sacrificed a broken hospital system for what was a non-system. This had serious consequences for their professional authority. Previously, psychiatrists would have fallen back on the mental hospital when faced with professional crisis or intensifying competition. In the state mental hospital system, their authority went unchallenged. It was theirs alone. They had created it, and they controlled it. Psychiatry's existence was secure as long as they could claim jurisdiction over the population of the chronically mentally ill. With deinstitutionalization and without a robust institutional replacement, however, psychiatry was left more vulnerable. It was bereft of an institutional base or an undisputed claim to any one patient population. When psychiatrists abandoned the hospitals, they abandoned their sickest patients in what activist Peter Sedgwick called an "almost unanimous abdication from the task of proposing and securing any provision for a humane and continuous form of care for those mental patients who need something rather more than short-term therapy for an acute phase of their illness."[149] In "the quixotic pursuit of ever more esoteric treatments and potential cures," psychiatrists had chosen to desert the very patients that justified their profession.[150] Going forward, future generations of psychiatrists would lack the professional security that the mental hospital had long afforded.

Community psychiatry had a second, less obvious, effect on the politics of ignorance. With its failure, psychiatrists had amassed a record of failed reforms that could not easily be ignored, nor swept under the rug. Failures were accumulating, suggesting a disturbing pattern if not handled well. As a result, by the 1970s, psychiatrists began to demonstrate a growing historical consciousness regarding the cyclical nature of the field's trajectory.[151] Collectively, they started to interrogate psychiatry's past. This is not to suggest that psychiatry lacked any sort of historical reflection prior to this time.[152] To the contrary, presidential addresses and periodic articles often commented on the profession's history. But this discussion was confined to occasional asides, observations of past curiosities, and moments of commemoration. Discussions of reforms rarely included historical analyses, aside from othering the past as a repository of error. Indeed, as late as 1959, many reformers were still claiming that psychiatry was "young,"[153] a claim that stretched credulity, given that American psychiatry was over a century old. Still, rhetorically it shielded psychiatrists from some of the responsibility for their ignorance. However, by the 1960s, these claims to youthfulness had dropped out of psychiatric discourse altogether. Encountering antipsychiatry criticisms, many of which were grounded in historical interpretations (e.g., Foucault), and mental hospitals, whose physical decay embodied the field's age, psychiatrists could no longer ignore its difficult history. New reformers called for the inclusion of history in the psychiatric curriculum, and a 1962 survey indicated broad support for such inclusion.[154] In 1978, psychiatrist David F. Musto asserted that historical consciousness "was a valuable tool in psychiatry," one that could reveal past errors, be mined for insight, insulate psychiatrists from "dogmatic certainty," and offer a guide to the future.[155] Subsequent reformers would heed this call, and a profession-wide interest in history would come to distinguish psychiatry from its medical peers.[156]

As this historical consciousness developed, the continuous cycles of reinvention were not lost on psychiatrists. A 1966 textbook identified this history as one "checkered with reforms and separated by periods of recession."[157] In 1967, psychiatrist Darold Treffert described this cyclical history: "What to one generation is a bandwagon, is to the next a scapegoat; only to be revived by still another generation as a new, revolutionary bandwagon."[158] Along this vein, Ames Fischer and Morton R. Weinstein declared that psychiatry has had "no rival among medical specialties in its susceptibility to fads and its readiness to board the newest bandwagon."[159] From the asylum to psychobiology to psychoanalysis to community psychiatry, psychiatry had invented and reinvented itself in an attempt to finally secure the knowledge of its object. But in this "cyclical process of death and rebirth, few changes have taken place,"[160] and few answers had been secured. Later this consciousness would be filtered through the rhetoric of "paradigm shift," and harnessed to justify yet another transformation (see chapter 5). For now, the emergence of this historical sensibility meant that, going forward, subsequent reformers would have to grapple with psychiatry's problematic history when articulating their future vision. To convince both their peers and the public that their program was not just another fad in a long history of fads, they would have to answer a new, vital question: Why should things be different this time around?

FIVE

Profession of the Book.

In 1970, protestors swarmed the typically staid annual meeting of the American Psychiatric Association. Energized by the Stonewall Riots the year before, gay rights activists descended upon the conference. There they deployed an array of guerilla theater tactics to make a single demand of psychiatrists—remove homosexuality from the *Diagnostic and Statistical Manual of Mental Disorders* (DSM).[1] Carrying placards declaring that "Psychiatry Kills," they condemned psychiatric "treatments" for homosexuality, such as electric shock aversion therapy—as barbaric. Activists did not want to be "cured." They railed against the "sickness theory" of homosexuality, arguing that it gave scientific cover for abusive treatments and discriminatory laws. Insisting their voices be heard, their message was firm: "Stop talking *about* us and start talking *with* us."[2]

The protests bewildered psychiatrists. That homosexuality was a mental disorder was psychiatric common sense at the time. Drawing on psychodynamic theories, psychiatrists argued that it arose from "stunted development caused by a faulty family constellation," and caused significant mental distress.[3] In their minds, this understanding of homosexuality as a mental disorder legitimized treatment; it was "an enlightened view in a society that regarded homosexuals as criminals to be punished for acting on their sexual inclinations."[4] Indeed, psychiatrists saw themselves as allies to their homosexual patients.[5] Rather than "sinners" to be condemned, they treated homosexuals as "patients" that could be helped, that could lead healthy, productive lives despite their deviations. For these reasons, psychiatrists were shocked by the protests. Confused as to why they had become targets, they mustered the meekest of responses: many insisted that the APA reimburse them for their conference expenses.

Over the next three years, activists dialed up the pressure. "We're rejecting you all as our owners," declared Franklin Kameny, who, along with Barbara

Gittings, coordinated the protests. "We possess ourselves and we speak for ourselves and we will take care of our own destinies."[6] The protests reached a dramatic climax during the 1972 meeting in Dallas. Responding to pressure, the APA granted activists a panel on the conference program. When the audience arrived for the panel, they discovered a masked man sitting at the dais. Referred to only as "Dr. H. Anonymous," the man was John Fryer, a gay psychiatrist from Philadelphia. Fearing professional ruin, Fryer agreed to participate under the condition of complete anonymity. Disguised in a wig and rubber mask and using a voice-distorting microphone, he recounted the discrimination he had endured as a homosexual psychiatrist. Once, when being fired after his sexual orientation had come to light, he was told by his supervisor, "If you were gay and not flamboyant, we would keep you. If you were flamboyant and not gay, we would keep you. But since you are both gay and flamboyant, we cannot keep you."[7] Fryer spoke to the double bind facing gay psychiatrists. "As psychiatrists who are homosexual," he stated,

> we must know our place and what we must do to be successful. If our goal is academic appointment, a level of earning capacity equal to our fellows, or admission to a psychoanalytic institute, we must make certain that no one in a position of power is aware of our sexual orientation or gender identity. Much like the black man with the light skin who chooses to live as a white man, we cannot be seen with our real friends—our real homosexual family—lest our secret be known and our dooms sealed.[8]

Not only did gay psychiatrists have to remain closeted at work, they often had to hide their professional identity in gay settings, lest they risk ostracism and opprobrium. They were pariahs in both psychiatric and homosexual circles.

While Fryer was giving his powerful testimonial, activists met behind the scenes with APA representatives. The threat that the disruptions would continue goaded the APA leadership into seeking a resolution. Leading the compromise efforts was Robert Spitzer, a young member of the APA's Committee on Nomenclature. Disillusioned with the dominance of psychoanalytic thinking, Spitzer had come to believe that psychiatry needed to hew closer to biomedicine, if it were to survive the assaults of antipsychiatry. The first step in this would be to get its diagnostic house in order. To Spitzer, the dispute over homosexuality was the result of years of neglecting diagnosis. This neglect was evident in the ambiguity regarding the very definition of a mental disorder. Adopting what would become his primary tactic in controversies, Spitzer sought to defuse the dispute through an act of classification. He developed and circulated a revised definition of mental disorder that defined it as a condition that "must either regularly cause subjective distress or regularly be associated with some generalized impairment in social effectiveness and functioning."[9] These two criteria provided a litmus test for diagnoses. Homosexuality was to be Spitzer's first test case. And it failed on both accounts—for many homosexuals, their sexual orientation caused no distress, nor did it inhibit them from leading fulfilling lives.

Wanting to dispense with the diagnosis of homosexuality with as little disruption as possible, Spitzer proposed a compromise. To appease activists, the diagnosis would be eliminated from the DSM. It would, however, be replaced with a new diagnosis of "sexual orientation disturbance" that applied "only to those homosexuals who are in some way bothered by their sexual orientation, some of whom may come to [psychiatrists] for help."[10] In December 1973, with activists more or less on board, the APA Board of Trustees endorsed the change.

However, a group of psychiatrists, mostly psychoanalysts, opposed the compromise and mounted a last-ditch effort to stop it. They invoked an obscure APA policy to force an association-wide vote on the issue. In the lead-up to the referendum, sides traded accusations of inappropriate politicking. Opponents of removing homosexuality argued that the APA had been cowed into submission by "militant homosexual organizations."[11] Supporters responded that in subjecting the nomenclature change to a vote, it was the opposition that was trying to adjudicate scientific questions by political means.[12]

With the outcome up for grabs, the vote was held. Over 10,000 members voted, with 58% in favor of removing the diagnosis. Homosexuality was no longer considered a mental disorder by the APA.[13] In a memorandum to fellow activists, Kameny cheekily proclaimed, "We have been 'cured'!"[14]

Significant in its own right, the controversy over homosexuality was a microcosm of psychiatric politics in the 1970s. During this period, psychiatry faced an existential crisis. Its future was in grave doubt. Buckling "under heavy fire" from antipsychiatry critics,[15] psychiatrists had been unable to muster an effective response. Psychoanalysis had staled and stalled. Community psychiatry had accomplished little more than dismantling the mental hospital system. The profession was left riven by internal divisions that "defy consensual cataloging."[16] Assessing the fractured field, Bertram S. Brown, NIMH director from 1970 to 1977, posed the questions that preoccupied psychiatrists: "What is the role of psychiatry? Does it even have a role, or is it, as some would have it, dead or dying?"[17]

Psychiatric ignorance had once again been exposed. "Basic semantic and philosophical issues still disturb many in the field," observed psychiatrist

Samuel B. Guze, exposing fundamental disagreements "concerning the definition of disease, the role of physicians, the nature of cause, the role of hereditary and social factors as causes, and the results of treatment."[18] After more than a century, the answers to these questions seemed as politicized as ever. Indeed, the profession had settled the homosexuality controversy, not through a demonstration of expertise but through backroom dealings, political machinations, and ultimately a referendum. Such a resolution seemed to confirm antipsychiatry suspicions that psychiatry created mental illnesses willy-nilly, based on the thinnest of evidence and rationales. If a mental disorder could be determined by a vote, what did psychiatry really know about the object of its purported expertise?

The controversy over homosexuality, however, was also a harbinger of where psychiatric politics were headed. It centered around the issue that would come to occupy psychiatric reformers for the next three decades—diagnosis. A new generation of psychiatric reformers, calling themselves "Neo-Kraepelinians," sought to shift psychiatry away from a psychoanalytic/psychodynamic model to a biomedical one. By reclaiming their identity as physicians, they believed that psychiatry could build a scientific research base that would solidify its professional authority and resolve its ignorance. The first and crucial step in this reinvention was to refashion psychiatric diagnosis. Reformers insisted that the myriad problems facing psychiatry were, at root, problems of diagnosis and classification. Fix diagnosis, fix psychiatry. Thus, for the next few decades, debates over the future of psychiatry were to be waged in the language of nomenclature. The war against psychiatric ignorance was to be combatted through proxy battles over classification, reliability, and validity. By resolving its diagnostic problems, argued reformers, psychiatry could expect to attain its long-sought goal: a somatic etiological explanation of mental illness.

Covering the period from 1980 to today, this chapter recounts psychiatry's most recent reinvention, the Neo-Kraepelinian revolution, situating it within the longer trajectory of the profession's dealings with ignorance. During this period, psychiatric reformers projected their ambitions onto nosology, the classification of mental disorders. The extent to which nosology became the focus of psychiatry's response to its ignorance is, on the surface, curious. Taxonomies are mundane and unobtrusive parts of the working infrastructure and "information environment" of institutions.[19] They dictate standards adhered to but rarely noticed. Yet, despite its prosaic-seeming character, classification is a political act. It involves an array of judgments and trade-offs among interested parties. It valorizes some points of views and silences others. There is great, if unassuming, power in delineating categories. If standardized, these categories can exert significant conceptual effects, remaking the world by defining its contours.[20] The first part of the chapter focuses on the revolutionary revision of DSM-III. To transform psychiatry through diagnostic reforms, Neo-Kraepelinian reformers sought to render mental disorders more legible.[21] Their neat, standardized classification system stood in stark juxtaposition to the mystery and opacity of mental distress under psychoanalysis. With their seeming transparency and scientific gloss, these classifications suggested a command over mental disorders that had long eluded psychiatry. Upon this appearance of mastery, Neo-Kraepelinians fashioned expectations that true scientific insight would follow from diagnostic reform.

Neo-Kraepelinian reformers harnessed diagnostic revisions to remake psychiatry. At the center of their reinvention, its most triumphant moments and its most wearisome conflicts, was the revision to DSM-III, a manual that defines the criteria for every mental disorder recognized by the APA. Today, DSM-III is viewed as a "paradigm shift" in which psychiatric reformers used the DSM as a vehicle to reconstitute psychiatry as a biomedical profession.[22] And in securing these diagnostic reforms, psychiatrists, for the first time, presented a conscious articulation of reinvention as a strategy. Unlike previous generations of reformers, they not only advocated a particular *vision* for psychiatry; they also justified reinvention as a general *strategy* for professional reforms.

The widespread adoption of DSM-III's classification system seemed to validate this strategy. However, despite the back patting of reformers, DSM-III has had ambiguous professional effects, especially in relation to psychiatric ignorance. Although psychiatry, through recent DSM editions, has achieved significant influence over how Americans—and increasingly the world—think and talk about mental illness, the etiology of mental disorders remains elusive. Reformers anticipated that the DSM revisions would lead to new developments in psychiatric research, specifically in genetic science and neuroscience. But research into the genetic mechanisms and neurological correlates of mental disorders has sputtered. The second half of this chapter focuses on these problems as they came to the forefront during the revision to DSM-5. It draws on interviews with participating psychiatrists to reconstruct the contentious revision process. The DSM-5 Task Force sought to right the wrongs of DSM-III. Dissatisfied with the DSM-III model, it called for a new "paradigm shift" to be achieved through DSM-5 revision. This effort generated intense controversy and ended in failure, leaving psychiatrists, once again, groping for a way forward. Despite the appearance of mastery conferred by DSM's tidy categorization of mental disorders, the unknown in psychiatry remains unknown.

DSM-III, a Revolution via Nomenclature

In the latter half of the 1970s, psychiatry was in a state of crisis, unsure how to proceed in response to its antipsychiatry critics. The broad program of community psychiatry had led to role blurring and further diluted its already weak professional identity. The fallout from the quick abandonment of community psychiatry was compounded by the lassitude surrounding psychoanalysis. Psychoanalysis was seen as reactionary and "increasingly conservative."[23] Its "mystique [was] not enough to sustain psychiatry."[24] Consequently, the profession became fractured at the precise moment when it was at its most vulnerable. Melvin Sabshin, who would serve as the medical director of the APA for two decades, warned of the "rapid segmentation of the psychiatric profession" that divided it "into significant ideological groupings."[25]

Once again, psychiatrists faced the question of "who we are and what we are or should be doing" without a clear answer.[26] Specifically, psychiatry was being torn between the sclerotic psychodynamic model and an emergent biomedical model. This division played out in many arenas, but perhaps none knottier than in the training of the next generation of psychiatrists. A sociological study on psychiatric training in the late 1970s revealed a profession grappling with acute questions over identity. "Constantly [vacillating] between psychological and physiological explanations of mental problems," psychiatry struggled with how to train residents.[27] The conceptual muddle forced residents into situations of untenable ambiguity. Trainees resolved this tension by committing to one school of thought over the other, a process more akin to ideological indoctrination than scientific exploration.

Into this void stepped an energetic group of reformers, who after decades of psychoanalytic dominance sought to reclaim a medical identity for psychiatry. Although previous reformers had laid claim to medicine, there was always something ill-fitting and half-hearted about these efforts. Historically, prominent psychiatric treatments displayed few, if any, medical qualities, and most that did had been revealed to be fraudulent and/or harmful. Simply put, the workaday world of psychiatry looked different than other medical specialties. Psychiatrists might insist on their medical identity, but they rarely displayed it in practice. Instead, their claims to medicine long served as "polemic shibboleth[s]" to secure credibility and legal protections.[28] Under psychoanalysis and community psychiatry, the connection to medicine had grown even more tenuous, as both of these reinventions promoted ontologies of mental distress that stressed its distinctiveness from physical illness. Thus, as late as 1984, it could be reasonably claimed, as it was by Nancy Andreasen, neuropsychiatrist and, later, editor in chief of the *American Journal of Psychiatry*, that among thousands of books on psychiatry, "oddly" almost none of them described it "from the medical perspective."[29] For psychiatry to survive, a new generation of reformers would have to re-claim "psychiatry's place in the medical sun" and recapture its "birthright."[30] Psychiatry had to move beyond shallow assertions that it was a medical specialty to actually become one.

Reformers also had pragmatic reasons for seeking to reconfigure psychia-try along the lines of biomedicine. With the rise of managed care and a shift in the political winds away from the activism of the 1960s to the more con-servative Reagan years, the "economic picture [had] changed," as funding for community interventions and service had "dried up."[31] New standards of evidence brought the inadequacy of psychiatric research into stark relief and heightened the otherness of psychoanalysis in medicine. If psychiatrists wanted to get paid for their services and secure research funding in such a climate, they would have to store their couches, come in from the com-munity, and don their white coats. Otherwise, psychiatry was "doomed as a discipline."[32]

To secure a future in medicine, the new Neo-Kraepelinian reformers turned to the past for inspiration. Just as psychoanalysts had a figurehead in Freud, so too did this new generation of reformers in Emile Kraepelin. A German psychiatrist and contemporary of Freud, Kraepelin is credited with importing the "clinical method" from other branches of medicine to the study of men-tal diseases.[33] Kraepelin adapted the tenets of the laboratory sciences to the clinic, stressing systematic and careful clinical observation as the bedrock for psychiatric knowledge. He emphasized diagnosis, developing a classification system based upon his ongoing observation of patients' symptoms and disease course. While Kraepelin's classification system achieved some influ-ence in the United States during the psychobiological period, it was never widely adopted. Once psychiatry became dominated by psychoanalysts in the 1950s, diagnosis was de-emphasized for depth psychology. Kraepelin became marginalized by American psychiatrists, his life's work reduced to that of a mere classifier. On the rare occasion when Kraepelin did come up, he was seen as "the Father of Descriptive Psychiatry and this, in turn, has in some quarters the connotation of an epithet."[34]

In the 1970s, Kraepelin was resurrected by a tight-knit group of psy-chiatric researchers centered in Washington University in St. Louis.[35] Neo-Kraepelinians were self-described "data-oriented" psychiatrists, who em-phasized research in a profession long neglectful of research. Considered outsiders—in the 1950s and 1960s, the NIMH refused to fund their grants for clinical studies—Neo-Kraepelinians saw opportunity in the turmoil of the 1970s.[36] And just as American psychoanalysts had done with Freud, Neo-Kraepelinians selectively adapted Kraepelin to articulate a particular vision for psychiatry. They de-emphasized Kraepelin's commitment to long-term observations of disease courses as well as his warnings that "there are no fixed, but only blurred borders between mental health and mental illness."[37] Rather, in their hands, Kraepelin became an uncompromising advocate of disease specificity and the priority of classification in the psychiatric endeavor.

As an alternative to psychoanalytic/psychodynamic psychiatry, Neo-Kraepelinians outlined a vision of psychiatry as a biomedical science. As described by psychologist Roger K. Blashfield, this program espoused nine core tenets:

1   Psychiatry is a branch of medicine;
2   Psychiatry should utilize modern scientific methodologies and base its practice on scientific knowledge;
3   Psychiatry treats people who are sick and who require treatment for mental illness;
4   There is a boundary between the normal and the sick;
5   There are discrete mental illnesses and it is the task of scientific psychiatry, as of other medical specialties, to investigate the causes, diagnosis, and treatment of these mental illnesses;
6   The focus of psychiatric physicians should be on the biological aspects of mental illness;
7   There should be an explicit and intentional concern for diagnosis and classification;
8   Diagnostic criteria should be codified, and a legitimate and valued area of research should be developed to validate such criteria by various techniques;
9   In research efforts directed at improving the reliability and validity of diagnosis and classification, statistical techniques should be utilized.[38]

These tenets reflected Neo-Kraepelinians' emphasis on psychiatric research. Indeed, they deemed psychiatric ignorance to be the result of psychiatry's lack of commitment to modern scientific research. Psychiatry had never invested enough in research, and during the psychoanalytic period had allowed the revolutions of medical science to pass it by. Refractory ignorance was the punishment for this grievous sin. To move beyond the particularistic interpretations championed by psychoanalysts or the vague sloganeering of community psychiatrists, Neo-Kraepelinians insisted that psychiatry pursue generalizable knowledge regarding mental illness using the tools of modern science. Only then would the profession escape the endless cycle of fads and reinventions.

Classification was the lynchpin of this vision. Without a standard classification, psychiatrists could never build the research infrastructure necessary to overcome their ignorance. Prior attempts at a standardizing classification, be it by the US Census, state legislatures, mental hospitals, or the military, had been motivated by interests outside psychiatry and pursued for bureaucratic reasons.[39] Psychiatrists looked askance at these attempts, eyeing them with suspicion. Meyer, for example, warned against the intellectual laziness induced by diagnostic labels. Psychoanalysts viewed diagnoses as shallow; since neurosis was particular to an individual's development, affixing a label to it offered little insight into the case. Diagnosis confounded more than clarified the case at hand. And community psychiatrists, attempting to extend psychiatry's reach, had stretched the notion of mental distress far beyond the bounds of medical diagnosis. Without buy-in from most psychiatrists, early classification systems failed to catch on.

To Neo-Kraepelinians, this classificatory status quo was unacceptable. It perpetuated ignorance by denying psychiatry the conceptual foundation necessary for collective, coherent science. Psychiatrist Robert Evan Kendell put the matter this way:

> Certainly the failure of both psychiatrists and psychologists to develop a satisfactory classification of their subject matter, or even to agree on the principles on which that classification should be based, is a most serious barrier to fruitful research into the aetiology of mental illness and even into the efficacy of therapeutic regimes. It is more exciting to develop explanatory theories, or to claim impressive results for this or that treatment, than it is to define the critical characteristics of the patients on whom one's research was based. It is probably more exciting to an architect to design parabolic canopies or baroque facades than it is to calculate the size and shape of the concrete slab on which his building will rest.[40]

Without classifications, without the unglamorous yeoman work of creating a standard system, psychiatry could not build a biomedical scientific research base. Thus, at a time when many psychiatrists were "extremely ambivalent about the whole notion of psychiatric diagnosis,"[41] Neo-Kraepelinians insisted that standardizing diagnosis was key to progress. Psychiatry's diagnostic problems should be met, they believed, not with indifference or surrender; ambivalence did not "indicate that diagnosis should be abandoned but that more precise criteria should be developed."[42] Led by John Feighner, Samuel Guze, Eli Robins, George Winkour, and Robert Woodruff, Neo-Kraepelinians concentrated their efforts on developing clear criteria for each mental disorder, consisting of concise descriptions of their symptoms, so that they could be identified and diagnosed with consistency. In 1972, the group published what became known as the "Feighner criteria," which operationalized the diagnostic criteria for fourteen psychiatric illnesses.[43] As a template for subsequent classification reforms, the Feighner criteria embodied the Neo-Kraepelinian vision for psychiatry. Feighner himself insisted that nosological revision would "form the basis for a better understanding of specific etiological mechanisms and greater specificity and efficacy in the treatment of patients suffering from psychiatric illness."[44]

Therefore, while often described as "biological psychiatry" or "biomedical psychiatry," the Neo-Kraepelinian reforms are best thought of as "diagnostic psychiatry."[45] Yes, they aspired to greater scientificity via a biological understanding of the causes of mental disorders. Yes, they expected that through biomedical science, psychiatrists' long-standing questions would be finally answered. But the means by which they sought to achieve this vision was through the standardization of psychiatric nosology. More than anything, the Neo-Kraepelinian vision asserted the significance of the diagnostic act.

Carving Mental Illness at Its Joints

Creating model criteria, citing each other, and nurturing an enclave of like-minded psychiatrists was one thing. Revolutionizing the entirety of psychiatry was another thing altogether. Neo-Kraepelinians needed a means to disseminate their vision and wrest psychiatry from the stranglehold psychoanalysts had on it. They found it in an unlikely place: the revision to DSM-III.

The DSM-III revision was overseen by Robert Spitzer, who would become the most influential member of the Neo-Kraepelinians. Spitzer spent his career at Columbia University and the affiliated New York State Psychiatric Institute. A product of the New York psychoanalytic scene, Spitzer had a personal relationship to the psychiatric school he would work so hard to supplant. His mother was a Jungian therapist, and Spitzer himself was trained in psychoanalysis (as most psychiatrists of his day were).[46] Early in his career, however, he became disenchanted with psychoanalysis and turned his attention to research. Always data-oriented, he developed an intense interest in what were then seen as the least glamorous topics in psychiatry: measurement, assessment, and diagnosis. He volunteered as a notetaker for the DSM-II revision and later joined the APA's Committee on Nomenclature. Although the Committee was viewed as something of a psychiatric backwater—after all, psychoanalysts had little interest in formal diagnoses and nomenclature—Spitzer found himself embroiled in three of psychiatry's most prominent controversies of the 1970s. In 1971, he was part of the team that published a watershed study that revealed significant disparities in the diagnostic conclusions drawn by English and American psychiatrists.[47] In 1973, he brokered the homosexuality compromise. And in 1975, Spitzer wrote a scathing review of Rosenhan's study that dismissed it as "pseudoscience."[48] "Stubborn, sometimes abrasive, and always eager," Spitzer was unafraid of controversy; in fact, he reveled in it.[49]

Spitzer applied his energies to improving psychiatric diagnosis. He developed structured diagnostic interviews and created one of the first computer software programs to assist in psychiatric diagnosis, DIAGNO I. With Jean Endicott and Eli Robins, he formulated the Research Diagnostic Criteria (RDC), which outlined "specified diagnostic criteria" for twenty-five common mental disorders.[50] The RDC, along with the Feighner criteria, established the template for standardized psychiatric classifications. But all these were mere preludes to what would become Spitzer's crowning achievement, DSM-III. Here, he left his mark. By the end of his career, he would be considered by many "the most influential psychiatrist of his time."[51] A *New York Times* obituary credited him with remaking psychiatry.

DSM had long been a marginal document, ignored by most clinicians and used primarily to serve bureaucratic functions. The official motive for the DSM-III revision was, on the surface, prosaic; the APA wanted to reconcile the DSM coding schema with an upcoming revision to the ninth edition of the *International Classification of Disease* (ICD-9). Few lobbied for the opportunity to head an obscure committee charged with such an unrewarding chore. But where most saw drudge work, Spitzer saw "an opportunity to make psychiatry more scientific."[52] He believed he could use the revision as a vehicle for psychiatric reform.

Given his career trajectory, as well as a lack of competition, Spitzer became the logical choice to chair the DSM-III revision. He quickly set to work overhauling psychiatry's diagnostic system. Using the wide discretion at his disposal—"I pretty much decided who was going to be on the committees"[53]—he staffed the Task Force with like-minded Neo-Kraepelinian peers. All those involved shared a consensus that DSM had to be totally revised.[54] Assessing psychiatry's predicament, they interpreted the multifaceted challenges as stemming from fundamental faults in how psychiatry defined and categorized its objects. Specifically, they focused their concerns on the lack of reliability in psychiatric diagnosis. Reliability pertains to the extent to which diagnostic criteria yield agreement among clinicians across contexts. The same patient should receive the same diagnosis regardless of the particular clinician he or she sees. For Neo-Kraepelinians, the lack of reliability in psychiatric diagnosis was a huge problem. If psychiatrists could not agree on basic diagnoses, psychiatry would never develop a coherent scientific research program.[55] Without reliability, researchers could not create homogeneous samples of subjects required by modern research design. Nor could they develop and test targeted treatments. Thus, nosological reform was critical to moving forward. It might not resolve psychiatric ignorance itself, but it was the crucial first step in doing so.

Thus, the Neo-Kraepelinians participating in DSM-III channeled their revolutionary aspirations into this seemingly technical task of how to construct classifications based on specified, operationalized criteria that could be standardized across contexts. Previous editions of DSM (DSM-I and DSM-II) were based on psychoanalytic/psychodynamic principles. As such, the texts reflected the indifference psychoanalysts and psychodynamic psychiatrists felt toward diagnosis. Treating mental disorders as continuous with normality and focused on the psychosocial development of individual patients, psychoanalysts just did not care all that much about delineating and categorizing specific diagnoses. This resulted in a certain looseness in DSM-I and DSM-II, as their "prose-based descriptions" were vague and theory-laden.[56] The DSM-III Task Force sought to replace the broad and continuous concepts of the previous DSM editions with a categorical system of classification.

The revised structure of classifications was intended to be as straightforward as possible. Each discrete DSM disorder would be defined by its phenotypic symptoms, with decision rules outlining the number of symptoms needed to meet a diagnosis. For example, major depressive disorder (MDD) was defined according to nine symptom criteria; to meet the threshold for an MDD diagnosis, a patient would have to demonstrate at least five of the symptoms. The criteria for each diagnosis were determined by expert consensus, what some derided as the "bogsat" method (the letters standing for *bunch of guys sitting around the table*). Spitzer chaired every committee. During meetings, he would compose diagnostic criteria on a typewriter, revising the language as the conversations progressed. Each of the manual's 494 pages bore his imprint.

DSM-III was advertised as atheoretical and agnostic toward schools of psychiatry. But the changes implicitly endorsed a medical model. This was most evident in the new diagnostic categories. DSM-III transformed fluid, dimensional neuroses into discrete disease-like entities.[57] In doing so, it reframed the ontology of mental disorders. The Task Force nevertheless held up the revised categories as necessary building blocks for rigorous biomedical research. Such research was to be organized around these diagnostic categories. The new diagnoses would be the targets of scientific inquiry. This gave away the game, revealing the "biological default" of the Neo-Kraepelinian approach.[58] Neo-Kraepelinians implied that the diagnostic categories reflected organic pathologies, however imperfect and provisional they might be.[59] To make psychiatry more medical, the DSM-III Task Force transformed the ontology of mental disorders—what mental disorders are understood to be—so as to address psychiatry's epistemological challenges—how to build a research program that would secure knowledge regarding mental disorders.

Sheltered as it was from scrutiny, the revision to DSM-III did not escape controversy altogether. When information regarding the changes leaked out, many psychiatrists, particularly those of the psychoanalytic/psychodynamic school, objected. At first, these objections focused on specific diagnostic categories as well as the manual's definition of mental disorder. Spitzer parried such objections by reducing them to semantic concerns. When pressed with a specific criticism, he channeled the discussion into questions of language. In doing so, he elided fundamental conceptual differences underlying the criticisms by focusing the discussion on rephrasing, clarifying, or removing problematic portions of the text. As such, DSM-III debates paid "an almost farcical attention to words."[60] Doing so allowed Spitzer to assert that the revisions operated on a descriptive level only. Invoking the "universally acknowledged" goal of reliability in diagnosis,[61] he insisted that the DSM-III manual could fit everyone's needs, regardless of school of thought, provided that the appropriate neutral language was found.

The façade of ecumenism, however, began to falter in the face of psychoanalytic opposition. Excluded from the process, psychoanalysts were caught off guard when the extent of the proposed revisions came to light late in the process. Voicing a number of criticisms (i.e., the lack of psychoanalytic representation on the Task Force, the absence of oversight, and the hostility of the Task Force to psychoanalytic/psychodynamic ideas, etc.), they directed most of their ire at the decision to eliminate "neurosis" from DSM-III. After all, neurosis was the bedrock of psychoanalytic thought and had been the organizing framework in understanding mental distress for decades. Psychoanalysts could neither envision nor countenance a psychiatric nosology without "neurosis" in it.

Spitzer tried to deflect the neurosis issue by treating it as symbolic, claiming that the word "neurosis" was a mere "shibboleth."[62] He justified its deletion on the basis that the term carried unproven etiological and theoretical baggage. It had no place in an atheoretical, descriptive nomenclature. In recalling the controversy decades later, Spitzer maintained his stated commitment to ecumenism: "I don't think we were itching for a fight. We looked forward to a vigorous debate. We didn't shy away from it. But also we always said DSM-III is not anti-psychoanalytic. You can be a psychoanalyst and use the thing."[63] Psychoanalysts countered that the etiological underpinning of neuroses was well established by decades of experience—not to mention mountains of writings on the topic—and its deletion reflected the Task Force's anti-psychoanalytic bias.[64]

The debate would find its way to the highest reaches of the APA leadership. However, its resolution in favor of the Neo-Kraepelinians was almost a foregone conclusion. Psychoanalysts had mobilized too late. By the time their disorganized challenge rounded into form in January 1979, it was mere months before DSM-III was scheduled to be voted on. The revisions had gained inexorable momentum. After a contentious back-and-forth, the APA Board of Trustees negotiated a compromise in which DSM-III would include neuroses in the parentheses following the relevant diagnostic categories (e.g., "Anxiety Disorder [or Anxiety Neurosis])." With little other recourse—and still unconvinced that DSM mattered all that much—psychoanalysts relented. In June 1979, the Board of Trustees approved the revisions.

Published in 1980, DSM-III outlined 228 diagnostic categories. Each category was assigned a diagnostic code, followed by a brief description of the disorder. Subsequent text marked out the disorder's characteristics with regard to its associated features, age of onset, course, impairment, complications, prevalence, and predisposing features, followed by a discussion of differential diagnoses from similar disorders. The core of each category, however, was the list of diagnostic criteria, set apart from the rest of the text in a gray background. Here, the features of each disorder, as well as the guidelines for diagnosis, were laid out in succinct and straightforward language.

DSM-III proposed a new ontology of mental disorders, one intended to move the profession in a medical direction away from the speculative flights of psychoanalysis. Although insisting "that there is no assumption that each mental disorder is a discrete entity with sharp boundaries,"[65] the organization of the diagnostic categories, with their discrete criteria, undermined this introductory qualifier. Each DSM-III diagnosis carried an assumption that it reflected an *actual* biological defect. But just as significant as its reframing of mental disorders was the appearance of competence that

DSM-III conveyed. Complex, mysterious, and idiosyncratic subconscious forces that preoccupied psychoanalysts were discarded for straightforward symptom lists and clear decision rules, wrapped in neutral technical prose. In doing so, DSM-III rendered mental distress more legible. Its content betrayed little of its messy origins in expert consensus or the arbitrary decisions that underwrote its diagnostic categories; in style and appearance, DSM-III suggested a confident, well-informed scientific grasp of mental illness, a physical embodiment of psychiatry in the scientific image.[66] Thus, DSM-III worked on psychiatric ignorance in two ways. It gave psychiatry a veneer of mastery understanding where there was little, while simultaneously promoting a coherent vision of a biomedical future in which this ignorance would be transcended. DSM-III mapped the entire universe of mental distress *and* supplied a road map for psychiatric research.

DSM-III Goes Viral

Today, the DSM-III revision is viewed as a watershed event in psychiatric history.[67] But for a brief time after its publication, psychiatrists remained uncertain of its relevance. For strategic reasons, Spitzer and the DSM-III Task Force never discussed the DSM-III revisions in revolutionary terms. To the contrary, they downplayed its ontological ramifications. Even in his more grandiose moments, Spitzer described the manual in neutral scientific language. For their part, psychoanalysts still remained skeptical of the importance of diagnosis and, by extension, DSM-III. As such, initial assessments of DSM-III minimized its importance for the Neo-Kraepelinian/psychanalyst struggle over the profession. Psychiatrists Allen Frances and Arnold M. Cooper tried to calm the backlash, insisting, "Psychodynamic psychiatrists need not be particularly alarmed or troubled by the descriptive approach of DSM-III."[68] Public reaction was similarly muted. DSM-III warranted only brief mentions in the press, and when it did, its significance was downplayed. The *New York Times* reported that DSM-III was "only catching up with current practices."[69]

Yet, these initial assessments quickly gave way to a more polarized interpretation. Psychoanalytic psychiatrists became the first to label DSM-III, derisively, as a paradigm shift. In 1982, the APA held a debate over DSM-III. Speaking in support of the revision were Spitzer and Gerald L. Klerman, head of the NIMH at the time. Two psychoanalysts, Robert Michels and George E. Vaillant, served as its critics. Klerman opened the exchange by lauding DSM-III as a "fateful point in the history of the American psychiatric profession." Even so, he portrayed it less as a revolution and more as a reclamation project, "a significant reaffirmation on the part of American psychiatry of its medical identity."[70] In his rebuttal, Michels disputed this interpretation, deeming the revisions a coup that "insist[ed] that a single paradigm encompass the entire nosology."[71] DSM-III endorsed the Neo-Kraepelinian paradigm as the *only* paradigm. Challenging the DSM-III Task Force's rhetoric of neutrality, Michels asserted that it "is not possible to be conceptually atheoretical unless one is mute."[72] In response, Spitzer stuck to the script: DSM-III was descriptive, agnostic, and could "be used by anyone, whether he or she is committed to a psychoanalytic, a biologic, a social learning, or some other theoretical paradigm."[73]

Spitzer's repeated declaration aside, it was Michels's interpretation that won the day. His portrayal of DSM-III as a paradigm shift stuck and set the terms for subsequent debates.[74] The "paradigm shift" interpretation gained acceptance among DSM-III's critics, and supporters of DSM-III responded in kind. They too embraced the attribution, but gave it a positive spin. The extensive diffusion of DSM-III categories was interpreted by supporters as confirmation that DSM-III was revolutionizing psychiatry along the lines of biomedical science.[75] For example, Sabshin deemed DSM-III the "turning point" in the effort to drag psychiatry in a scientific direction.[76] Once an epithet, the attribution of paradigm shift assumed a positive valence. It was transformed by Neo-Kraepelinians into a narrative of scientific progress.

DSM-III dissemination, however, was propelled more by institutional fit than intellectual innovation. The manual's power came less from its intrinsic merits and more from the manner in which it intersected with, and complemented, specific trends affecting the mental health field. As discussed in chapter 3, in the 1970s, a confluence of actors began to demand greater transparency of psychiatry. The standardized DSM-III diagnoses were poised to meet this demand.

Pharmaceutical companies were the primary engine in this regard. Their role in facilitating psychiatry's reinvention along biomedical lines in the last decades of the twentieth century cannot be overstated. At the time of DSM-III's publication, the use of psychopharmaceutical drugs in the treatment of mental disorders was neither novel nor groundbreaking, as evidenced by the popularity of Thorazine. Additionally, minor tranquilizers like meprobamate (marketed as "Miltown"), marketed as "mothers' little helpers," became the first blockbuster psychotropic drugs when introduced in the mid-1950s.[77] In the 1960s, diazepam (Valium) and other benzodiazepines replaced Miltown as the drug of choice to treat anxiety, and by 1970, 20% of American women were using minor tranquilizers and sedatives.[78] Therefore, while drug treatments were in tension with the previous psychoanalytic/psychodynamic framework in theory, their extensive use indicates pre-DSM-III psychiatry was not opposed to drug treatment in practice.

Two developments led to an explosion in the market of psychotropic drugs. First, in 1987, the FDA approved Prozac (fluoxetine), the first of a new generation of psychopharmaceutical drugs in the class of selective serotonin reuptake inhibitors (SSRIs). Within a year, Eli Lilly was garnering $350 million in annual sales from Prozac.[79] Prozac became something of a cultural touchstone, fodder for best-selling books,[80] popular memoirs,[81] and abundant media attention. Prozac was followed by other top-selling drugs like Zoloft (sertraline) in 1991, Paxil (paroxetine) in 1992, and serotonin and norepinephrine reuptake inhibitors (SNRIs) like Effexor (venlafaxine) in 1993. Perceived as having fewer side effects than the previous generation of psychopharmacological agents, these drugs were heralded as scientific breakthroughs. They promised a new era of biological psychiatry when targeted, effective, and safe treatments could make people, in the words of psychiatrists and Prozac enthusiast Peter Kramer, "better than well."[82] Second, in 1997, the FDA changed its guidelines regarding the advertisement of pharmaceutical drugs. It allowed drug companies to market their products directly to the consumer, through direct-to-consumer advertisements (DTCAs). The onslaught of advertisements that followed not only promoted the drugs, but in "selling the disease to sell the pill" also promoted the disease model of mental disorders.[83]

The new drugs, and the ads promoting them, drew their rationale from what is known colloquially as the "chemical imbalance theory." The chemical imbalance theory holds that mental disorders are related to dysfunctions in the brain, specifically an imbalance in neurotransmitters (serotonin, dopamine, norepinephrine, and epinephrine). SSRIs are purported to work by preventing the "uptake" of these neurotransmitters, increasing the level of, say, serotonin in the brain and thereby alleviating the prominent symptoms of, say, depression. Ad campaigns portrayed this theory as a novel, revolutionary discovery, but it dates back to the 1960s.[84] Subsequent research has challenged its claims, indicating that the theory is, at best, limited or, at worse, flat-out wrong.[85] Even defenders of "the molecular foundations of psychiatry" have copped to these shortcomings, acknowledging that given the current state of research, "it is difficult to argue that putative neurotransmitter and receptor abnormalities provide insight into the pathophysiology of psychiatric disorders, rather than being consequences that may be quite far removed from the disease etiology in the chain of connections."[86] But these qualifications have not stopped pharmaceutical companies from promoting the chemical imbalance theory as sound, solid, and scientifically objective.

Instead of gatekeepers guarding against the expansive claims of pharmaceutical companies, psychiatrists became willing accomplices in propagating them. For psychiatric reformers, the chemical imbalance theory, and the false certainty of pharmaceutical advertisements through which it was promoted, served their professional interests. It solidified their claims to medical science and legitimated the reinvention of psychiatry "from the study of the 'troubled mind' to the 'broken brain.'"[87] "Psychiatry, like the prodigal son, has returned home to its place as a specialty within the field of medicine," asserted Andreasen in her well-regarded book *The Broken Brain*. "Psychiatry now recognizes that the serious mental illnesses are *diseases*. Mental illnesses are diseases that affect the brain, which is an organ of the body just as the heart or stomach is."[88] Although more circumspect than the typical DTCA commercial, Andreasen, like her medically inclined peers, endorsed the chemical imbalance theory, stressing the "excesses and deficits in the chemical transmission between neurons."[89] Thus, the chemical imbalance theory was convenient for psychiatrists. If mental disorders were problems of the brain, treatable through drug agents, psychiatry was poised to reconstitute its fledgling authority through medicine. Medication management became "the last bastion of authority, the last fortress of uncontested decision making."[90] While there are debates as to how much psychiatrists promoted the chemical imbalance theory,[91] at the very least they were complicit in its spread by holding their tongues.

DSM-III locked psychiatry in a symbiotic relationship with the pharmaceutical companies. For drug companies, DSM provides a compendium of possible markets and new drug targets, a universe that has grown with each subsequent revision. If a pharmaceutical company happens to develop a drug similar to one already on the market, it can reposition the drug as a treatment for one of DSM's many other disorders.[92] DSM also facilitates and standardizes drug research and development. To produce evidence of efficacy and secure FDA approval, new drugs need a specific target. DSM provides these. The diagnostic categories enable randomized controlled trials (RCTs), the gold standard of drug development and approval, by allowing researchers to construct samples organized around discrete diagnostic entities. For their part, psychiatrists accrue professional benefits from their ties to pharmaceutical companies. Depending on one's perspective, DTCAs either raise awareness of existing problems related to mental illness or medicalize more and more problems as illnesses demanding medical treatment. Either way, the ads reinforce the need for psychiatric expertise. Because of regulations on prescribing medications, the demand for psychopharmaceutic treatments seems to ensure psychiatry's relevance, for among mental health professionals, it is psychiatrists, as MDs, who control the practice of prescribing.

DSM-III also gained influence through other developments external to the profession, some scientific, some economic. First, the publication of DSM-III intersected with new developments in genetic science and neuroscience. The launch of the Human Genome Project in 1990 fueled visions of a revolution in medicine, promising genetic understandings of diseases, gene therapies, and personalized medicine. In popular discourse, the gene has become an icon, with many articles announcing the latest discovery of the "gene for x."[93] Like the rest of medicine, psychiatric reformers have been caught up in this exuberance, leading to predictions that psychiatry would be "transformed by genetic research" that would "reveal much about the etiology and pathogenesis of mental illness."[94] A similar enthusiasm inflects neuroscience. President George H. W. Bush declared the 1990s the "Decade of the Brain," instigating an interagency promotion of neuroscience. Technological developments in imaging, notably functional magnetic resonance imaging (fMRI), promised transparent access into the workings of the brain that would "blow away old barriers to knowledge."[95] Visions of transforming psychiatry into a "clinical neuroscience" proliferated.[96] Indeed, today the medical model, promoted by Neo-Kraepelinians, has taken a molecular turn; psychiatrists have come to see "the potential of brain imaging, molecular genetics, neurobiology, and immunology research [as] phenomenal."[97] The programs for neuroscience and genetic research are organized according to DSM diagnoses, which provide the targets for genetic markers and neural correlates.

Finally, DSM-III received an institutional lift through changes in the payment for health care. During the 1960s, health insurance companies began to cover psychotherapy, but "had little actuarial ability to forecast future expenditures."[98] The increasing cost of health care combined with legislation, passed in 1996, that required insurers to maintain parity in the coverage of mental health increased insurance companies' desire for greater oversight and cost control. Under such conditions, the opacity, mystique, and prolonged treatment of psychoanalysis were no longer acceptable. Indeed, insurers would help kill off psychoanalysis by refusing to pay for it. Third-party insurers demanded accountability, and DSM-III contained a coding system that could be adapted for the purposes of monitoring treatment. DSM codes became required for coverage and are now used by insurers to assess patient progress and make determinations on coverage. Even psychiatrists opposed to DSM must use its codes if they want reimbursement. Psychiatrists might resent the formulaic "zeal" with which insurers seized on DSM-III, recognizing that it gives off a misleading "image of precision and exactness" and threatens clinician autonomy.[99] But they cannot ignore it. Nor can they deny that this adoption by insurance companies represents something of a victory for Neo-Kraepelinians' medical aspirations. Psychiatrists are to be compensated like other physicians, thus solidifying their medical identity.

Therefore, the success of DSM-III was driven by a confluence of events. And a startling success it was, far beyond the imaginations of even its most fervent proponents. DSM-III and its subsequent editions (DSM-III-R, DSM-IV, and DSM-IV-TR) have achieved ubiquity. DSM-III-R sold 1.1 million copies in just six years,[100] earning the APA $16.65 million in profits.[101] Recent editions, DSM-IV and DSM-IV-TR, have sold over 800,000 copies.[102] DSM's reach extends beyond the borders of the United States; increasingly, DSM is being exported, affecting how mental distress is understood globally.[103] This success has been interpreted by many within the profession as a validation of psychiatric expertise generally, and as an endorsement of the Neo-Kraepelinian revolution specifically. DSM-III helped displace the hegemony of psychoanalysis, contributing to "the changing power base" that installed "biomedical investigators as the most influential voices in the field."[104]

The crisis of the 1970s appeared resolved. DSM-III, recalled Spitzer, was "terrific for the self-esteem for psychiatry." He went on, "Psychiatry felt, 'Now we've got something. Look at this thing. It's scientific.'"[105] It gave "assurance to the public (and to funding agencies) that psychiatry is a clinical science and not a belief system or religion."[106] Naming and classifying the universe of mental disorders conveyed a degree of mastery and comprehension at a time when psychiatry's ignorance threatened its very existence. Intertwined in all facets of the mental health system, DSM-III made psychiatry the de facto arbiter of what constitutes mental illness. Psychiatrists still lacked a basic understanding of mental disorders, but DSM-III stabilized things. "Much more than a list of disorders," DSM-III represented "a program to place the mental health professions on a firm conceptual footing" after decades of virulent and often embarrassing criticism.[107]

By cataloging and defining mental disorders in DSM, psychiatrists seemingly controlled them. Psychiatry became a profession of the book.

The Tragedy of History Repeating

In a 1991 article in the *American Journal of Psychiatry*, David Reiss, Robert Plomin, and E. Mavis Hetherington made an astute observation about psychiatry's past and present.[108] Throwing cold water on their peers' optimism toward genetic science, they noted that as a "precarious discipline," psychiatry "derives a remarkable portion of its self-image from pictures of its future."[109] By appealing to the future, psychiatrists deflect criticisms of their inadequate knowledge, over and over. But these visions never materialize. Overzealous optimism collapses, gives way to disappointment, and the cycle repeats. The molecular vision, warned Reiss, Plomin, and Hetherington, appeared to be following the same script.

From the start, the promise of DSM-III was never just nosological. Rather, Neo-Kraepelinian reformers saw standardizing diagnosis as the first necessary step in a research revolution that would resolve psychiatry's most vexing questions. Reliability was accompanied by great expectations. Reformers believed that better reliability would lead to validity, an understanding of the specific etiological mechanisms of mental disorders and, in turn, more effective treatments. Despite charges to the contrary,[110] the DSM-III Task Force claimed success in its objective of increasing reliability,[111] a claim that most in the profession accept. With reliability taken care of, an etiological understanding of mental illness would follow short on its heels, or so claimed reformers.

However, thorny issues have arisen in the proposed leap from reliability to validity. DSM-III focused on creating standard, reliable categories with the idea that these would inevitably lead to greater validity. Validity, the extent to which diagnoses describe actual existing diseases, was always the long-term goal. But reliability in and of itself does not ensure validity. People can adopt consistently reliable criteria that are not valid, thus ensuring that they are consistently wrong. If standard categories possess little verisimilitude with reality, the effects of their use, in research and clinical practice, will be misleading and problematic. Researchers, using the same problematic categories, might reproduce flawed sample groups or pursue research objects that are mere mirages. Clinicians, using the same flawed criteria, might reach the same misguided diagnostic conclusions. Validity involves an understanding of the causes and underlying nature of mental disorders. The DSM-III Task Force argued that the new standardized categories would serve as the springboard to this understanding. But there was never any logical warrant to believe this was guaranteed.

In the heady days of the 1980s and 1990s, understanding of mental disorders seemed right around the corner. However, by the turn of the millennium, doubt began to creep in. It has grown since. Decades into DSM-III, basic questions regarding mental disorders remain. Genetic science and neuroscience have produced few answers and, if anything, reveal far greater complexity than psychiatric reformers anticipated. In 2005, Ken Kendler put this lack of progress into stark relief: "We have hunted for big, simple neuropathological explanations for psychiatric disorders and have not found them. We have hunted for big, simple neurochemical explanations for psychiatric disorders and have not found them. We have hunted for big, simple genetic explanations for psychiatric disorders and have not found them."[112] The "project to ground our messy psychiatric categories in genes" is, he argues, in "fundamental trouble."[113] Genetic research has certainly not been kind to discrete DSM categories. For example, recent research suggests that disorders as different as autism, schizophrenia, bipolar disorder, depression, and alcoholism share common genetic patterns, thus throwing into question the classification logic of DSM-III.[114] Likewise, neuroscience has faltered; it has "failed to identify a single neurobiological marker."[115] As psychiatrists began to ponder what might be causing this lack of progress, they attributed some of it to the complexity of the brain, genetic expression, and mental disorders themselves. But they also turned a critical eye toward the diagnostic classification system inherited from DSM-III.

While psychiatrists began to criticize DSM, social scientists were subjecting it to withering scrutiny. Social scientists worry about DSM's facilitation of medicalization, defined as the process by which nonmedical problems become transformed, defined, and treated as medical illnesses.[116] Echoing previous concerns over labeling, critics of medicalization argue that DSM pathologizes more and more behaviors as mental illnesses, either through diagnostic creation—the inclusion of new categories in each subsequent edition—or diagnostic expansion—altering the criteria of existing diagnoses to include more cases under its purview.[117] Subsequent DSM editions have grown in size. From the 228 diagnoses described in DSM-III's 494 pages, the manual swelled to 383 diagnoses delineated in 943 pages of text in DSM-IV-TR.[118] Medicalization, as facilitated by DSM, is blamed for the misguided transformation of normal behaviors into pathological entities—shyness into social anxiety disorder, normal sadness into major depressive disorder, menstruation into premenstrual dysphoric disorder, and classroom fidgeting into ADHD.[119] DSM categories have also been implicated in the creation of false, or at least overstated, epidemics by inflating prevalence rates.[120] These criticisms raise questions about the validity of psychiatric diagnosis and, in turn, the edifice of psychiatric knowledge claims. Can psychiatrists distinguish harmful conditions due to internal dysfunctions from non-disordered problems in living? If not, does DSM-III actually represent progress?

On the surface, it appears that these criticisms have done little to compromise the authority of DSM or psychiatry as a profession. DSM provides the framework and language through which Americans make sense of mental disorders; just as psychoanalysts reaped credibility from the diffusion of its ideas into elite popular culture, so too have Neo-Kraepelinians with the cultural diffusion of DSM. Dig deeper, however, and psychiatry is more compromised than it appears. In the rush to renounce its psychoanalytic past and embrace medication, psychiatrists have ceded psychotherapy to their competitors, chiefly psychologists and social workers.[121] The percentage of visits to psychiatrists that included psychotherapy dropped from 44% in 1996–1997 to 29% in 2004–2005.[122] Psychiatry's distinct expertise is increasingly limited to medication management. While this may distinguish psychiatrists from their mental health competitors, it exposes them to competition from other physicians. Indeed, general practitioners are now responsible for the majority of prescriptions for psychopharmaceutical drugs.[123] As such, medication management has not been the solution to psychiatry's professional threats. Finally, the efficacy of antidepressants and other psychopharmaceutic drugs has come under increasing scrutiny. Meta-analyses, conducted by Irving Kirsch, a Harvard psychology professor, suggest that when unpublished studies are included, antidepressants provide little benefit over a placebo, especially for moderate cases of depression.[124] Such claims fuel critics who believe that psychiatrists and Big Pharma have colluded to foist untested drug treatments upon an unwitting public via the unfounded chemical imbalance theory.[125] Whether one believes Kirsch and his peers or not,[126] current research demonstrates that, at the very least, SSRIs are not as effective or as harmless as pharmaceutical companies and their advocates portray them to be. In their efforts to make psychiatry more medical, Neo-Kraepelinian reformers unintentionally narrowed the scope of their expertise and reduced their professional jurisdiction to managing treatments of questionable efficacy. The legacy of DSM-III has been an ambiguous one.

By the early planning stages for the DSM-5 revisions in 1999, the specter of crisis once again gripped the profession. Although these worries were not as intense or prevalent as they had been in the 1970s, some psychiatrists had grown impatient with the status quo. They were not ready to give up on the biomedical dream embodied in DSM-III altogether; in fact, they wanted to double down on this vision. But they could not accept staying the diagnostic course. Instead, seeking a significant revision, a group of reformers attempted to repeat the feat of DSM-III, using the DSM-5 revision as a vehicle to affect another "paradigm shift." In doing so, they stirred passionate debate over the future of psychiatry, one that pitted the new DSM-5 Task Force against previous DSM Task Force chairs, exposed fault lines between researchers and clinicians, and ended in failure. The DSM-5 controversy not only tarnished psychiatry's public image; it also brought into stark relief the limits of psychiatry's habit of reinvention.

From its inception, the DSM-5 Task Force embraced DSM-III as the template for how to reform psychiatric knowledge. In laying out its objectives, the DSM-5 Task Force framed its agenda in terms of "paradigm shift." This framing first appeared during a DSM-5 planning conference, the contents of which were later published in an edited volume.[127] While many of the conference's specific proposals were later abandoned, it established the Task Force's priority to "fundamentally alter the limited classification paradigm now in use."[128] In so doing, the Task Force linked its ambitions to DSM-III (rather than to the conservative revision of DSM-IV). This time, however, the Task Force adopted validity, rather than reliability, as a goal. DSM-5 would tackle "the goal of validating these syndromes and discovering common etiologies," which in "the more than 30 years since the introduction of the Feighner criteria by Robins and Guze" had remained "elusive."[129] By these means, the Task Force would nudge psychiatry out of ignorance.

While recognizing DSM-III was a "brilliant advance," the Task Force insisted that "it is now time to move on."[130] Evaluating the lack of progress in psychiatric research, it identified DSM-III itself as "*the* major factor in how little we yet know of the causes and cures of mental disorders."[131] DSM-III categories might be reliable, but they were mere heuristics. Kendler summarized the problems associated with the unquestioned acceptance of DSM:

> Many of us trained in the past two generations in psychiatry, especially those under the influence of the "DSMs," have come to consider our major diagnostic categories to be obvious and even "natural." They have become a part of our world view. However, the formulations of the categories in use have been heavily influenced by specific "expert" opinion, which, though certainly clinically informed, has been heavily influenced by a priori factors. In this situation, we are vulnerable to these historical contingencies, to arbitrary features of our heritage that reflect much better a particular essential view of psychiatric disorders rather than the empirical reality out there in the world.[132]

In short, DSM fostered reification; the constructed categories have all too often been treated as real diseases.[133] Critics argued that "in the hands of naive biological reductionists," its categories have been "oversold as diseases and worshiped as false icons."[134] The vicious combination of the wholesale reorganization of psychiatric research under DSM categories, when combined with the tendency to treat the heuristic categories as real diseases, has impeded the search for a mechanistic understanding of mental distress.

Instead, researchers target "arbitrary chimeras."[135] As one Task Force member stated in an interview, "If you and I were talking in 1980, we would have been sure that by this time that psychiatry would be primarily etiological. But it didn't happen. And it did not happen because of what DSM-III did."[136] Another member of the Task Force argued, "The field for sure has wasted a lot of its energy studying things at the syndrome level that are not likely to pay off at the syndrome level."[137] Rather than placing psychiatry on track to better research, DSM-III waylaid it.

With DSM at a "crossroads," reformers called for "another 'radical' new taxonomic paradigm" that focused on validity.[138] The DSM-5 Task Force signaled from the start that it would pursue changes on the magnitude of DSM-III. Committees were encouraged to "come up with native ideas," and they bought into the belief that "anything was possible."[139] Optimism abounded; one Task Force member recalled, "The way that this was all addressed in the warm-up was 'we're going to create a new valid taxonomy. And we're going to keep our eye on the prize.'"[140]

The Task Force hoped to replace the phenomenological diagnostic categories with a system based on the neurological/genetic mechanisms that cause particular symptoms. However, it was quickly determined that research in these fields had not progressed far enough to support such an ambition. "But when we got down to specific points and looked at the literature, there wasn't nearly as much we could go on because the studies have small numbers and they were often done with different techniques," noted a Task Force member. "The findings are rather fragmentary, suggestive but fragmentary, but certainly not enough to base huge changes on, from the standpoint of biology."[141] Retreating from this plan, the DSM-5 Task Force turned to dimensionalization as the means to achieve a paradigm shift.

The DSM-III diagnostic schema posited a categorical understanding of mental disorders. They were conceptualized as discrete conditions analogous to physical illnesses, defined by clusters of symptom manifestations. Such a categorical understanding constructs a rigid boundary between normality and pathology. However, mounting research favors a dimensional view of mental distress over a categorical model.[142] The DSM-5 Task Force reached "a growing realization that until we have dimensional measures we're not going to figure [mental illness] out."[143] To correct for what it perceived to be a "myth of discontinuity,"[144] it sought to dimensionalize DSM: "We have decided that one of the major—if not the major—differences between DSM-IV and DSM-5 will be the more prominent use of dimensional measures in DSM-5."[145] Dimensionalization entailed replacing the categorical logic of DSM-III with a classification system that recognized the continuous character of mental disorders, as divergences on spectra between normality and pathology. Rather than an either/or categorical assessment, patients would be assessed along a spectrum, with diagnoses expressed numerically. Mental disorders, formally conceived as *qualitatively* distinct, would be construed as *quantitatively* different, a difference in magnitude, not in kind.

In its most ambitious form, dimensionalization might have represented a paradigm shift. It might have reconceptualized the contemporary understanding of mental disorders. However, in response to internal resistance, the Task Force moderated its goals. Rather than a wholesale reconfiguration of the DSM categories, it settled on introducing a dimensional logic into DSM-5 through the inclusion of two types of quantitative scales—a general, cross-cutting dimensional scale to screen all prospective patients, and severity scales for each diagnosis. By introducing numerical scales, the Task Force hoped to encourage psychiatrists to begin to think about mental disorders in a more dimensional way. Yet, even as it narrowed its proposals, the DSM-5 Task Force never moderated its rhetoric. It continued to promote DSM-5 as a paradigm shift. The mundane-seeming scales would be the lever by which they would raise the profession.[146]

The Revolution Will Not Materialize

As the revision proceeded, some within the profession balked at the DSM-5 Task Force's pretenses to paradigm shift. Led by the two chairs of previous DSM revisions, Spitzer and Allen Frances (DSM-IV), this opposition grew concerned that the Task Force was acting rashly. They mobilized to rein it in. Frances, in particular, relished the role of DSM-5's chief critic, maintaining a regular blog on the *Psychiatric Times* website attacking the DSM-5 Task Force.

Critics' initial objections to DSM-5 were wide ranging, encompassing everything from accusations of incompetence to inappropriate ties to the pharmaceutical industry, from lack of transparency to bad writing. In 2009, Spitzer and Frances published a letter to the APA laying out their many concerns.[147] The APA leadership responded by painting Frances and Spitzer as disingenuous, arguing that their efforts were motivated by financial and reputational concerns.[148] Such interpersonal conflicts would color the debate over DSM-5. Over time, critics' varied complaints coalesced into a focus on the Task Force's paradigm shift strategy. In their criticism, opponents interpreted the state of psychiatry differently. Whereas the Task Force framed the current moment as one of "crisis," imbuing it with urgency that could only be resolved by another paradigm shift, opponents did not see things as dire. Although delayed, the Neo-Kraepelinian revolution was not in crisis. DSM-III may have been taking longer to yield its payoff than anticipated, but thirty years was not an unreasonable amount of time to wait for progress. The sense of urgency felt by members of the DSM-5 Task Force was a by-product, not of impending professional calamity, but of their unrealistic expectations. In truth, psychiatry was nowhere near as compromised as it had been in the 1970s, when the dominant paradigm had proved to be insolvent. Thus, to the Task Force's insistence that it was time for a paradigm shift, opponents retorted that "the DSM-V goal to effect a 'paradigm shift' in psychiatric diagnosis is absurdly premature."[149] For DSM-5's critics, there was no need for changes on the level of DSM-III.

Additionally, DSM-5 opponents believed that the aspirations for paradigm shift distorted the revision process itself. It led to disorganization, confusion, and an unnecessary cutting of corners. Indeed, the revision process was plagued by setbacks. Deadlines and benchmarks were missed. Delays forced the Task Force to cancel an entire second round of field testing, fueling complaints that the changes had not been properly vetted or assessed. In the rush to effect a revolution, "the work on DSM-V suffers from the unfortunate combination of being heavy on ambitious goals for change and light on the methodological rigor necessary to avoid the many problems that such change may cause once the system is in wide use," argued Frances.[150] The Task Force supplied the work groups with only the vaguest of guidance, particularly with regard to dimensionalization and the construction of the scales. One critic complained, "When I speak to friends on the various work groups, it doesn't seem to me, or to them, that there are specific directions coming from the Task Force about how this should be done and each of the workgroups is sort of thinking about different ways of approaching dimensionality diagnoses."[151] Once the "grand ambition to provide a 'paradigm shift' in psychiatric diagnosis, based on the identification of biological markers," was determined to be unattainable, the Task Force should have abandoned any pretense of a paradigm shift, critics argued.[152] Instead, it doubled down, entertaining ideas for which there was no obvious consensus or demand. The scope of the proposed change—the dangers when "everything is on the table"—and its pace—"claiming too much too soon"—resulted in poor execution and changes that were likely to create "havoc."[153]

In opposing the Task Force's *invocation* of paradigm shift by the DSM-5 Task Force, critics were not necessarily disputing the logic of reinvention as a professional strategy altogether. They too recognized DSM-III as a watershed event and a legitimate transformation; after all, DSM-5's most vocal opponents were associated with the previous editions. But they questioned whether the current situation necessitated such dramatic action. In the minds of DSM-5 detractors, paradigm shifts should be treated as rare events. It was foolhardy to try "to jump-start a paradigm shift" before its time had come.[154] "We know that the system we have now doesn't map onto reality," argued one critic, "but since we don't know what reality is, we have no idea what the paradigm shift might be."[155] By acting prematurely, the Task Force was inviting "a backlash against psychiatry."[156] Constant dramatic changes might "poison the reputation"[157] of DSM and, by extension, psychiatry. To be considered scientific, "classifications have to stay relatively stable."[158] Thus, to the Task Force's insistence that it "was now time" to change course, opponents argued that the Task Force was rushing something that, by nature, took time. Patience, not panic, was coached.

Over the course of the revisions, however, this defense of the status quo and the questionable timing of DSM-5 morphed into something more fundamental. The dispute evolved in such a way as to put the whole question of reinvention in the crosshairs of critics. Some began to raise epistemological questions regarding *how* psychiatric knowledge should proceed. This involved an acknowledgment of psychiatry's history of reinvention and a confrontation with its implications. The continual recourse to dramatic change seemed, well, flaky. Disturbed by psychiatry's constant pursuit of revolution and paradigm shift, DSM-5's criticism countered with a commitment to incrementalism.

In a 2010 article, Kendler and Michael First described the DSM-5 debate as involving two distinct visions of psychiatric thought: "the 'iterative model' of the opponents, in which incremental changes are made while retaining the fundamental assumptions of the existing model, and the 'paradigm shift model' of the DSM-5 Task Force, where the underlying paradigm is discarded in favor of a fundamentally new approach."[159] The iterative model "assumes that using increasingly rigorous empirical methods, each subsequent revision of our diagnostic system will produce improvements over its predecessor."[160] Under epistemic iteration, science evolves in a cumulative fashion. Epistemic iteration does not require that the initial foundations are sound or even accurate. A discipline needs to start somewhere. But initial assumptions would be held lightly with the understanding that they would be revised "through successive stages of scientific research toward a better and better approximation of reality in 'a spiral of improvement.'"[161]

The commitment to epistemic iteration did not mean rejecting the narrative of DSM-III as a paradigm shift. Nor did it mean rejecting psychiatry's past reinvents out of hand (although these were perceived as indicators of psychiatry's immaturity and lack of scientific rigor). Rather, it meant resisting *future* reinventions as a strategy going forward. Psychiatry had been there, tried that, to no avail. This was joined with an interpretation of DSM-III as a singular event, the reinvention to finally end the cycle of reinvention. While imperfect, DSM-III had provided a foundation for scientific psychiatry. It should be allowed to unfold according to its own pace. Psychiatrists ought to focus their efforts on the incremental development of this foundation, not its dismantling. Thus, iteration carried with it an implied critique of psychiatry's history. Reinvention after reinvention had not tamed ignorance. Given this checkered history, perhaps it would be more prudent to commit to a paradigm instead of being enticed, once again, by the next new thing.

To transform epistemic interaction into an actionable strategy, opponents of DSM-5 lobbied the APA to create an independent committee to check potential overreach. In 2010, responding to negative publicity and a chorus of complaints, the APA established the Scientific Review Committee (SRC) to review the scientific justification for every proposal and ensure "the rigor and consistency of the DSM review process."[162] Although the SRC was limited to an advisory role to the APA president and the Board of Trustees, it exercised tremendous influence on the revision, since the board had final approval over the revisions. To head the committee, the APA chose Kendler, a fortuitous choice for the opposition, given his sympathies for epistemic iteration. The SRC imposed more onerous standards on proposed revisions, insisting that they had to be justified by empirical research. This prohibited the work groups and Task Force from making significant changes. They were caught in a catch-22. It was difficult, if not impossible, to locate research justifying significant changes to DSM when the overwhelming bulk of existing research is designed around DSM categories. By these means, the SRC effectively handcuffed the DSM-5 revisions. Those on the Task Force and work groups who aspired for significant changes complained that the SRC had "moved the goal posts in the middle of the game."[163] But these complaints fell on deaf ears. While the SRC rejected fewer than half of the proposals it evaluated, this number underestimates its effect, as the Task Force withdrew an unknown number of revisions before ever being assessed, in anticipation that they would not meet the SRC's standards. In this manner, the SRC imposed incrementalism upon the revision process.

While significant, the SRC was not solely responsible for DSM-5's failure. In many ways, this failure was overdetermined. As soon as the DSM-5 Task Force uttered the words "paradigm shift," it exposed itself to heightened expectations. These expectations served to mobilize forces for the status quo before the revision could gain momentum. DSM-5 faced vested interests like insurers, drug companies, and patient groups that risked losing something should the manual be radically revised. Intertwined and built into the mental health system, DSM categories had become "locked in," accruing significant inertia.[164] The very success of DSM-III made it difficult to change the manual in any sort of significant way. Moreover, the predominance DSM had gained after the DSM-III revision ensured that any subsequent revision would be highly scrutinized. Unlike the DSM-III revision, which had operated in obscurity, the DSM-5 revision was a major news event that intensified the pressure on the Task Force. With every change adjudicated in the public sphere, the Task Force was constantly distracted by public relations.

The spirited controversy over DSM-5 culminated at the APA's annual meeting in May 2012. During this meeting, two events occurred that finally derailed any pretense the DSM-5 Task Force had of achieving a paradigm shift. First, the Task Force announced the results of its field trials. The findings regarding reliability of the proposals were underwhelming.[165] DSM-5 did not appear to be an improvement over DSM-III. The lackluster results only fueled criticisms that the revision was unnecessary, unwarranted, and premature. Second, and more significantly, the APA Assembly voted at the meeting to reject the Task Force's severity scales. The scales had assumed great symbolic importance as the Task Force's last shot at dimensionalization. As such, they became a flashpoint of controversy, not only between the Task Force and its critics, but between psychiatric researchers and clinicians over the issue of clinical utility. While DSM "tries to be all things to all people,"[166] clinical utility has long been held to be DSM's primary goal. Despite this avowed emphasis, psychiatric researchers have controlled the revision process since DSM-III. To clinicians, it seemed that utility often long took a backseat to the interests of researchers in the revisions.[167] Now assessing the clinical utility of the scales, the Assembly, composed primarily of clinicians, found them wanting. Their "level of sophistication has been achieved at the cost of a simple approach that clinicians are going to be able to use in their daily practice."[168] The scales might be useful for researchers (e.g., they might standardize the measurement of severity, ensuring consistent data collection across contexts), but their hasty construction and divergent logics promised little to clinicians, other than more paperwork. The Assembly voted unanimously to relegate any dimensional scales to the appendix, citing their lack of utility and the undue burden they placed upon clinicians. Although the Assembly resolution was nonbinding, the Task Force could not risk outright revolt among the APA's rank and file. In the end, the Task Force abandoned the very scales that, for better or worse, had become the centerpiece of the revision.

Rebuked, the Task Force began to walk back its paradigm-shifting rhetoric, adopting the incremental language resonant with that of their most vehement critics. In its own introduction, DSM-5 is defined as a transitional document: "The DSM-5 Task Force overseeing the new edition recognized that research advances will require careful, *iterative* changes if DSM is to maintain its place as the touchstone classification of mental disorders."[169] While the manual has been reorganized and includes important changes to specific categories (i.e., the elimination of Asperger's syndrome), care has been taken so that continuity was "maintained with previous editions of the DSM."[170] And while the introduction endorses dimensionality as a goal, it defers revisions along these lines to the future.[171] The categorical logic of DSM-III endures. In fact, the APA's formal letter announcing DSM-5 did not even mention the dimensionality.[172] DSM-5 is being sold as a "living document," a status symbolically represented in a change in the manual's naming convention from Roman numerals (i.e., DSM-IV) to Arabic numerals (i.e., DSM-5), which can be regularly updated (i.e., DSM-5.1, DSM-5.2, etc.). The APA will no longer undertake major revisions every decade or so, but will amend it as needed. Epistemic iteration has won the day for now.

Conclusion

Mere days before DSM-5's publication, the NIMH announced that it would be moving away from research oriented around DSM categories. In doing so, NIMH director Tom Insel stated bluntly, "We [researchers] cannot succeed if we use DSM categories as the 'gold standard,'" and for this reason the NIMH "will be re-orienting its research away from DSM categories."[173] In its place, the NIMH is promoting an alternative classification system, Research Domain Criteria (RDoC), as its preferred framework. RDoC rests on firm assumptions regarding the ontology of mental disorders. Mental disorders are brain disorders, and "the dysfunction in neural circuits can be identified with the tools of clinical neuroscience."[174] RDoC intends to develop a new classification system based not on phenotypic symptoms but on underlying neurobiological mechanisms. Consistent with the NIMH's more general pivot to neuroscience, the NIMH hopes that RDoC will jump-start future translational research.

The timing of the NIMH announcement spoke volumes. Amid what was supposed to be DSM-5's triumphant unveiling, the NIMH stole the spotlight to announce a significant shift in psychiatric nosology *away* from DSM. More significantly, RDoC signaled that the aspiration to achieve a universal classification system for all would no longer be the motive force driving psychiatric nosology. Unlike DSM, which claims to serve all interests, RDoC decouples research needs from clinical concerns to develop a classification system constructed for research purposes only.[175] With its substantial institutional backing, RDoC indicates that the era of a one-size-fits-all nosology is over.

The DSM-5 Task Force scrambled to minimize the fallout from the announcement, circulating a joint press release with the NIMH that insisted on the complementary relationship between the two classifications. But on the tail of the contentious revision, the NIMH's announcement could only be interpreted as a hit on DSM's reputation. The symbolic impact of RDoC eclipses its practical implications. It does not end DSM's relevancy—the manual will continue to serve important clinical and institutional purposes— but it does bring to an end its hegemony over psychiatric nosology.

RDoC also reveals a growing dissatisfaction with the Neo-Kraepelinian vision. As mundane parts of working infrastructures, classifications rarely garner consideration for those who use them, much less attract media attention. DSM is no typical classification manual. It has become the symbol of a paradigm shift, of a profession striving to reinvent itself as a hard biomedical science. Its dry prose belies its revolutionary significance; written between its lines are the hopes of a profession. Any challenge to DSM, therefore, strikes at the heart of contemporary psychiatry.

DSM-III was lauded by Neo-Kraepelinians as securing the reliability crucial to the development of a robust research base. But its effects on alleviating psychiatric ignorance have been minimal. While DSM-III may have improved reliability, the question is, at what cost? Standardization carries risks. If non-valid, albeit reliable, diagnostic classifications became standardized and widely adopted, they risk setting an entire research program on the wrong path. DSM-III may have committed psychiatry to classifications of dubious worth. The lack of research progress in psychiatry suggests to many exactly this. More than three decades in, psychiatry remains ignorant of the mechanisms of mental disorders. Neuroscience and genetic research have not clarified the workings of the mind. With the payoff of this research elusive, some "wonder whether anything has been learned to warrant all of the efforts put into these studies."[176] Psychiatry bet on DSM-III. The bet has not paid off. Consequently, a malaise has once again descended upon the profession. Psychiatry "finds itself at a crossroad" (again).[177] The hopes that drove the Neo-Kraepelinian revolution have not been extinguished altogether, but like the reinventions that preceded it, optimism is running out.

The setbacks for psychiatry go beyond research. Despite the cultural influence of DSM-III, psychiatry's jurisdiction has shrunk since its publication. Compared to previous generations, contemporary psychiatrists *do* less. Psychiatrists' role in the field of mental health has been largely reduced to medication management. Even this reduced role is precarious. Questions regarding the efficacy and safety of drug treatments have gained increasing traction, as has skepticism toward the "pill-and-neuron story" upon which such treatments are rationalized.[178] Furthermore, psychiatrists' control over medication management is being threatened. Primary care physicians, not psychiatrists, prescribe most of the psychopharmaceutical drugs in circulation, and the legal protections that grant psychiatrists a monopoly over prescribing medication are being challenged by clinical psychologists in state legislatures.[179] The insecurity and anxiety that accompany this shrinking jurisdiction manifest in a professional paranoia. "We have enemies," warned APA president Nada Stotland, enemies who "refuse to believe that psychiatric illnesses are serious," who "say that psychiatric treatments are not 'scientific,'" and who insist "that psychiatric disorders aren't real because we have not discovered specific etiologies for them."[180] The DSM-III revolution was supposed to provide the answers to psychiatry's vexing questions and quell such criticisms. It did not. Its descriptive categories were supposed to provide the foundation for research leading toward valid diagnoses. They have not. While DSM-III changed how mental disorders are thought about in the United States, it has not translated into secure professional authority.

These very concerns led the DSM-5 Task Force to pursue its own paradigm shift.[181] In its rhetoric, the DSM-5 Task Force invoked DSM-III. It sought to repeat its history. But the deck was stacked against DSM-5 from the start. Classification, as sociologists have shown, can confer great power upon certain ways of seeing; when institutionalized, these frameworks become privileged as part of the common sense by which individuals segment and divide the world.[182] However, the power of classification is derived in great part from being under the radar as a mundane and invisible aspect of information infrastructure. When classifications become visible, so too do the politics of their construction. DSM-III benefited from its marginality and obscurity. Few psychiatrists anticipated that revolutionary change could be affected via diagnostic reform. Indeed, the idea would have struck most psychodynamic psychiatrists as preposterous. As a result, Spitzer and the Task Force were able to gain momentum before anyone realized what was happening. The DSM-5 Task Force enjoyed no such luxury. Their revisions took place under the glare of intense scrutiny and media focus. Those committed to the status quo had plenty of advance warning and fought proposals every step along the way. Of course, the Task Force did not do itself any favors with its lack of subtlety. To its discredit, it spoke the language of paradigm shift publicly and prominently. This too put the forces for the status quo on alert, leaving the Task Force vulnerable to attacks that it was being rash.

Still, more than anything the DSM-5 Task Force did, the DSM-5 revision was undermined by historical developments that preceded it. The Task Force was always at a disadvantage, due to the very success of DSM-III. DSM-III success raised the bar for changes as well as the public scrutiny the DSM-5 Task Force would have to face. For while a massive overhaul of classification can convey mastery the first time, any subsequent revision of similarly radical aspiration can betray a lack of mastery, a nervous fiddling. This invites questions as to whether the whole exercise might be arbitrary. In short, the historical success of DSM-III made revolutionary changes through DSM-5 unlikely.

With DSM imbricated in all aspects of mental health care, any changes risked significant disruption. They would not be accepted without a fight. DSM-5 faced the headwind of the forces for the status quo, and the Task Force was never able to navigate these winds. Indeed, the DSM-5 Task Force did not foresee these challenges. And in a sense, who can fault them? After all, psychiatry has spent the better part of 150 years reinventing itself. Who can blame the DSM-5 Task Force for thinking they could carry on this august tradition?

DSM-5's failure demarcates a crucial moment in the history of psychiatry's reinvention. For the first time, reformers, through the language of paradigm shift, explicitly endorsed reinvention as a legitimate means to address ignorance. For the first time, they consciously articulated what had long been psychiatry's habitual response to professional crisis. And for the first time, reinvention was roundly rejected. The historical consciousness that developed in the wake of community psychiatry reached a full flowering in the DSM-5 controversy. Through its use of paradigm-shifting rhetoric, the DSM-5 Task Force invoked reinvention, adopting an interpretive framework consistent with reinventions in the past. The profession was in crisis; as in the past, the proposed solution was reinvention. However, unlike previous eras, these efforts were met with a countermobilization against reinvention itself. DSM-5's critics, aware of psychiatry's checkered past, questioned aloud whether the best course forward was another reboot. Beyond the specific debates over the merits of particular reforms, psychiatrists in the DSM-5 debate grappled with a deeper epistemological question as to how psychiatric knowledge *ought* to proceed. Embracing the way psychiatric reform had always been done, the DSM-5 Task Force held up reinvention as a strategy. It explicitly endorsed the epistemological assumptions upon which psychiatric reformers had long been acting, but which had remained prethematic and in the background. Just as previous generations of reformers had, the DSM-5 Task Force sought reinvention. It just was not shy about it.

The explicitness with which the DSM-5 Task Force embraced reinvention provided the discursive opportunity to dissect its merits. Critics responded, challenging not just the legitimacy of *this* paradigm shift, but of paradigm shifts (or reinvention) as a general strategy. They articulated, for the first time, an alternative approach to psychiatric ignorance—epistemic iteration. Rather than repeat the cycle of reinvention-crisis-reinvention, critics advocated staying the course and allowing knowledge to grow incrementally. Psychiatric ignorance had never been fixed by forging clear breaks from the past and adopting a new program. Perhaps it was time to try a different approach.

In the end, epistemic iteration won out in the controversy over DSM-5. Whether psychiatry will maintain a commitment to epistemic iteration going forward—whether it has escaped its cyclical trajectory—remains to be seen. Old habits die hard. However, regardless of how things play out, the mere articulation of epistemic iteration as an alternative is a significant development for the politics of ignorance. It indicates an increasing unease with the habit of reinvention. Faced with a history of accumulated failures, of overzealous commitment fueled by misplaced optimism, some psychiatrists ponder whether there might be a better way to manage their ignorance.

Conclusion

Psychiatry has been shaped less by the knowledge it has secured and more by the ignorance that it cannot resolve. Indeed, the most striking feature of psychiatry's history is how little progress it has made in resolving its basic questions. That psychiatry has changed, there can be no doubt. But how far has it really come? Confessions of ignorance in the past eerily echo those of today. Philippe Pinel, considered a founder of psychiatry, observed centuries ago, "Mental disease appears to tax the attention of good observers because it presents itself to us as a mixture of incoherence and confusion."[1] This statement still rings true. Psychiatry remains as enveloped in ignorance as ever.

Today, once again, psychiatrists are coping with the precariousness that accompanies its stubborn ignorance. Today, once again, there are calls to rethink the psychiatric enterprise. In the past fifty years, psychiatrists have narrowed their jurisdiction and reduced the scope of their expertise. Backing deinstitutionalization, they displaced patients with serious mental illness from the center of their concerns. Inpatient treatment of this population endures—albeit in a far more limited scope—but psychiatrists direct their aspirations elsewhere. Additionally, in the rush to jettison outmoded Freudian thought, psychiatrists have ceded concerns of the mind to their competitors. Psychotherapy has become the province of psychologists and social workers.

Contemporary psychiatrists have largely reduced their professional authority to medication management. Their professional identity is "now closely bound up with its monopoly over the prescribing of drugs."[2] But psychopharmaceutical drug treatments are being assailed on multiple fronts. With meta-analyses suggesting mixed benefits and fueling suspicions that these drugs are little more than placebos,[3] skepticism grows. The current generation of psychopharmaceutical drugs no longer appear to be the magic bullets they were promoted as. This fuels accusations that psychiatrists have become willing conspirators with pharmaceutical companies, that they have sold out, sullied their reputations, and enabled drug companies' insatiable pursuit of profit.[4] The fraught alliance between psychiatry and pharmaceutical companies has grown more tenuous as drug companies face their own challenges, including a drying pipeline for new psychopharmaceutical drugs[5] and high-profile lawsuits for misleading claims regarding antidepressants.[6] At the same time that the psychiatric drug treatments are losing their allure, psychiatrists' monopoly over prescribing them is being challenged. As noted in the previous chapter, most prescriptions are written by physicians other than psychiatrists,[7] and clinical psychologists have won the right to prescribe in five states. Add these developments together and psychiatrists find themselves in a weakened state. The victories of the Neo-Kraepelinian reinvention, like those of reinventions before it, have been scant.

By no means do these developments suggest that psychiatry is doomed. History is littered with premature declarations and smug prophecies of psychiatry's death, only to see psychiatry resurrected, phoenix-like, on the promises of the next new reinvention.

Neuroscience is the most recent candidate for such a reinvention. Like many other fields, psychiatry has been swept up in "neuroscientific hype" driven by breathless media coverage and the mystique of fMRI.[8] Recent developments evince a "neuro-turn" in psychiatry, particularly in its aspirational, research wing. This neuro-turn champions "neurobiological conceptions of personhood," namely, that we are our brains.[9] Scrambling to adapt fMRI to research mental disorders, psychiatry increasingly embraces "a zeitgeist increasingly conceptualizing neuropsychological dysfunctions as being at the root of psychological problems."[10] If mind can be reduced to brain, it follows that psychiatrists should focus on the brain to explain madness. They must become applied neuroscientists.

External forces are pushing psychiatry in this direction. Despite President George H. W. Bush's designation of the 1990s as the "Decade of the Brain," the past ten years more aptly fit this designation. In 2013, President Barack Obama announced the BRAIN initiative (Brain Research through Advancing Innovative Neurotechnologies), a public/private research initiative seeking "to revolutionize our understanding of the human mind and uncover new ways to treat, prevent, and cure brain disorders like Alzheimer's, schizophrenia, autism, epilepsy, and traumatic brain injury."[11] With an initial $100 million in funding allocated, BRAIN is big science on a scale comparable to the Human Genome Project. In conjunction with BRAIN, the NIMH has shifted its priorities to neuroscience. Tom Insel, NIMH director from 2002 to 2015, overhauled its research portfolio to steer most of its $1.5 billion budget to neuroscience, primarily to RDoC-inspired research and the Human Connectome Project, a five-year effort to build a network map ("connectome") of the functioning human brain.[12] In 2012, just 10% of NIMH's overall research funding went to clinical research.[13] Joshua Gordon, Insel's successor, is continuing this course. He is enthralled by optogenetics, a method that combines techniques from optics and genetics to trace the activities of individual neurons.[14] The NIMH's most recent Strategic Plan asserts that "fundamental to our mission is the proposition that mental illnesses are brain disorders expressed as complex cognitive, emotional and social behavioral syndromes" and that "progress [in psychiatric research] depends on advances in basic behavioral science and fundamental neuroscience."[15] Critics object to these developments, accusing leadership of transforming the NIMH into "exclusively a brain institute," one that neglects clinical research on psychotherapy and mental health services.[16] But, like other scientific fields, research psychiatry is undergoing what sociologist Sara Shostak calls "molecularization."[17] Doubling down on the search for the neural correlates of mental distress, psychiatry seeks the resolution of its ignorance at the submicroscopic level.

One can raise legitimate questions as to whether the neuro-turn represents a unique reinvention or merely a renewed commitment to the last Neo-Kraepelinian one. But it is certainly being promoted as novel and revolutionary. The grandiose rhetoric surrounding psychiatry's embrace of neuroscience induces vertiginous déjà vu. "Legions of dedicated scientists and over 60 dedicated professional societies worldwide" stand poised at the ready "to understand mental disorders in terms of the biological function of the nervous system."[18] Scientific opportunities, "unprecedented in human history," are there for the taking, awaiting only psychiatry's full commitment. Once again, we hear promises of new, more effective treatments, this time under the rubric of "precision medicine."[19] Once again, psychiatry is proclaimed to be "at a crossroad" in need of rejuvenation. Once again, we see reformers generating expectations that psychiatry's issues will be resolved, once and for all. Once again, psychiatric ignorance is framed as a temporary problem with a clear fix. This rhetoric is eerily reminiscent of that of the asylum, and of psychobiology, and of psychoanalysis, and of community psychiatry, and of diagnostic psychiatry. Neuroscience is playing a similar role in managing ignorance for psychiatry today as past reinventions did for previous generations of psychiatrists. The hopes are the same; they are just dressed in a different cloak. Psychiatry is a profession that writes lavish promissory notes. And yet.

The parallel with previous reinventions does not mean the neuroscientific vision of psychiatry will necessarily fail, that it will succumb to the same fate of its predecessors. It is far too early to tell. Tomorrow a neuroscientific breakthrough might occur. Revelatory fMRI images might illuminate the mysteries of the mind. Psychiatry's long, tortured relationship with ignorance might finally come to an end. It might all have been worth it. I don't know. Nor am I interested in indulging such oracular exercises. As I noted in the introduction, from the standpoint of today, we have no way of knowing whether psychiatry's ignorance is temporary or permanent, whether it is an issue of epistemology—we have not yet figured out *how* to understand mental distress—or an issue of ontology—that, as a matter of property, we *can't* know it. Still, count me as guardedly skeptical, less about neuroimaging as an interesting tool for research and more about the hype of neuroscience as psychiatry's savior. Steeped in psychiatry's history of failures, I have my suspicions. But they amount to just that—suspicions. History need not repeat. This time could very well be different. Failure is not inevitable, but neither is success.

In pressing forward, we should heed the lessons of psychiatry's history. Under conditions of uncertainty and ignorance, caution is warranted, for all parties involved. Psychiatrists should not repeat the mistake of believing its own hype and overcommitting prematurely to the newest shiny thing. And for those of us on the outside of psychiatry, looking in, we should cast a skeptical eye toward this latest round of bullish predictions. The protean character of mental distress should disabuse us of dreams of easy explanations and warn us away from efforts that pursue a monocausal account of mental illness. We have been here, done that before.

To conclude this book, I adopt a wider lens in the service of two distinct tasks. First, speaking to fellow social scientists, I advocate for a research program on professional politics—and politics generally—that maintains an abiding appreciation of the role of ignorance in these processes. From the case of psychiatry, I extract and identify an array of tactics available to professions (and collective actors in general) to manage and mitigate the effects of ignorance. The resulting classification of tactics is intended to provide an effective language for future research. My hope is that such research will expand our understanding of the breadth, scope, and diversity by which ignorance is managed. Once we acknowledge ignorance as a fundamental feature—and not merely a bug—of professions and elevate it to the appropriate place in our analyses, we can begin to unearth the many ways in which it drives professional politics and practice.

In the second section of the conclusion, I take up the sticky question that is hinted at but not explicitly addressed throughout the book. Why do we keep accepting psychiatry's reinventions? If these reinventions repeatedly fail, why do we continue to go along with them? We might mock psychiatrists in *New Yorker* cartoons and deride them as doctors who are not quite legitimate (or worse, quacks). We might vocalize antipsychiatry sentiments and express dismay toward particular psychiatric treatments. But we continue to endorse the profession's authority. We seek psychiatrists' counsel when we or our loved ones succumb to mental distress. What's more, we pour energy and resources into supporting psychiatry's inclinations and transformations. Why? Surely, part of the explanation lies in the efficacy of the tactics psychiatric reformers have adopted in response to ignorance. But this explanation only gets us so far in understanding psychiatry's persistence. It is wrong to view psychiatric power as a conspiracy foisted upon an unwitting public. We choose to buy what psychiatrists are selling. Our enduring support cannot be explained by psychiatrists' magical capacity to fool us.

To begin to understand why psychiatry maintains our support, we must first appreciate that the ignorance regarding mental distress is not the sole property of psychiatry alone. We all share it. However, unlike psychiatry, most of us would rather not grapple with it. Psychiatry endures, I argue, through a combination of inertia and societal indifference toward those with serious mental illness. Madness, insanity, mental illness, or whatever one calls it undermines our most cherished perception of ourselves as reasoned, rational creatures. It reveals our collective fragility, presents us with inconvenient truths, and induces a terror that most of us cannot face. We would rather turn a blind eye or a deaf ear than accept madness as a possibility for ourselves. Once psychiatrists took the responsibility of the mad away from families and local communities, we as a society have been more than willing to allow them to resume the responsibility, absent a viable alternative. We have abdicated our duty to those with serious mental illness. They have become psychiatry's problem. For this reason, historian Jack Pressman has deemed psychiatry "a field demarcated by our collective helplessness."[20] Ignorant, impotent, and unsure of what to do, we willingly pass the buck to psychiatrists, despite their obvious failings.

Recognizing our collective ignorance and culpability not only helps explain psychiatry's endurance; it should clarify our criticisms of it by shifting the locus of responsibility onto us all. This is not to declare psychiatry innocent or excuse its failings; rather, it is to see psychiatry as a symptom of a more widespread societal illness. For too long, we have allowed psychiatry to play the all-too-easy role of scapegoat. Yes, psychiatry has deserved much of the opprobrium thrown its way. But in our haste to point a wagging finger elsewhere, we obscure the true source of the problem—ourselves. What if psychiatry's true function is not to resolve ignorance, but rather to make apparent good-faith gestures in trying to do so, so that we can delude ourselves into thinking we are doing something? What if psychiatry's role is to become the repository for our fears of madness so we can carry on without the burden? What if we are willing accomplices in the deception of reinvention? What if we get the psychiatry we deserve? What if we demanded more?

When Knowing Is Not an Option

Social scientists have had a blind spot when it comes to ignorance, displaying "a certain sociological ignorance of ignorance."[21] For example, the sociology of professions has focused on the production, accumulation, and contests over knowledge. This understandable emphasis has led to a neglect of the unique and specific dynamics that surround the professional politics of ignorance.[22] However, a small group of researchers, operating under the banner of ignorance studies,[23] is countering this oversight by recognizing ignorance as a vital topic of social scientific study in its own right. Rather than viewing ignorance as the mere absence of knowledge or as a deviant state to be overcome, these researchers begin from the premise that ignorance is an omnipresent feature of social life. By doing so, they open promising vistas for research, the potential of which has only begun to be tapped.

Much research remains to be done in order to understand the interplay between ignorance and professional power. Indeed, professions have a complicated relationship with ignorance. On the one hand, professional power *depends* on ignorance, specifically outsiders' ignorance. Professions are granted autonomy and control over their work because their expertise is deemed to be of such a specialized character that only professionals themselves can understand it.[24] In turn, only they can organize their work in a rational fashion. Lay outsiders cannot effectively regulate that which they do not understand. Thus, the ignorance of nonprofessionals justifies the very privileges afforded to professions to determine their own course. Their ignorance sustains the "professional mystery" that underwrites professional autonomy.[25] Knowledge that becomes too codified, transparent, or available voids the rationale for professional autonomy. Ignorance, therefore, has its professional uses.

On the other hand, as we have seen, ignorance within a profession can threaten to undermine its authority. The public is willing to grant professions some leeway here; after all, these are complicated topics and tasks with which professions must grapple. But if ignorance becomes too evident or if it is perceived as too extensive, professions risk losing their authority. Therefore, ignorance is a potential problem for every profession, one that must be negotiated and mitigated if professional authority is to be maintained. Because this authority is dependent on claims to expertise and because all human knowledge is limited and imperfect, all professions must negotiate, overcome, or elide that which they do not know. Their very existence is premised on maintaining the perception that they have overcome ignorance, or at least that they can manage it and prevent it from negatively affecting their work. As such, all professions must delicately balance that which they do know and that which they do not.

Consequently, ignorance has a Janus-faced character for professions. It is a source of professional authority and a potential source of weakness. It can both serve a function *and/or* present thorny, existential problems. The one thing it cannot be is entirely eliminated. Fallible and without access to perfect knowledge, humans everywhere must make do with imperfect knowledge. But the stakes are raised when it comes to professions.

The specific balance between knowledge and ignorance differs for each profession. Generally speaking, the dilemmas posed by ignorance are more acute for "consulting professions"[26] than scientific professions. For the latter, ignorance lacks a certain urgency. To the contrary, even, ignorance can provide the motivation and justification for scientists' continued work; it spurs calls for more research and a redoubling of efforts.[27] This contrasts with the situation facing consulting professions. Professions, like engineering, law, and medicine, are called upon to act, to provide services to clientele that display some sort of efficacy despite the gaps in their knowledge base. They are asked not just to *know something*, but to *do something*—often with an audience. Implored to act on their knowledge, consulting professions continuously risk the exposure of their ignorance in the concrete results they obtain (or fail to). For these professions, ignorance can mean the difference between recognition and rejection, legitimacy and irrelevance, a job or unemployment, and even life or death.

Psychiatry, however, grapples with its ignorance to an extent unseen in other consulting professions. Its failings have been dramatic and public; its successes, rare, disputed, and mainly pyrrhic. Psychiatry lacks a basic understanding of its object. This troubling state introduces instability in the very framing of mental distress—notice its changing ontology—and, by extension, psychiatrists' very identity—evidenced in the wholesale reimaginings of psychiatry. Sociologist Rose Laub Coser observes that while "in every specialty the practitioner learns to act in the face of some degree of uncertainty; in psychiatry that uncertainty can hardly be ignored."[28] Unlike other medical specialties, psychiatry possesses very few unmistakable triumphs it can point to as indications that it is on the path to knowing.

Unable to deny or ignore its ignorance, psychiatry has maintained its authority by delicately negotiating it. This negotiation has hinged on how psychiatric ignorance is understood. When it comes to ignorance, perceptions matter. Psychiatrists have attempted to put the field's ignorance in the best possible light. This has involved framing its characteristic features in such a way as to minimize the significance of their ignorance and manage its effects. First, psychiatrists have had to attend to the nature of their ignorance, specifically its source and origins. Is ignorance a result of psychiatrists' failings (e.g., psychiatrists are bad/uninterested/neglectful researchers)? Or does it reflect something about the character of its object (e.g., is mental distress itself resistant to explanation)? Second, psychiatrists have had to grapple with perceptions regarding the scope and magnitude of their ignorance. Is this ignorance all-encompassing and thus damning, suggesting the need for an alternative? Or is it contained and controllable, suggesting that the reasonable response is to stay the course? Third, psychiatrists have had to speak to the motivations behind their ignorance. Is it intentional and willful (e.g., psychiatrists perpetuate false theories to secure power)? Or unintentional and involuntary (e.g., they want to understand but cannot)? Finally, psychiatrists have had to address the temporal character of their ignorance. Is it temporary? Or permanent? If a profession can demonstrate a modicum of progress and a record of success, it is granted some benefit of the doubt and the requisite breathing room to resolve its ignorance. If not, if its ignorance is perceived as permanent, a matter of property, substantial in scope, or even if its resolution is taking too long, a profession is susceptible to existential challenges. Such has been the fate of psychiatry.

Primarily, the contentious process of framing of the character of psychiatric ignorance has focused on a basic question with which generations of psychiatrists have grappled. Is mental illness "unknown *but* knowable" or "unknown *and* unknowable"? Dealing with this question has required constant policing on the part of psychiatrists. The very existence of their profession is at stake. Why accord the professional benefits—autonomy, authority, prestige, and so on—to a group that cannot know its object and thus uphold their end of the professional bargain? Why vouchsafe their credibility and grant them protections if their ignorance is recalcitrant? To justify their profession's continued existence, psychiatrists have had to affirm the "knowability" of mental illness or, at the very least, delay others from refuting it.

Reinvention

The unique depth and persistence of psychiatry's ignorance has led generations of reformers to pursue the atypical course of reinvention. Whenever a crisis arises, whenever psychiatry's ignorance begins to seem unresolvable, reinvention comes to the rescue, resetting things and changing the benchmarks by which progress is assessed. Through reinvention, psychiatric reformers reframe ignorance that might be considered unknowable into something potentially knowable provided the right reforms are adopted. This reorients the assessment of psychiatry away from past and present failings toward future promises. The credibility of psychiatry becomes tied to ex ante anticipations of psychiatric reforms, rather than ex post facto assessments of its disappointments. Psychiatry is reconstituted in a future idiom. As long as psychiatry's patrons can be convinced that the new direction is promising, psychiatrists can avoid the professional fallout from their ignorance. Reinvention serves a delaying function, deferring the final reckoning to some ever-receding future.

Therefore, at root, reinvention is about rescuing hope from the ashes of failure. By its means, generations of psychiatric reformers have promulgated expectations that psychiatric ignorance will be resolved, and they have done so precisely at the moments in which it has appeared intractable. Future expectations and promises are crucial to understanding social action, for they provide the dynamism and momentum for new endeavors.[29] To garner support for reforms, to generate the hype necessary for buy-in, and to build the needed infrastructure and networks to pursue them, reformers articulate expectations of where the reforms will lead.[30] The future is transformed from an empty neutral space to one populated with promise and vision. In this way, expectations are performative and constitutive; they produce "the incentives and obligations that will be necessary to mobilize the necessary resources for a particular aspiration to be realized."[31] The actions that hype spurs are more important than its outcomes. Indeed, it matters little whether the hype ever comes to fruition. This is a simple matter of timing. The investment in hype, by necessity, antedates the assessment of the fruits of this investment. Thus, even highly misleading and ultimately disappointing hype can have significant effects.

Via expectations, psychiatry has wrested professional success from knowledge failures. Indeed, generation after generation of reformers have transformed these failures into moments of possible liberation. Heightened expectations keep everyone interested, engaged, and compliant. Sociologist

Andrew Scull argues that psychiatrists are "like the poor folks waiting for Godot (who, as it happens, were quite possibly waiting for a madman)," awaiting the arrival of "those mysterious and long-rumored" explanations of the causes of mental distress.[32] It is the expectations promulgated by reformers that have kept psychiatry alive, and us waiting.

Consequently, reinvention performs crucial *time work* for psychiatrists. Time work involves the reframing of time, particularly past and future, so as to chart a course of action in the present. In terms of the past, reinvention involves the construction and reconstruction of interpretations through narratives. Trying to "work the past" in a way favorable to one's objectives,[33] actors engage in "mnemonic battles"[34] to secure favorable readings of the past[35] Throughout psychiatry's history, reformers have offered alternative readings of psychiatry's past in order to forge a temporal discontinuity from it. As sociologist Niklas Luhmann puts it, "modern society produces its own newness by way of stigmatizing the old."[36] Cleaving time into a before and an after, psychiatric reformers "other" their predecessors as hopelessly ignorant. This type of time work contains the fallout from ignorance by relegating it to the past and treating it as a by-product of a previously wrong way of thinking. And it has an added benefit of creating the illusion that psychiatrists have learned from their mistakes. With regard to the future, time work involves "projectivity," or the construction of imagined futures that suggest actions in the present.[37] Psychiatric reformers articulate the future resolution of ignorance through the expectations they proffer and the promises they make. Indeed, promissory practices abound in all of psychiatry's reinventions; reformers accrue authority by heralding a brighter future of insight. Promissory practices simultaneously downplay the contingency of the future—expectations are presented as certain provided reforms are adopted—as well as eliding the significance of present ignorance by "jettisoning uncertainties and empirical tests into the future."[38] In their reinventions, psychiatric reformers want us to discard the past failures, downplay the present uncertainty, and keep our attention trained on a future of great expectations.

Over time, reinvention has become a habit encoded in psychiatry. Subsequent generations of reformers have returned to it time and time again when the professional pressures caused by ignorance grow too intense. For most of psychiatry's history, reinvention has operated in an almost knee-jerk-like fashion, entailing a low level of conscious reflection and little deliberation. Each generation of reformers has arrived at it through specific responses to their current situations and the particular crisis in front of them at the time. While the underlying habit repeats, each reinvention differs in character: in the tactics by which it is secured, in the particular ideas and epistemological assumptions it promotes, in the definitions of mental distress it endorses, and in the professional identity it imagines. But despite these differences, all of psychiatry's reinventions have had the same overarching goal—to overcome ignorance by insisting on its temporary character.

With each successive iteration, however, this habit has become a topic of reflection and interrogation in its own right. As reinventions have accumulated, reformers and critics alike take note of them. Greater deliberation · surrounds each new reinvention. Thus far, this growing consciousness has reached its apogee in the DSM-5 debate over epistemic iteration versus paradigm shift, where, for this first time, critics expressed explicit concern not just over the *content* of reforms but over the *form* they assumed. It remains to be seen how much this conscious reflection will affect reforms moving forward, but one can expect that subsequent reinventions will have to meet a higher bar of scrutiny in response to psychiatry's mounting record of failure.

Reinvention is a drastic act, rarely pursued. For most professions, it remains a rare, infrequent event, often a singular one. For example, medicine proper can count one reinvention in the last century, the laboratory revolution by which it solidified professional authority at the turn of the twentieth century.[39] Over the same period, psychiatry has burned through five transformations. The general rarity of reinvention reflects the abundant risks it carries. Because it plays with the very identity of a profession and raises questions about its core mission, the conversations over reinvention can get away from reformers and aggravate the very existential problems reinvention is meant to address. But there are other, less existential risks to which reinvention is particularly susceptible as well. First, reinvention can set a profession off on the wrong path by prematurely overcommitting to a particular direction. We might call this the "all-eggs-in-one-basket" problem. This was the concern of DSM-5 proponents, for example, who worried that the DSM-III paradigm shift locked psychiatry into a problematic path, absorbing its limited resources and energies in the process. Second, the necessarily inflated hype that accompanies each new reinvention can induce unjustified hubris on the part of its most committed reformers. Psychiatry's worst abuses—for example, psychosurgery, lobotomy, and forced sterilization—can be traced to the inflated hype used to sell particular reinventions. These abuses have been perpetrated in the name of innovation by individuals driven by an undue faith in the rightness of the new program. Finally, reinvention, as a professional move, seems to have inherent limits. Over time, as failed reinventions accrue, those who continue to pursue them are susceptible to what we might deem the "going to the well one too many times" critique. Each new reinvention, when situated within psychiatry's boom-bust cyclical past, threatens to give the game away. Psychiatry's professional history itself—its lurchings from paradigm to paradigm, its ebbs and flows of optimism and despair—threatens to become a reflection of its ignorance. With this history in mind, it becomes that much harder to argue that *this* time things will be different.

Professional Tactics to Manage Ignorance

For professions reluctant to indulge in radical reinvention, there are other ways to manage ignorance. While the degree to which ignorance presents a problem for professions varies, it nevertheless is an inescapable problem for all. As such, each profession must police its ignorance and manage its repercussions in its own way, according to its own needs. While psychiatry might be an outlier, the tactics by which its reinventions were obtained reveal a diverse tool kit by which professions—and other groups as well—deal with ignorance.

What follows is a working classification of tactics for the collective management of ignorance drawn from the case of psychiatry. This is not an exhaustive list; rather, it is an elaboration of the tactics most central in psychiatry's tumultuous history with ignorance. Undoubtedly, future research of different cases will illuminate other tactics. Moreover, the tactics identified below are by no means unique to professions. Because professional power is so intimately bound up with claims to knowing, professions provide an excellent place to investigate the management of ignorance. But these tactics crop up in other arenas of social life and among different kinds of collective actors. Wherever people make knowledge claims, there are corresponding maneuvers aimed at protecting the claimants against ignorance.

The tactics by which psychiatrists have managed ignorance can be roughly categorized into two kinds—those that are primarily cultural in aim and those that are primarily organizational. Cultural tactics seek to influence processes of meaning-making (e.g., framing, identity formation, public discourse, boundary work, etc.). Involved in "the politics of cognition,"[40] they seek to steer the *interpretation* of ignorance in ways that are favorable to the profession. Organizational tactics address a more traditional sense of politics. They are aimed at shoring up power (e.g., governance, organizational formation, creating networks, forging alliances, etc.). This distinction between cultural and organizational tactics should not be reified or taken too literally; in practice, the two kinds of tactics are intertwined and inextricably linked. I adopt this distinction for heuristic purposes only, to highlight that the management of ignorance assumes a diversity of forms with different targets and objectives.

Cultural tactics attempt to shape how ignorance is perceived. However, before even acknowledging ignorance as something in need of framing, it is important to acknowledge that a profession might engage in *denial*, refusing to even entertain the existence of ignorance. Given the obvious failures of psychiatry, denial has not been all that viable as a tactic. There were elements of denial in the founding period of psychiatry, when superintendents, puffed up by exaggerated cure rates, adopted a posture of certainty. But once these rates were exposed as fraudulent and psychiatric ignorance was laid bare, subsequent reformers were prohibited from engaging in outright denial, as evident in the prevalent discussions of ignorance in psychiatric discourse. Still, despite its relative lack of relevance for psychiatry, denial is a feasible tactic for professions with a clearer record of success. In fact, it is likely the most common one.[41]

Unable to sweep ignorance under the rug, psychiatric reformers have adopted other tactics to frame ignorance in a way commensurate with their professional aspirations. As mentioned above, central to this has been the time work by which psychiatrists have deflected concerns that psychiatric ignorance is permanent, that there is something ineffable about mental distress. It would not be a stretch to argue that *all* of reformers' cultural tactics have focused on defining psychiatric ignorance as "unknown but knowable" rather than "unknown and unknowable," as temporary rather than permanent. This, in turn, creates the expectations that ignorance *can* and *will* be resolved.

In addition to time work, psychiatric reformers have deployed a number of other tactics to manage the impression of ignorance. These include:

Appeal to exemplars: If a profession is mired in ignorance, it can appeal to accomplishments in order to shore up its credibility. Exemplars of things that have become known imply that other, currently unknown, things share a similar destiny. By appealing to an exemplar, ignorance is framed as temporary. Moreover, exemplars endorse particular ways of knowing. The exemplar becomes a stand-in for all puzzles facing the profession, suggesting that they too can be explained by deploying the same reasoning or techniques. It becomes the embodiment of a paradigm and the fulfillment of its expectations. For example, early twentieth-century somatists held up neurosyphilis, a rare medical success for psychiatry, as an exemplar to support their commitment to sepsis theories of mental illness (and, in turn, appropriating the prestige of the germ theory revolution). Later, Freud's famous psychoanalytic case studies served a similar purpose for the psychoanalytic reinvention. However, given the lack of clear cases of psychiatric success, the appeal to exemplars has been perhaps less evident in psychiatry than it might be for other professions.

Appropriation: Reformers can deflect attention away from their own ignorance by adopting and adapting ideas from outsiders who are already accepted as legitimate knowers. Appropriation involves importing external ideas and claiming them as your own. The most important instance of appropriation in psychiatry occurred at its onset, when psychiatrists seized moral therapy and the asylum from lay reformers, rebranding these efforts as medical in character and thus establishing psychiatric jurisdiction over the population of inpatient mental health treatment. In many ways, the profession owes its existence to this successful appropriation. But beyond its origins, appropriation has been a common tactic for psychiatric reformers. Psychobiological reformers appropriated ideas from pragmatist philosophy and evolutionary theory, psychoanalytic reformers appropriated Freud, community psychiatrists appropriated antipsychiatry criticisms toward the mental hospitals to promote community care, and Neo-Kraepelinian reformers appropriated Emile Kraepelin's emphasis on classification and transformed it into diagnostic psychiatry.

Bandwagoning: Bandwagoning entails forging conceptual links with ideas and/or respective outside groups that possess pre-established cachet. Often done in conjunction with appropriation, this tactic is an attempt to bask in the glow of others' prestige, capturing some of their authority through a perceived association or relationship. Bandwagoning has also been rampant in the history of psychiatry. Psychobiological reformers of a somatic bent claimed an association with the germ theory revolution and its newsworthy discoveries. Psychoanalysts drew on the cultural prestige and perceived erudition of Freudian ideas to effect a takeover of psychiatry. Current psychiatrists are attempting to hitch their future to neuroscience and the cultural hype surrounding fMRI research. However, the most common target of psychiatry's bandwagoning has been medicine proper, which has been far more stable, institutionalized, and even revered. Throughout psychiatry's history, psychiatric reformers have sought to link their various programs to medicine so as to shore up their own professional legitimacy.

Boundary work: Like science more generally,[42] psychiatric reformers have engaged in boundary work, constructing rhetorical boundaries between legitimate approaches to understanding mental distress and non-legitimate, pseudo-scientific means. To promote their reinventions, reformers at various times have wielded the attribution of science as a weapon, portraying previous generations and/or competitors as non-scientific and thus unworthy of consideration. Insofar as psychiatric reformers can locate their efforts within science, ignorance presents itself as less of a problem. Indeed, it can even be construed as a functional and necessary motivator for research. Such boundary work has been present throughout psychiatry's reinventions, as the definition and understanding of what constitutes "science" has been malleable and made to fit a diverse array of intellectual programs. Two concrete examples include psychobiologists' appeal to norms of science to differentiate their psychotherapy from lay and religious therapies of the period, and Neo-Kraepelinian reformers' insistence that psychoanalysis is inherently unscientific and thus bankrupt as a means of foundation for psychiatry.

Deflecting blame onto the object: In response to charges of ignorance, psychiatrists have often argued that their ignorance results not from their own failings, but is a reflection of the object they are tasked with understanding. Specifically, they have framed the mind/brain as dizzyingly complex. As a result, psychiatry has lacked recourse to the kind of easy explanations available to other medical specialties. Such deflection may be done out of a fit of self-pity or worn as a badge of honor, but in all cases, it locates the explanation of ignorance in the object itself. For example, psychobiologists elevated complexity to the center of their program and used it to explain away the lack of psychiatry's progress when compared to other branches of medicine. Psychoanalysts also pointed to the mysteries of the mind—most importantly, its subconscious features—as justification for an alternative way of approaching the "medical" treatment of psychotherapy. And increasingly, this discourse of complexity erupts in explaining the challenges facing genetics and neuroscience. However, there is a limit to which reformers can resort to deflection, for if done too vehemently or regularly, it can risk the perception that mental distress is fundamentally unknowable. Consequently, reformers have insisted that while it is *hard* to understand mental distress, it is not *impossible*. The complexity of mental distress demands extra patience, not the abandonment of psychiatry altogether.

Mystification: Mystification, or obscurantism, involves the practice of rendering expertise inaccessible and opaque to outsiders, so as to insulate it from criticism. If professional knowledge is too transparent and codifiable, the need to defer to expert authorities becomes less pressing. To maintain their authority, professions withhold elements of their expertise, shrouding them in mystery. Mystification allows professions to control the perceptions surrounding their ignorance. It thwarts external assessment, for without an understanding of a profession's knowledge base, critics cannot identify its gaps. Professional power gets reduced to blind trust. As a tactic, mystification was most central to the psychoanalytic reinvention, when reformers cordoned off psychiatric expertise in the space of the psychoanalytic encounter and grounded their expertise in obscure theories and enigmatic interpretations. Such mystery underwrote their authority and made it hard, at least for a while, for outsiders to assess what they knew and what they did not.

Naming the object: An underappreciated tactic in conveying understanding and mastery is classification. Naming an object implies some dominion over it. Classification takes complex reality and organizes it into neat, discrete categories. It obscures that which is not known by masking disorder and incomprehension. Classification not only conveys a sense of comprehension; it also surreptitiously valorizes some ways of knowing over others.[43] If reformers can get others to adopt their classifications and speak their language, they can disseminate the thinking that is embodied within these. This tactic has been crucial in the current era of diagnostic psychiatry. As a totem of psychiatric expertise, DSM catalogs and organizes the universe of mental distress so as to project a sense of understanding where there is little. The welter of mental distress gets domesticated in discrete diagnostic classifications created by psychiatrists.

Rescaling the object: Faced with identified ignorance at one level, reformers can change the scope of their inquiry, broadening or narrowing its purview, to reorient the field to a new conceptual scale. A change in scale forces a change in assessment of claims to knowledge. Both psychoanalytic reformers and community psychiatrists drastically rescaled the scope of psychiatric expertise. In psychoanalysis, the object of inquiry was scaled down to the micro level, reduced to the individual psyche, and even further to the role of subconscious forces in producing mental distress. This limited psychoanalytic claims to the level of individual patient; idiosyncratic and specific, such claims were hard to assess generally. Community psychiatrists shifted the scale in the opposite direction. They broadened the purview of psychiatry's concerns appreciably, orienting psychiatry away from the individual to macro social factors (and everything in between). This broadening of scale sought to manage psychiatric ignorance by essentially diluting it across various levels of analysis. Spread afield, its size and scope became obscure.

Shifting the object: Like rescaling, shifting the object manages ignorance by replacing old standards for new ones. Here, reformers shift the focus of their inquiry away from an object that has been the subject of failed investigations onto something else. As evident in the changing ontological understanding of mental distress over time, this tactic recurs throughout psychiatry's history. Mental distress has been variously considered as frazzled nerves disturbed by the pressure of modern society, as maladaptations to the functional demands of one's life, as diseases caused by infectious agents, as neuroses resulting from unconscious conflicts and familial complications, as socially patterned responses to large-scale societal forces, as disorders resulting from neurotransmitters not reuptaking, and so on. Every time psychiatry has come to an impasse, reformers have redefined its object, sometimes slightly, sometimes drastically. Ignorance gets reinterpreted not as a failure of psychiatry itself, but as the result of the wrong way of thinking about the object.

By some combination of these cultural practices, generations of psychiatric reformers have set the terms by which this ignorance has been interpreted, and set them in such a way as to ensure psychiatry's perpetuation. Ignorance gets transformed into something that psychiatry, more or less, has under control.

Problems of ignorance, however, cannot be managed by cultural tactics alone. Professional power rests on both persuasion and force, cultural and organizational authority.[44] It has not been enough for reformers to explain ignorance; they have had to build an organizational infrastructure to withstand the assaults to its authority. Organizations confer solidity and endurance upon a profession whose existence is under attack. They can also be mobilized in "trials of strength,"[45] providing the resources to promote and disseminate particular viewpoints and ideas against competitors.

Over its various reinventions, psychiatric reformers have engaged in a number of organizational tactics. They have adopted traditional professional tactics, like creating a professional society (APA), establishing educational and training standards, lobbying for favorable legislation, controlling licensing and certification, and establishing and maintaining professional norms through a code of ethics. These common professional tactics are important, but they have not been sufficient for psychiatry. The unique persistence of psychiatric ignorance has forced psychiatric reformers to resort to additional organizational tactics.

These organizational tactics complement the typical ways in which professions shore up institutional authority, but have been pursued with the express intent of minimizing the potential consequences of ignorance. Three of these are of particular note:

· *Retrenchment:* Whenever antipsychiatry sentiment has reached a fever pitch, psychiatry has withdrawn to its institutional strongholds, a practice called *retrenchment.* Just as armies retreat behind fortress walls when faced with an advancing foe, so too have psychiatrists retreated to organizations in which their authority is secure when faced with advancing critics. For more than a century, whenever things got too dicey, psychiatrists withdrew to the mental hospital, where they held unquestioned jurisdiction over patients with serious mental illness. Indeed, the resistance to psychiatry has been greatest when it has tried to extend its jurisdictional reach beyond these walls. Despite their myriad problems and the professed ambivalence psychiatrists felt toward them, mental hospitals had enduring relevance. They long protected embattled psychiatrists and provided a floor to psychiatry's authority. The common recourse to retrenchment and its conspicuous absence today underscores the great significance of deinstitutionalization. Deinstitutionalization took retrenchment to the mental hospital off the table, leaving psychiatrists more vulnerable in the process. Psychiatrists helped dismantle the one place in which their authority went more or less unquestioned. Today, psychiatry is dependent upon its associations with medicine proper, for without medicine's endorsement, psychiatrists have nowhere to go, nowhere to work.

Forging new alliances: Psychiatric reformers have also attempted to limit the negative consequences of ignorance by securing new allies and forging new connections. The construction of new alliances is the organizational dimension of the cultural practices of bandwagoning and appropriation discussed above. As things get tough and as previous alliances fray, reformers look for outside support elsewhere by constructing new alliances. For example, psychoanalytic reformers forged crucial connections to the military during the two world wars. These connections provided psychiatrists new opportunities and institutional supports for their labors. In the current period, Neo-Kraepelinian reformers have cultivated a mutually beneficial relationship with pharmaceutical companies. Most significant in this regard, however, have been the continual, but never fully successful, attempts on the part of psychiatrists to establish organizations that both look like, and connect it to, medicine proper.

Shifting arenas: Finally, when one arena proves unfavorable, collective actors seek out alternative arenas in which to assert their authority.[46] By shifting arenas, psychiatric reformers have sought out more favorable contexts for their arguments, or at least new places to argue when old arenas become too hostile. Specifically, they have sought audiences less familiar with psychiatry's failings and therefore more likely to accept reformers' framing of ignorance. Here, psychiatry has benefited from American federalism. As state legislatures became increasingly hostile and therefore resistant to funding psychiatry, psychiatrists shifted their attention to the federal government. Whereas once it secured most of its funding from state coffers, psychiatry now gets most of its support from federal agencies.

As these multiple tactics indicate, when it comes to the management of ignorance, it is not a matter of *either* cultural *or* organizational means, but a matter of *both/and*. Out of necessity, psychiatric reformers have created a diverse arsenal of tricks to manage their ignorance.

Ignorance is a potential problem for all professions—for really all claims makers, be they experts, corporations, government institutions, or social movements. Given the complex politics of ignorance, there is no one magical, foolproof solution to the difficulties it poses, only a host of possible tactics to be desperately pursued in the quest for survival.

Shared Ignorance, Collective Failure

Knowing *how* psychiatry has managed its ignorance does not answer a crucial question: Why do we accept psychiatry's constant reinventions? Put differently, why do we continue to recognize psychiatry's authority, given its dubious history?

Professional authority is both captured and conferred. This book has focused on explaining how psychiatrists have captured authority despite the field's persistent ignorance. Each reinvention has reset psychiatry's historical chronometer. In pursuing a new direction with new standards, new measures of success, reformers reboot things and, in the process, buy the profession more time to resolve its knowledge gaps. Psychiatric authority, sullied by a record of failure, gets renewed on the basis of a forecast of a brighter future to be obtained by a new package of reforms. However, there would seem to be an inherent limit to this maneuver. How many times can one resort to reinvention before people start to grow skeptical of yet another round of promises? As reinventions accumulate and as both critics and reformers become conscious of the hype/disappointment cycle of psychiatry, one would think that people would grow wary of psychiatry and seek alternatives. And yet, this point has not been reached. Why?

Addressing this question pushes me into the admittedly more speculative terrain of cultural critique. Here, my argument is informed by empirical data, but to formulate it and flesh it out, I must make some leaps. I have reservations about this. However, given the importance of the question at hand, it would be irresponsible of me not to venture an explanation.

Before laying out my argument as to why I think psychiatry's reinventions are accepted over and over, it is important to qualify the question a bit. While psychiatry has endured, acceptance of it has never been without reservations. We have not awarded professional authority easily or uncritically. Instead, we granted it grudgingly. Our reservations reflect the fact that psychiatry has been constantly imperiled. This is evident in the repeated flowerings of antipsychiatry sentiment, the aspersions we repeatedly cast toward the psychiatric project, and the constant drumbeat of complaints we direct psychiatry's way. It is evident in our mocking humor in which the bumbling "shrink" is the butt of the joke. It is evident in polling, where psychiatrists consistently poll behind their medical and professional peers when it comes to perceptions of honesty, ethics, and trust.[47] And it is evident in the lack of esteem with which other physicians hold psychiatry.[48] Aside perhaps from a brief moment at the start of the asylum period, psychiatric authority has always been fragile and conditional, granted with an asterisk.

Nevertheless, psychiatry survives. For nearly two centuries, American society has continued to defer to psychiatry on matters related to mental illness. This feat, I argue, is the by-product of a combination of inertia and collective indifference. Collectively, we are stuck in a rut when it comes to dealing with mental illness, and thus far, we have not cared enough to get out of it.

A disconcerting amount of human behavior is motivated by the ease and convenience of doing things as they have always been done. Sociologist Howard Becker recognizes the sheer power of the status quo.[49] Most tasks can be accomplished in many ways. When presented with options, people tend to embrace the existing package of practices and relationships rather than investing the labor and resources required to create new ones. Innovation is possible, but it is costly and laborious. Inertia works against it, for without significant impetus, people tend to fall back on what is already available by default. Thus, once a way of doing something is established, it is just easier to maintain the status quo. Seeking out psychiatric expertise and assistance has become the default option when encountering mental illness. We have turned to psychiatrists before, so we will turn to them again. We are, after all, creatures of habit. This inertia confers upon psychiatry what Max Weber calls "the dignity of oughtness."[50]

Once we appreciate the power of inertia, the enduring significance of psychiatrists gaining control over the asylum nearly two hundred years ago becomes evident. The various historical contingencies and accidents that led to psychiatry's capture of the asylum have shaped its fate ever since. This is a simple path-dependency argument. Decisions that arose in response to specific dilemmas got locked in over time, narrowing and determining the path forward. When psychiatrists won control over the asylum system, they established themselves as wardens of patients with serious mental illness. Despite all the subsequent challenges they have faced, psychiatrists' claim over the jurisdiction of serious mental illness has never been seriously threatened. The capture of the asylum foreclosed other possibilities and alternatives. It established psychiatry as a relevant force. We can only imagine alternate histories, a series of what-ifs that might have yielded different outcomes. What if Dorothea Dix had not been so effective in building up the asylum system? What if early superintendents had failed to wrest asylums from lay reformers? What if neurologists had mounted a stronger challenge at the turn of the century? Had these things turned out differently, psychiatry may never have existed or may no longer exist. But such counter-factuals are the province of fiction. In reality, psychiatrists seized a robust institutional system and used it as a foundation upon which to construct their professional authority. Once they did so, they secured a place at the mental health table. They became the custodians of patients with serious mental illness, a job for which there was frankly little competition. Without a viable alternative, they have remained at the table. Consequently, the echoes of the asylum system reverberate to this day in the persistence of psychiatry, even though this system has long been dismantled.

That those with serious mental illness need psychiatrists is never disputed. They have no alternative, really. But that psychiatrists are just as dependent upon those with serious mental illness often goes underappreciated. Psychiatrists need patients with serious mental illness to justify their profession's existence. Moreover, time and time again, these patients have rescued psychiatry from oblivion. When its overambitious reinventions go astray, when its aspirational attempts to extend their authority over less severe forms of mental distress are repelled, and when its indissoluble ignorance is exposed, psychiatrists fall back into their awkward embrace with the seriously mentally ill. The irony of psychiatric power is that it relies upon the very patient population that psychiatry has spent the better part of its history trying to escape.

The irony of this mutual dependence has not been lost on psychiatrists. To the contrary, it has wormed its way into the profession's mythology. Take for example a story, likely apocryphal, told by Gregory Zilboorg.[51] The story involves Philippe Pinel during the French Revolution. As a medical reformer, Pinel was sympathetic to the ideals of the French Revolution. Indeed, his symbolic unchaining of the mad served as an apt metaphor for the revolution, which sought to break the chains of monarchial oppression. But Pinel was no revolutionary ideologue; he was moderate, conservative, and [gasp] aristocratic in demeanor. These qualities left him vulnerable to suspicion, and as the political fervor heightened, the revolutionary mob turned on him. Rumors circulated that Pinel was harboring priests, émigrés, and other enemies of the revolution in his hospital. Revolutionaries demanded his head for this supposed crime. One day, a mob surrounded Pinel in the street, seized him, and proceeded in the direction of a nearby lamp post to lynch him. At the last second, a former patient of his named Chevigné intervened, rescuing Pinel from the clutches of the mob and aiding his escape. For Zilboorg, this moment carries great insight into the relationship of psychiatry with its most troubled patients:

> This incident may be viewed as a symbol of the historical vicissitudes of psychiatry. It was the doctor who had to annex psychiatry to medicine—almost forcibly. It was the patient who protected the new domain. It was society, or at least the populace, which still threatened to conquer the doctor and to recapture territory on which it had no moral and less scientific right.[52]

Just as Pinel was (supposedly) saved by his patient from the collective mob, so too has psychiatry been saved, countless times, from antipsychiatry sentiment, societal hostility, and professional irrelevance by the population of patients with serious mental illness over whom it maintains its jurisdiction. Without the protection this population affords, psychiatry would likely be extinguished.

The inertia underwriting psychiatric power, however, is not without its limits. In cases when a viable alternative has emerged, we have been quick to abandon psychiatry. When biological knowledge of a condition under psychiatry's purview is obtained, this condition is promptly removed from psychiatry and placed under the care of other medical specialties. In other words, the moment when a psychiatric condition becomes explained by a somatic cause, "both the disease and patients are shifted to the province of a different specialty."[53] General paresis, long a major focus of psychiatry, was taken from psychiatry once its bacteriological cause was identified and an effective treatment was discovered. Psychiatry has lost stroke to neurologists, mental retardation to pediatricians, and neurosyphilis to internists.[54] Vitamin deficiency, thyroid disorders, and pellagrous insanity were similarly confiscated. This phenomenon is not lost on contemporary psychiatrists wary of the neuro-turn. They point out a contradiction at the heart of efforts to reconstitute psychiatry as clinical neuroscience: If psychiatry helps develop a comprehensive neurological account of mental illness and thus convinces everyone that mental disorders are brain disorders, wouldn't it make sense to hand them over to neurologists, who possess greater expertise on the brain? These limits reveal that the inertia psychiatry has accrued, while certainly powerful, is not invulnerable.

Although crucial, inertia alone is not sufficient to account for psychiatry's survival. After all, the lack of viable alternatives might very well reflect a lack of motivation to seek out and cultivate such alternatives. In addition to inertia, psychiatry has benefited from societal indifference toward mental illness, or more specifically to those with serious mental illness. We have demonstrated a ruinous lack of concern for these patients in particular, and this indifference, when combined with inertia, has kept psychiatry going.

Running parallel to the history of ignorance in psychiatry is a quieter history of collective complicity, a willingness of the state, the public, and family members of those with serious mental illness to relieve themselves of responsibilities and the vexing challenges posed by this population. The motivations behind this willing abandonment are murky and complex, rooted as they are deep in our history and collective psyche. Michel Foucault argues that during the Renaissance, the mad were perceived as bearers of a type of wisdom.[55] But during the Age of Reason, the mad posed an existential threat. They had to be separated from reason so as to define and protect its contours. This separation had a conceptual dimension—the mad were redefined as the "other"—and an institutional dimension—they were confined in institutions and consigned to marginality. Exiled from society and placed under the charge of psychiatry, madness was transformed into a distinct object of analysis and target of discipline. Thus, Foucault's story is an Enlightenment tragedy, in which the modern understanding of madness was born from the insecurities of reason and a desire to banish the concerns that madness presented. "In the serene world of mental illness," he writes,

> modern man no longer communicates with the madman: on the one hand is the man of reason, who delegates madness to the doctor, thereby authorizing no relation other than through the abstract universality of illness; and on the other is the man of madness, who only communicates with the other through the intermediary of a reason that is no less abstract, which is order, physical and moral constraint, the anonymous pressure of the group, the demand for conformity. There is no common language: or rather, it no longer exists; the constitution of madness as mental illness, at the end of the eighteenth century, bears witness to a rupture in a dialogue, gives the separation as already enacted, and expels from the memory all those imperfect words, of no fixed syntax, spoken falteringly, in which the exchange between madness and reason was carried out. The language of psychiatry, which is a monologue by reason *about* madness, could only have come into existence in such a silence.[56]

This rupture in dialogue was accompanied by a collective forfeiture of responsibility for the mentally ill. The mad became the province of the disciplinary regime of psychiatry so that the rest of us could go about ignoring them.

Foucault is known for playing fast and loose with the historical record. He paints vivid pictures and provocative arguments, but often at the expense of rigor. Yet, while we might doubt Foucault the historian, Foucault the cultural critic has captured something of the essence of Western society's dealings with madness. The mad embody a species-wide terror, revealing what happens to our status as reasoned beings when we lose our minds. Frightened, we want madness controlled, confined, and kept out of view. And we want this because madness terrifies us in its incomprehensibility.

Of course, Foucault does not have a monopoly over observations of our collective fear, incomprehension, and marginalization of those with serious mental illness. Goffman speaks of the "havoc" attributed to those whose symptoms are "specifically and pointedly offensive" to polite society.[57] Sociologist Thomas Scheff sees mental illness as a category of "residual deviance," a flexible catchall label we affix to behaviors that lie outside the bounds of our understanding and existing normative mechanisms.[58] This convenient label allows us to assert arbitrary control over those who make us uncomfortable. And historian Charles Rosenberg argues that psychiatry's true role is to preside over the uncanny. To it, we have allocated conditions that reside on the boundary between "disease and willed misbehavior or culpable self-indulgence," for which we have little understanding and little recourse.[59] As "the designated trustee of those social and emotional dilemmas that can plausibly—and thus usefully—be framed as the product of disease,"[60] psychiatry allows us the luxury of recoiling from the raving delusions of the schizophrenic, the cheerless gloom of the depressed, the nervous jittering of the anxious, and the tumultuous mood swings of the manic.

The fear and discomfort toward mental illness is met with a number of cultural coping mechanisms. The first and most common is avoidance. We do everything in our power to try to avoid thinking about or considering the fates of those with serious mental illness. Avoidance is buttressed by compassion fatigue. The plight of those with serious mental illness is so consistently miserable that those of us who might be otherwise sympathetic have become overwhelmed by the scope and intensity of their suffering. Witness the half-life of the outrage that meets psychiatric exposés; after a short period of hand wringing and weak calls for reform, we return to our lives and our fragile status quo. As the Joint Commission on Mental Health and Illness argued fifty-five years ago, the public does not mobilize in response to exposés, because patients with serious mental illness "lack appeal."[61] "People do seem to feel sorry for [the mentally ill]," the report goes on, "but in the balance, *they do not feel as sorry as they do relieved to have out of the way persons whose behavior disturbs and offends them."*[62] Our sensibilities overloaded and the limits of our empathy reached, we remove ourselves from their trials. Second, we construct "empathy walls" around individuals with serious mental illness, obstacles to a deep understanding of another person that solidifies our indifference to their plight and can induce hostility.[63] This cordoning off is achieved through othering. Stigma supplants empathy and understanding. Finally, when forced to face serious mental illness among our loved ones, we can lash out and project our insecurities in the form of constant reproach. As a culture, Americans tend to display high levels of expressed emotion toward family members with mental illness. Our frustrations boiling over, we hector them into relapse and decompensation.[64]

The collective indifference *felt* toward individuals with serious illness, in and of itself, is hard to observe directly. Few outright espouse it, especially in polite company. However, the collective indifference *displayed* and *acted upon* certainly is not. The evidence for it is everywhere, manifold and damning. Our indifference is revealed in the persistence of stigma. Even today, despite the hope that medicalization—and specifically the pivot to genetic/neurological accounts of mental disorders—would alleviate stigma by taking personal responsibility out of the equation, we still want to maintain our social distance from those diagnosed with mental illness.[65] Our indifference is also revealed in our popular culture, where negative stereotypes of patients with serious mental illness abound.[66] We represent the mentally ill as violent and dangerous, justifying and reinforcing our fear of them in the process. And indifference is revealed in those rare moments when mental illness penetrates popular discourse. Today mental illness only registers on the public agenda during the aftermath of mass shootings. Even then, the proposed solution is not more robust mental health care, but rather better screening to prevent those with serious mental illness from legally obtaining guns.[67] Nearly our entire public discussion of mental illness is built on the faulty premise that those with mental illness are dangerous. In truth, they are far likelier to be victims of violent crimes than perpetrators.[68]

The most damning evidence of our indifference, however, comes from how we invest our resources, or more accurately, how we decide not to. The United States lacks anything resembling a functional institutional response to mental illness. Deinstitutionalization has virtually eliminated inpatient care as a viable health care option. For those in need of such care, there are few resources available; in 2010, there were only fourteen psychiatric beds per 100,000 Americans, and in some states, like Arizona, Iowa, and Minnesota, there were fewer than five per 100,000.[69] After a half-hearted attempt at community-based care, we have thrown our hands in the air and decided to leave those most in need of mental health care to fend for themselves.

With no place to go, many with serious mental illness find their way either to the street or to prison. Although data can be hard to come by, it is estimated that 46% of the chronically homeless population suffers from serious mental illness and/or a substance use disorder.[70] The sight of the homeless mentally ill has become a staple of urban experience, but it is important to remember that it is a relatively recent phenomenon dating from the 1980s.[71]

Individuals with serious mental illness, languishing on the street with nowhere to turn, invariably encounter law enforcement. The criminal justice system has become the de facto institution charged with handling those with serious mental illness. More than 1.8 million people with serious mental illness are jailed every year. In forty-four states, a jail or prison holds more individuals with mental illness than the largest state hospital, and the three institutions holding the largest population of mentally ill individuals are Cook County Prison in Illinois, Los Angeles County Jail, and Rikers Island in New York.[72] Of those incarcerated in jails and prisons, an estimated 20% have a serious mental illness.[73] As police and prison officials find themselves having to deal with the specific needs of this population, some are taking proactive measures, whether it be crisis intervention training for police officers or programs aimed at hiring more mental health professionals to work in prisons. Although laudable, these programs are inadequate. Simply put, authorities in the criminal justice system are not up to the task we have foisted upon them. About one in four fatal police encounters involves a victim with mental illness, and individuals with mental disorders are sixteen times more likely to be killed in a police incident than other civilians.[74] Behind these statistics are individual stories of policing gone wrong, like the shootings of James Boyd and Christopher Torres in Albuquerque, or incarceration turned ugly, as in the death of Darren Rainey, a prisoner in Florida's Dade Correctional Institute, who died after being locked in a hot shower for two hours, his skin peeling and molting from the scalding water.[75] A "nonsystem" as callous and ineffective as this can only exist when supported by a deep and abiding indifference to those that we force to endure it.

Historically, psychiatry's authority has been constructed upon the backs of patients with serious mental illness. As a population, they have comprised its most secure jurisdiction. And in a curious fashion, the malevolent neglect of this population by society translates into a type of benign neglect for psychiatry. In his analysis of stigma, Goffman notes the phenomenon of "courtesy stigma," or stigma by association imposed on those close to the stigmatized group.[76] For psychiatry, however, courtesy stigma works in a complex fashion. On the one hand, psychiatry suffers in prestige, especially in comparison to other medical professions, as a result of its patient population. On the other hand, this courtesy stigma comes with a real courtesy, namely, professional survival. The existence of a stigmatized population of individuals with serious mental illness perpetuates the existence of psychiatry as a profession. We accept its repeated reinventions. We let psychiatrists do what they may without asking too many questions, all in exchange for allowing us to avoid our own fears and ignorance toward serious mental illness. We are willing to endure psychiatrists' ignorance because they take on our collective responsibility for not knowing. We can sit on our hands and continue to wait for some sort of resolution, for someone else to address the problem. Even if this waiting is misguided and perpetual, it serves its purpose. It allows us to maintain the façade that we are doing something. It transforms our indifference into seemingly steadfast patience. It gives us the false sense of security that the authorities will take care of it. But we aren't, it isn't, and they won't. Rather than confronting our ignorance and compassionately caring for those whom we do not understand, we have chosen the easier, more convenient course.

Out of inertia and indifference, we serve as psychiatry's enablers. We endorse a profession whose true function is not to solve mental illness or even to treat it effectively. Rather, psychiatry functions as a repository of our collective angst felt toward madness and the puzzles it creates. Frightened of the implications that mental illness has for our pretenses to reason, we farm out our terror. We wrap up our insecurities regarding mental illness and gift them to psychiatry in the form of professional authority. At least when things go awry, we have somewhere to point our fingers. Ignorance is not just built into the role of psychiatry; psychiatry is premised on it.

Consequently, psychiatry's perseverance, and the litany of abuses that have accompanied it, cannot be understood by examining psychiatrists alone. The causes run deeper and wider. Once psychiatrists captured a place at the mental health table, barring a viable alternative, they have been allowed to remain without enough scrutiny or oversight. They reap the benefit of our collective fear and uncaring neglect of those with serious mental illness. Therefore, while rightly critical of psychiatrists, a history that appreciates the centrality of ignorance should not lead us to demonize them. We should hold psychiatrists to account, but in doing so, we should avoid turning them into easy scapegoats for what is a broad collective failure. We must acknowledge our own culpability. Psychiatry does not have a monopoly over the ignorance of mental distress. We all share in it. But unlike psychiatrists, most of us do not struggle with this ignorance, attempt to over-come it, or work to manage its fallout. Instead, we have been all too eager to delegate the responsibility. So yes, we should criticize psychiatry's failings, particularly when it causes harm to those entrusted in their care. But we should not fool ourselves into thinking that the blame lies with them alone.

We are all complicit.

NOTES

INTRODUCTION

1. John Charles Bucknill, "The Pathology of Insanity," *American Journal of Psychiatry* 14, no. 3 (1858): 29.
2. John E. Tyler, "Tests of Insanity," *American Journal of Psychiatry* 22, no. 2 (1865): 141.
3. August Hoch, "On the Clinical Study of Psychiatry," *American Journal of Psychiatry* 57, no. 2 (1900): 283.
4. Harold I. Gosline, "A Physiological and Anatomical Approach to a Classification of Mental Diseases," *American Journal of Psychiatry* 79, no. 2 (1922): 235.
5. Thomas W. Salmon, "Presidential Address," *American Journal of Psychiatry* 8, no. 1 (1924): 3.
6. George S. Sprague, "Etiology of Mental Disease, a Changing Concept," *American Journal of Psychiatry* 100, no. 7 (1944): 795.
7. Steven Reiss, "A Critique of Thomas S. Szasz's 'Myth of Mental Illness,'" *American Journal of Psychiatry* 128, no. 9 (1972): 1082.
8. Roberto M. Unger, "A Program for Late Twentieth-Century Psychiatry," *American Journal of Psychiatry* 139, no. 2 (1982): 155.
9. Ibid.
10. Martin Roth and Jerome Kroll, *The Reality of Mental Illness* (New York: Cambridge University Press, 1986), 72.
11. Michael B. First and Mark Zimmerman, "Including Laboratory Tests in DSM-V Diagnostic Criteria," *American Journal of Psychiatry* 163, no. 12 (2006): 2041.
12. Kenneth S. Kendler, "Toward a Philosophical Structure for Psychiatry," *American Journal of Psychiatry* 162, no. 3 (2005): 434–35.
13. Gerald Grob, "Psychiatry's Holy Grail: The Search for the Mechanisms of Mental Diseases," *Bulletin of the History of Medicine* 72, no. 2 (1998): 189–219.
14. Andrew Abbott, *The System of Professions: An Essay on the Division of Expert Labor* (Chicago: University of Chicago Press, 1988); Eliot Freidson, *Professional Powers: A Study of the Institutionalization of Formal Knowledge* (Chicago: University of Chicago Press, 1986).
15. Eliot Freidson, *Professionalism: The Third Logic* (Chicago: University of Chicago Press, 2001).
16. Eliot Freidson, *Profession of Medicine: A Study of the Sociology of Applied Knowledge* (Chicago: University of Chicago Press, 1988).

17. Abbott, *The System of Professions*, 9.

18. See for example Richard L. Jenkins, "Psychiatry at the Crossroads," *American Journal of Psychiatry* 106, no. 5 (1949): 358–61; Allan Beigel, "Psychiatric Education at the Crossroads: Issues and Future Directions," *American Journal of Psychiatry* 136, no. 12 (1979): 1525–29; Robert O. Pasnau, "Psychiatry in Medicine: Medicine in Psychiatry," *American Journal of Psychiatry* 144, no. 8 (1987): 975–80; James H. Shore, "Psychiatry at a Crossroad: Our Role in Primary Care," *American Journal of Psychiatry* 153, no. 11 (1996): 1398–1403; Kenneth B. Wells, "Treatment Research at the Crossroads: The Scientific Interface of Clinical Trials and Effectiveness Research," *American Journal of Psychiatry* 156, no. 1 (1999): 5–10.

19. See J. L. Moreno, "The Role Concept, a Bridge between Psychiatry and Sociology," *American Journal of Psychiatry* 118, no. 6 (1966): 518; Ransom J. Arthur, "Social Psychiatry: An Overview," *American Journal of Psychiatry* 130, no. 8 (1973): 846; Thomas Detre, "The Future of Psychiatry," *American Journal of Psychiatry* 144, no. 5 (1987): 625; Robert K. Schreter, "Coping with the Crisis in Psychiatric Training," *Psychiatry* 60, no. 1 (1997): 51–59; Paul S. Appelbaum, "Response to the Presidential Address—The Systematic Defunding of Psychiatric Care: A Crisis at Our Doorstep," *American Journal of Psychiatry* 159, no. 10 (2002): 1638–40.

20. Psychiatry's repeated reformulations of its object present a writing problem, namely, how to refer to this object without endorsing one perspective over another. The names given to this object are enmeshed in the very politics I wish to elucidate. Sensitive to this issue, I use the generic term "mental distress" when discussing this object generally. When referring to specific eras or discussing particular psychiatric paradigms, I adopt the terminology of that period (i.e., mental illness, mental disorder, maladjustment, neuroses, etc.).

    Additionally, when discussing the population of patients with more severe manifestations of mental distress—variously termed "chronic mental illness," "severe and persistent mental illness," "severe and/or chronic mental illness," "serious and persistent mental illness," "severe mental illness," and so on—I follow the current convention of the Substance Abuse and Mental Health Services Administration (SAMHSA) and use the term "serious mental illness." See SAMHSA's National Registry of Evidence-Based Programs and Practices, "Behind the Term: Serious Mental Illness," https://nrepp-learning.samhsa.gov/sites/default/files/documents/behind_the_term /pdf_07_26_2017/Behind_the_Term_SMI_7.2017.pdf. SAMHSA makes a further distinction between serious mental illness (SMI) and serious and persistent mental illness (SPMI). While important, this distinction is not as relevant for my analysis. Rather, the crucial historical distinction is between those patients with severe manifestations of mental distress and patients with less severe manifestations (previous generations of psychiatrists called these patients "neurotic"; today they are often referred to colloquially as the "worried well"). I argue that the care and responsibility of the population of patients with *serious mental illness* has been psychiatry's primary mandate. For much of this history, these patients were treated in long-term, inpatient care facilities, first asylums and then mental hospitals. Psychiatrists, I argue, have maintained clear jurisdiction over these individuals, and it is to this population that the profession owes both its existence and endurance.

21. Gabriel Abend. "Styles of Sociological Thought: Sociologies, Epistemologies, and the Mexican and US Quests for Truth," *Sociological Theory* 24, no. 1 (2006): 1–41.

22. Ian Hacking, "Styles of Scientific Reasoning," in *Post-Analytic Philosophy*, ed. John Rajchman and Cornel West (New York: Columbia University Press, 1985), 145–65.

23. Andrew Scull, *Social Order/Mental Disorder: Anglo-American Psychiatry in Historical Perspective* (Berkeley: University of California Press, 1989), 22.

24. Today, the most vocal critics of psychiatry are Scientologists. In an effort to ensure that this book is not hijacked by Scientology, let me be exceedingly clear. I consider Scientology to be a fraudulent pyramid scheme that deploys cultish beliefs in order to make use of tax loopholes and enrich its leadership. My unequivocal rejection of Scientology includes its antipsychiatry critique, which is intentionally misleading. Psychiatric history is problematic enough as it is; one need not resort to the exaggerated, misguided drivel proffered by Scientologists. For those interested in learning more about Scientology, I recommend the book *Going Clear: Scientology, Hollywood, and the Prison of Belief* by Lawrence Wright (2013).

25. Grob, "Psychiatry's Holy Grail," 216–17.

26. Erving Goffman, *Asylums: Essays on the Social Situation of Mental Patients and Other Inmates* (Chicago: Aldine Publishing, 1962); Gregory Zilboorg, *A History of Medical Psychology* (New York: W. W. Norton, 1967); Tracy M. Luhrmann, *Of Two Minds: An Anthropologist Looks at American Psychiatry* (New York: Vintage Books, 2001); Nikolas S. Rose, *Governing the Soul: The Shaping of the Private Self* (New York: Routledge, 1990); Elizabeth Lunbeck, *The Psychiatric Persuasion: Knowledge, Gender, and Power in Modern America* (Princeton, NJ: Princeton University Press, 1996); Thomas J. Scheff, *Being Mentally Ill: A Sociological Theory*, 3rd ed. (New York: Aldine de Gruyter, 1999).

27. Jerome M. Schneck, *A History of Psychiatry* (Springfield, IL: Charles C. Thomas, 1960); Michel Foucault, *Madness and Civilization: A History of Insanity in the Age of Reason* (New York: Vintage Books, 1988); David J. Rothman, *The Discovery of the Asylum: Social Order and Disorder in the New Republic* (Hawthorne, NY: Aldine de Gruyter, 1971); Nancy Tomes, *A Generous Confidence: Thomas Story Kirkbride and the Art of Asylum-Keeping, 1840–1883* (New York: Cambridge University Press, 1984); Andrew Scull, *The Most Solitary of Afflictions: Madness and Society in Britain, 1700–1900* (New Haven, CT: Yale University Press, 2005); Elaine Showalter, *The Female Malady: Women, Madness, and English Culture, 1830–1980* (New York: Pantheon Books, 1985).

28. Lest this bipolar categorization be taken too far, it should be noted that many historical accounts are more nuanced than the extreme brushes with which their critics paint them. Some historians intentionally stake out an explicit middle ground between these extremes. For example, see Gerald N. Grob, *From Asylum to Community: Mental Health Policy in Modern America* (Princeton, NJ: Princeton University Press, 1991); Gerald N. Grob, *Mental Institutions in America: Social Policy to 1875* (New Brunswick, NJ: Transaction Publishers, 2008); Jack D. Pressman, *Last Resort: Psychosurgery and the Limits of Medicine* (New York: Cambridge University Press, 2002).

29. For example, see Michel Foucault, *History of Madness*, trans. J. Khalfa (New York: Routledge, 2013); Phyllis Chesler, *Women & Madness* (New York: Avon Books, 1973); Jonathan Metzl, *Prozac on the Couch: Prescribing Gender in the Era of Wonder Drugs* (Durham, NC: Duke University Press, 2003); Jonathan Metzl, *The Protest Psychosis: How Schizophrenia Became a Black Disease* (Boston: Beacon Press, 2010).

30. Stephen Toulmin, *Cosmopolis: The Hidden Agenda of Modernity* (Chicago: University of Chicago Press, 1992).

31. Linsey McGoey, "The Logic of Strategic Ignorance," *British Journal of Sociology* 63, no. 3 (2012): 554.

32. John Rawls, *A Theory of Justice* (New York: Oxford University Press, 1999).

33. Robert Proctor and Londa L. Schiebinger, eds., *Agnotology: The Making and Unmaking of Ignorance* (Stanford, CA: Stanford University Press, 2008); Matthias Gross, "The

Unknown in Process: Dynamic Connections of Ignorance, Non-Knowledge and Related Concepts," *Current Sociology* 55, no. 5 (2007): 742–59; McGoey, "The Logic of Strategic Ignorance"; Matthias Gross and Linsey McGoey, *Routledge International Handbook of Ignorance Studies* (New York: Taylor & Francis, 2015).

34. Throughout the book, I use the term "ignorance." My reasons for doing so are two-fold. First, I find the idea of "non-knowledge" susceptible to one of the very problems that the "turn to ignorance" seeks to correct; namely, the treatment of ignorance as the simple obverse of knowledge. Second, I believe that calling it "ignorance" retains the critical thrust of this line of research.

35. Michael Smithson, "Toward a Social Theory of Ignorance," *Journal for the Theory of Social Behaviour* 15, no. 2 (1985): 151–72.

36. Gross and McGoey, *Routledge International Handbook*, 4.

37. A sample of the types of ignorance catalogued by researchers: "epistemologies of ignorance" (Charles W. Mills, *The Racial Contract* [Ithaca, NY: Cornell University Press, 1997]; Nancy Tuana, "Coming to Understand: Orgasm and the Epistemology of Ignorance," *Hypatia* 19, no. 1 [2004]: 194–232), or the active construction of a worldview organized around willful ignorance on the part of the powerful to deny or ignore the reality of their power; "nescience" (Gross, "The Unknown in Process") or "meta-ignorance" (Smithson, "Toward a Social Theory"), which is the complete absence of knowledge to the extent that the absence is unrecognized (Matthias Gross, *Ignorance and Surprise: Science, Society, and Ecological Design* [Cambridge, MA: MIT Press, 2010]); "negative knowledge" (Karin Knorr-Cetina, *Epistemic Cultures: How the Sciences Make Knowledge* [Cambridge, MA: Harvard University Press, 1999]), or knowledge about the limits of knowledge; "specified ignorance" (Robert K. Merton, "Three Fragments from A Sociologist's Notebooks: Establishing the Phenomenon, Specified Ignorance, and Strategic Research Materials," *Annual Review of Sociology* 13, no. 1 [1987]: 1–29), or recognition of what is not yet known but needs to be known in order to lay the foundation for yet more knowledge; "knowledge-gaps," or "organizationally circumscribed domains of unrealized knowledge" (Scott Frickel and M. Bess Vincent, "Katrina's Contamination: Regulatory Knowledge Gaps in the Making and Unmaking of Environmental Contention," in *Dynamics of Disaster: Lessons on Risk, Response, and Recovery*, ed. B. Allen and R. Dowty Beech [New York: Routledge, 2011], 12); "selective ignorance," or ignorance that results when producers disseminate specific sorts of information while failing to produce or emphasize others (Kevin Elliot, "Selective Ignorance in Environmental Research," in Gross and McGoey, *Routledge International Handbook*, 165–73); "forbidden knowledge," or knowledge that is too dangerous or taboo to investigate (Joanna Kempner, Jon F. Merz, and Charles L. Bosk, "Forbidden Knowledge: Public Controversy and the Production of Nonknowledge," *Sociological Forum* 26, no. 3 [2011]: 475–500); Roger Shattuck, *Forbidden Knowledge: From Prometheus to Pornography* [Wilmington, MA: Mariner Books, 1997]); "unknown unknowns," that is, ignorance that individuals are unaware of and cannot anticipate, most famously "black swans" (Nassim Nicholas Taleb, *The Black Swan: The Impact of the Highly Improbable Fragility* [New York: Random House Publishing Group, 2010]); forgotten knowledge, or "structural amnesia" (Mary Douglas, *How Institutions Think* [Syracuse, NY: Syracuse University Press, 1986], 70); "concerted ignorance," or ignorance intentionally produced to avoid policing during cover-ups (Jack Katz, "Concerted Ignorance: The Social Construction of Cover-Up," *Urban Life* 8, no. 3 [1979]: 295–316); and "undone science," or potential research that for some reason is not pursued (Scott Frickel et al., "Undone Science:

Charting Social Movement and Civil Society Challenges to Research Agenda Setting," *Science, Technology & Human Values* 35, no. 4 [2009]: 444–73).

38. Merton, "Three Fragments," 10.

39. For example, see McGoey, "The Logic of Strategic Ignorance"; Robert Proctor, *Cancer Wars: How Politics Shapes What We Know and Don't Know About Cancer* (New York: Basic Books, 1995).

40. See Stuart Firestein, *Ignorance: How It Drives Science* (New York: Oxford University Press, 2012). Indeed, one of the crucial insights of ignorance studies is the crucial role of ignorance in science. The more insights gained, the more questions raised. Thus, science, widely acknowledged as our greatest tool in producing knowledge, not only depends on ignorance for its motivations and its methods; it is also a primary producer of ignorance.

41. Readers will likely note the similarities between my concept of reinvention and Thomas Kuhn's notion of "paradigm shift" (Thomas S. Kuhn, *The Structure of Scientific Revolutions*, 3rd ed. [Chicago: University of Chicago Press, 1996]). Both are posited as involving revolutionary changes that alter the knowledge production of a collective. However, I have decided to use the more general term "reinvention," out of an appreciation of important differences between the two processes. First, Kuhn's analysis is restricted to scientific fields, whose primary responsibility is the production of knowledge. The pressures on psychiatry are broader; as a consulting profession (Freidson, *Profession of Medicine*), it is tasked with both understanding its object *and acting upon this understanding*. This difference is significant when it comes to the dynamics related to ignorance. For science, ignorance can serve as a motivation for research and a justification for the knowledge-producing endeavor (Firestein, *Ignorance*). For a consulting profession, ignorance presents a problem and takes on a more negative valence. Tasked with doing something, consulting professions cannot be perceived as knowing little. Second is the matter of degree of crisis implied. Kuhn's paradigm shifts are posited as emerging from the accumulation of anomalies that create dissatisfaction with a paradigm over time. Psychiatry's crises are driven by something more fundamental, not by anomalies within a particular paradigm but by a persistent ignorance that cuts across all paradigms. Finally, reinventions encompass more fundamental epistemological changes than Kuhn's paradigm shift. Scientific fields undergoing a paradigm shift retain basic epistemological assumptions regarding the nature of scientific inquiry. They might posit new theoretical models to make sense of facts, but they do not involve a reconsideration of what is considered a fact. Not so for psychiatry's reinventions. Here, we witness changes in basic epistemological assumptions. Given these differences, I use "reinvention" to highlight the distinct politics of psychiatry's transformations.

42. Especially those interested in technological innovation; see Harro van Lente and Arie Rip, "The Rise of Membrane Technology: From Rhetorics to Social Reality," *Social Studies of Science* 28, no. 2 (1998): 221–54; Paul A. Martin, "Genes as Drugs: The Social Shaping of Gene Therapy and the Reconstruction of Genetic Disease," *Sociology of Health & Illness* 21, no. 5 (1999): 517–38; Adam M. Hedgecoe, "Terminology and the Construction of Scientific Disciplines: The Case of Pharmacogenomics," *Science, Technology, & Human Values* 28, no. 4 (2003): 513–37; Brigitte Nerlich and Christopher Halliday, "Avian Flu: The Creation of Expectations in the Interplay between Science and the Media," *Sociology of Health & Illness* 29, no. 1 (2007): 46–65; Nik Brown and Brian Rappert, *Contested Futures: A Sociology of Prospective Techno-Science* (London: Taylor & Francis, 2017).

43. Nik Brown and Mike Michael, "A Sociology of Expectations: Retrospecting Prospects

and Prospecting Retrospects," *Technology Analysis & Strategic Management* 15, no. 1 (2003): 4.

44. Mike Fortun, *Promising Genomics: Iceland and deCODE Genetics in a World of Speculation* (Berkeley: University of California Press, 2008); Grégoire Mallard and Andrew Lakoff, "How Claims to Know the Future Are Used to Understand the Present," in *Social Knowledge in the Making*, ed. Neil Gross, Charles Camic, and Michèle Lamont (Chicago: University of Chicago Press, 2012), 339–77.

45. Mads Borup et al., "The Sociology of Expectations in Science and Technology," *Technology Analysis & Strategic Management* 18, nos. 3–4 (2006): 285–98.

46. Harro van Lente, *Promising Technology: The Dynamics of Expectations in Technological Developments* (Chicago: Eburon, 1993), 238.

47. Brown and Michael, "A Sociology of Expectations."

48. Borup et al., "The Sociology of Expectations."

49. Adam Hedgecoe and Paul Martin, "The Drugs Don't Work: Expectations and the Shaping of Pharmacogenetics," *Social Studies of Science* 33, no. 3 (2003): 327–64; Cynthia Selin, "The Sociology of the Future: Tracing Stories of Technology and Time," *Sociology Compass* 2, no. 6 (2008): 1878–95.

50. Eviatar Zerubavel, *Time Maps: Collective Memory and the Social Shape of the Past* (Chicago: University of Chicago Press, 2003), 91.

51. Underlying this argument is a view of human agency, both collective and individual, taken from Emirbayer and Mische. They conceive agency as a "temporally embedded process of social engagement, informed by the past (in its 'iterational' or habitual aspect) but also oriented toward the future (as a 'projective' capacity to imagine alternative possibilities) and toward the present (as a 'practical-evaluative' capacity to contextualize past habits and future projects within the contingencies of the moment)." The interaction between the past, present, and future in social action comprises a "chordal triad." While all social actors are embedded within each of these temporalities at once, they can be oriented toward one more than the other at any given moment. Psychiatric reformers, I will argue, have been oriented primarily toward the future in managing their ignorance. Hence the central importance of expectations in my analysis. See Mustafa Emirbayer and Ann Mische, "What Is Agency?" *American Journal of Sociology* 103, no. 4 (1998): 962–1023.

52. Here, I draw on an understanding of habit derived from American pragmatist philosophy. Pragmatism harbors an abiding appreciation of the role of habit in human thought and action. Pragmatism begins from the premise that thought and action are inextricably linked and that the purpose of ideas is to accomplish real-world practical ends. Thus, appealing to the American pragmatist tradition, sociologist Neil Gross defined collectively enacted habits as "ways that groups of individual actors, including those who comprise collective actors of various kinds, have of working together to solve problems" ("A Pragmatist Theory of Social Mechanisms," *American Sociological Review* 74, no. 3 [2009]: 370–71).

53. John Dewey, *The Quest for Certainty: A Study of the Relation of Knowledge and Action* (New York: Minton, Balch & Co., 1929), 42.

54. The depth to which this habit permeates psychiatry is reflected in the fact that the hype/disappointment cycle is reproduced at lower levels in disease fads (see Ian Hacking, *Mad Travelers: Reflections on the Reality of Transient Mental Illness* [Cambridge, MA: Harvard University Press, 2002]; Allan V. Horwitz and Jerome C. Wakefield, "The Epidemic in Mental Illness: Clinical Fact or Survey Artifact?," *contexts* 5, no. 1 [2007]: 19–23; Elizabeth Lunbeck, *The Americanization of Narcissism* [Cambridge,

MA: Harvard University Press, 2014]; Richard Noll, *American Madness* [Cambridge, MA: Harvard University Press, 2011]) and treatment trends (see Pressman, *Last Resort*; Elliot S. Valenstein, *Great and Desperate Cures: The Rise and Decline of Psychosurgery and Other Radical Treatments for Mental Illness* [New York: Basic Books, 1986]). The manifestation of this pattern at different levels reflects a fractal-like relationship (Andrew Abbott, *Chaos of Disciplines* [Chicago: University of Chicago Press, 2001]) with the more general professional transformations.

55. Charles E. Rosenberg, "Contested Boundaries: Psychiatry, Disease, and Diagnosis," *Perspectives in Biology and Medicine* 49, no. 3 (2006): 407–24.

56. I adopt an agnostic position common to social constructionist analyses of science. Given the politics of mental illness, especially as they have emerged among antipsychiatry activists who argue that mental illness is a myth, any sociological analysis of psychiatry and mental illness invariably must address the bugaboo of social constructionism. Much of the literature on social construction offers a false choice: that one either accepts the reality of mental illness or rejects it as purely socially constructed. This forced choice betrays a lack of humility toward our basic ignorance of mental disorders. Too much remains uncertain to justify a firm commitment either way. Under such conditions, it seems to me that the most prudent *analytical* position is the least *politically* satisfying one; that is, avoiding a commitment to final judgment one way or the other.

57. Harry C. Solomon, "The American Psychiatric Association in Relation to American Psychiatry," *American Journal of Psychiatry* 115, no. 1 (1958): 1.

58. Pace sociologist of science Bruno Latour (*The Pasteurization of France* [Cambridge, MA: Harvard University Press, 1988], 19), I view these articles as "little machine[s] for displacing interests, beliefs, and aligning them in such a way as to point the reader, almost inevitably, in a particular direction." As such, I focus on the persuasive rhetoric and performative aspect of scientific writing (Stephen Hilgartner, *Science on Stage: Expert Advice as Public Drama* [Stanford, CA: Stanford University Press, 2000]).

59. Interviews focused on topics related to psychiatry today, specifically as they pertain to the *Diagnostic and Statistical Manual of Mental Disorders* (DSM). The sample included mostly psychiatrists (and a couple of psychologists) who participated in the DSM-5 revision or acted as public critics of the revision. Research subjects were identified primarily through a snowball sample. The interviews were conducted by phone or in person when possible and lasted approximately one hour. The interviews were semi-structured so that the pertinent topics were addressed but in a manner that allowed respondents a degree of flexibility in formulating their answers. The interviews covered two main sets of questions. The first section asked respondents about their general views on DSM as well as their use of the manual. The second section focused specifically on the proposed revisions to DSM-5. Data from these interviews is anonymized so as to protect the research subjects from any liability or professional risks.

60. Of particular help has been the research by Gerald Grob, Nathan Hale, Allan Horwitz, S. D. Lamb, Elizabeth Lunbeck, George Makari, Richard Noll, Roy Porter, Jack Pressman, Charles Rosenberg, David Rothman, Andrew Scull, Edward Shorter, and Eli Zaretsky, to name a few. I take responsibility for any confusions or misinterpretations that may arise in my discussion of the research of others.

61. Noll, *American Madness*, 8.

62. Ian Gold and Joel Gold, *Suspicious Minds: How Culture Shapes Madness* (New York: Free Press, 2015), 230–34. The notion of aspirational psychiatry underscores the role that reformers perform in articulating visions of psychiatry's future and its aspirations.

These often become the dominant face of the profession, despite the fact that this face might not reflect the reality of psychiatric practice.

63. Joao Biehl, *Vita: Life in a Zone of Social Abandonment* (Berkeley: University of California Press, 2005).

64. Pressman, *Last Resort*, 438.

CHAPTER ONE

1. The terms "psychiatry" and "psychiatrist" did not become part of general use in the United States until the twentieth century. See Norman Dain, *Concepts of Insanity in the United States, 1789–1865* (New Brunswick, NJ: Rutgers University Press, 1964).

2. David Gollaher, *Voice for the Mad: The Life of Dorothea Dix* (New York: Free Press, 1995), vii.

3. Dorothea Lynde Dix, *Conversations on Common Things: Or, Guide to Knowledge. With Questions. For the Use of Schools and Families. By a Teacher* (Boston: Munroe and Francis, 1824).

4. Gollaher, *Voice for the Mad*, 112.

5. Dorothea Lynde Dix, *Memorial to the Legislature of Massachusetts* (Boston: Directors of the Old South Work, 1843), 3, 4.

6. Ibid., 7.

7. Ibid., 5.

8. Ibid., 5, 6.

9. Ibid., 4.

10. Gollaher, *Voice for the Mad*, 133.

11. Without suffrage, petitioning was one of the only means by which women could participate in political life.

12. Thomas J. Brown, *Dorothea Dix: New England Reformer* (Cambridge, MA: Harvard University Press, 1998), 122.

13. General Assembly of the State of Illinois, *Reports Made to the Senate and House of Representatives of the State of Illinois, Regular Sessions* (Springfield, IL: George R. Weber, public printer, 1846), 81.

14. Gollaher, *Voice for the Mad*, 192.

15. This vast body of literature includes Alex Beam, *Gracefully Insane: The Rise and Fall of America's Premier Mental Hospital* (New York: Public Affairs, 2009); Ellen Dwyer, *Homes for the Mad: Life Inside Two Nineteenth-Century Asylums* (New Brunswick, NJ: Rutgers University Press, 1987); Foucault, *Madness and Civilization*; Lynn Gamwell and Nancy Tomes, *Madness in America: Cultural and Medical Perceptions of Mental Illness before 1914* (Ithaca, NY: Cornell University Press, 1995); Lawrence B. Goodheart, *Mad Yankees: The Hartford Retreat for the Insane and Nineteenth-Century Psychiatry* (Amherst, MA: University of Massachusetts Press, 2003); Gerald N. Grob, *The State and the Mentally Ill: A History of Worcester State Hospital in Massachusetts, 1830–1920* (Durham: University of North Carolina Press, 1966); Grob, *Mental Illness and American Society, 1875–1940* (Princeton, NJ: Princeton University Press, 1983); Grob, *Mental Institutions in America*; Peter McCandless, *Moonlight, Magnolias & Madness: Insanity in South Carolina from the Colonial Period to the Progressive Era* (Durham: University of North Carolina Press, 1996); Roy Porter and David Wright, *The Confinement of the Insane: International Perspectives, 1800–1965* (New York: Cambridge University Press, 2003); Benjamin Reiss, *Theaters of Madness: Insane Asylums and Nineteenth-Century American Culture* (Chicago: University of Chicago Press, 2008); Rothman, *The Discovery of the Asylum*; Andrew Scull, *Madhouses, Mad-Doctors, and Madmen: The Social*

History of Psychiatry in the Victorian Era (Philadelphia: University of Pennsylvania Press, 1981); Scull, *Decarceration: Community Treatment and the Deviant: A Radical View* (New Brunswick, NJ: Rutgers University Press, 1984); Tomes, *A Generous Confidence*; Edwin R. Wallace and John Gach, *History of Psychiatry and Medical Psychology* (New York: Springer, 2008); Carla Yanni, *The Architecture of Madness: Insane Asylums in the United States* (Minneapolis: University of Minnesota Press, 2007); Katherine Ziff, *Asylum on the Hill: History of a Healing Landscape* (Athens: Ohio University Press, 2012); and Zilboorg, *A History of Medical Psychology*.

16. For example, see Zilboorg, *A History of Medical Psychology*.

17. Historians are divided on how effective asylum treatment was. Grob (*The State and the Mentally Ill*) is bullish. Citing research conducted by Dr. John G. Park in the late 1800s, he concludes that while superintendents' cure rates were inflated, moral treatment appeared to have helped about half of the patients treated. Others, including Scull (*Social Order*), are less confident. The nineteenth-century asylum statistics are so shot through with problems that it is unlikely the efficacy question will ever be resolved.

18. See Foucault, *Madness and Civilization*, 60; Scull, *Social Order*, 50.

19. Grob, *The State and the Mentally Ill*.

20. Rothman, *The Discovery of the Asylum*.

21. George Miller Beard, "Neurasthenia, or Nervous Exhaustion," *Boston Medical and Surgical Journal* 80, no. 13 (1869): 217.

22. Alexis de Tocqueville, *Democracy in America*, trans. A. Goldhammer (New York: Library of America, 2004), 628.

23. Daniel Walker Howe, *What Hath God Wrought: The Transformation of America, 1815–1848* (New York: Oxford University Press, 2007).

24. Karen Halttunen, *Confidence Men and Painted Women: A Study of Middle-Class Culture in America, 1830–1870* (New Haven, CT: Yale University Press, 1982).

25. While similar reforms occurred in other countries, the particular combination of lay and medical influence varied across contexts. However, nonmedical reformers were important to all these efforts. This fact should caution against narrowly viewing the emergence of psychiatry as a discretely medical phenomenon. Indeed, the role of nonmedical persons in the establishment of the mental health system seems noteworthy today only because we have grown accustomed to viewing the problems of mental distress through the lens of medicine.

26. Samuel Tuke, *Description of the Retreat* (reprinted, London: Process Press, [1813] 1996), 141.

27. Scull, *Social Order*, 99–100.

28. Quoted in Dora B. Weiner, "Philippe Pinel's 'Memoir on Madness' of December 11, 1794," *American Journal of Psychiatry* 149, no. 6 (1992): 730.

29. Philippe Pinel, *A Treatise on Insanity: In Which Are Contained the Principles of a New and More Practical Nosology of Maniacal Disorders than Has Yet Been Offered to the Public* (Sheffield: W. Todd, 1806), 4; quoted in Weiner, "Philippe Pinel's 'Memoir on Madness,'" 731.

30. Pinel, *A Treatise on Insanity*, 4.

31. Andrew Scull, *Madness in Civilization: A Cultural History of Insanity, from the Bible to Freud, from the Madhouse to Modern Medicine* (Princeton, NJ: Princeton University Press, 2015), 190.

32. Grob, *Mental Institutions in America*, 87.

33. Rothman, *The Discovery of the Asylum*, xviii.

34. Grob, *Mental Institutions in America*.

35. Amariah Brigham, "The Moral Treatment of Insanity," *American Journal of Psychiatry* 4, no. 1 (1847): 1.

36. Ibid., 10.

37. Reiss, *Theaters of Madness*, 4.

38. For example, Foucault (*History of Madness*, 504) argues: "It was not as a scientist that *homo medicus* gained authority in the asylum, but as a wise man." See also Rothman, *The Discovery of the Asylum*.

39. Paul Starr, *The Social Transformation of American Medicine* (New York: Basic Books, 1982); Owen Whooley, *Knowledge in the Time of Cholera: The Struggle over American Medicine in the Nineteenth Century* (Chicago: University of Chicago Press, 2013).

40. Benjamin Rush, *Diseases of the Mind* (reprinted Birmingham, AL: Classics of Medicine Library, [1812] 1979), 17.

41. Quoted in Rothman, *The Discovery of the Asylum*, 112.

42. Tomes, *A Generous Confidence*; Dain, *Concepts of Insanity*.

43. George Makari, *Soul Machine: The Invention of the Modern Mind* (New York: W. W. Norton, 2015).

44. Amariah Brigham, "Definition of Insanity: Nature of the Disease," *American Journal of Psychiatry* 1, no. 2 (1844): 105.

45. Ibid., 97.

46. Ibid., 99.

47. Eric Carlson, "The Influence of Phrenology on Early American Psychiatric Thought," *American Journal of Psychiatry* 115, no. 6 (1958): 535–38.

48. Rothman, *The Discovery of the Asylum*, 110.

49. Grob, *Mental Institutions in America*, 154.

50. Bucknill, "The Pathology of Insanity," 357–58.

51. Ibid., 348.

52. Isaac Ray, *A Treatise on the Medical Jurisprudence of Insanity* (Boston: Freeman and Bolles, 138), 65.

53. Managers of the State Lunatic Asylum, *First Annual Report of the Managers of the State Lunatic Asylum* (Utica, NY: reprinted at the Asylum, 1844), 1.

54. Ibid., 25.

55. Quoted in Walter Barton, *The History and Influence of the American Psychiatric Association* (Arlington, VA: American Psychiatric Publishing, 1987), 39.

56. Henry Alden Bunker, "American Psychiatric Literature During the Past One Hundred Years," in *One Hundred Years of the American Psychiatric Association*, ed. American Psychiatric Association (New York: Columbia University Press, 1947), 195–272.

57. Nancy Tomes, "A Generous Confidence: Thomas Story Kirkbride's Philosophy of Asylum Construction and Management," in *Madhouses, Mad-Doctors, and Madmen*, 123.

58. Pliny Earle, "The Psychopathic Hospital of the Future," *American Journal of Psychiatry* 24, no. 2 (1867): 123.

59. Thomas Story Kirkbride, *On the Construction, Organization, and General Arrangements of Hospitals for the Insane* (Philadelphia: Lindsay & Blakiston, 1854), 42.

60. Ibid., 2.

61. Ibid.

62. Ibid., 7.

63. Ibid., 9.

64. Ibid., 11–12.

65. Ibid., 16.

66. Ibid., 16–17, 21.

67. Brigham, "The Moral Treatment of Insanity," 1.
68. Grob, *Mental Institutions in America*, 168.
69. Tomes, *A Generous Confidence*.
70. Kirkbride, *On the Construction*, 37.
71. Managers of the State Lunatic Asylum, *Sixth Annual Report of the Managers of the State Lunatic Asylum* (Albany, NY: Weed, Parson and Co., 1849), 55.
72. Managers of the State Lunatic Asylum, *Twenty-Sixth Annual Report of the Managers of the State Lunatic Asylum* (Albany, NY: Argus, 1868), 17.
73. Kirkbride, *On the Construction*, 37.
74. Ibid., 58.
75. Earle, "The Psychopathic Hospital," 124.
76. Kirkbride, *On the Construction*, 62.
77. Reiss, *Theaters of Madness*, 78.
78. Isaac Ray, "Shakespeare's Delineations of Insanity," *American Journal of Psychiatry* 3, no. 4 (1847): 328, 289.
79. Dain, *Concepts of Insanity*, 139.
80. Mary Poovey, *A History of the Modern Fact: Problems of Knowledge in the Sciences of Wealth and Society* (Chicago: University of Chicago Press, 1998).
81. Theodore Porter, *Trust in Numbers: The Pursuit of Objectivity in Science and Public Life* (Princeton, NJ: Princeton University Press, 1996).
82. Steven Kelman, "The Political Foundations of American Statistical Policy," in *The Politics of Statistics*, ed. William Alonso and Paul Starr (New York: Russell Sage Foundation, 1987), 275.
83. Porter, *Trust in Numbers*.
84. Albert Deutsch, "The Cult of Curability, Its Rise and Decline: A Page from Psychiatric History," *American Journal of Psychiatry* 92, no. 6 (1936): 1261–80.
85. Theodore Porter, "Funny Numbers," *Culture Unbound: Journal of Current Cultural Research* 4 (2012): 585–98.
86. Pressman, *Last Resort*, 154. Using the metaphor of a turnstile, Pressman demonstrates that if even a few admitted patients are not discharged in a timely matter, over time a "fatalistic logic" takes hold. The accumulation of even a small percentage of chronic cases would overrun mental hospitals in the long run.
87. Grob, *Mental Institutions in America*, 190.
88. Grob, *Mental Illness and American Society*, 180–95.
89. Historian Edward Shorter attributes some of this growing demand to an actual increase in the prevalence of mental illness, particularly for neurosyphilis, alcoholism, and schizophrenia. It is hard to assess these claims, given all the problems with statistical data on mental illness in this period. Shorter might be on to something regarding neurosyphilis and alcoholism, but I find his case of the rising prevalence of schizophrenia unconvincing. See Edwin Shorter, *A History of Psychiatry: From the Era of the Asylum to the Age of Prozac* (New York: John Wiley & Sons, 1997), 53–64.
90. These were later published in 1887, in a book entitled *The Curability of the Insane: A Series of Studies*. Pliny Earle, *The Curability of Insanity: A Series of Studies* (Philadelphia: J. B. Lippincott Co., 1887).
91. Pliny Earle, *A Glance at Insanity and the Management of the Insane in the American States* (Boston: Franklin Press, 1879), 6.
92. Ibid., 7.
93. Earle, *The Curability of the Insane*, 18.
94. Earle, *A Glance at Insanity*, 5.

95. John M. Galt, "The Farm of St. Anne," *American Journal of Psychiatry* 11, no. 4 (1855): 352–57.
96. Rothman, *The Discovery of the Asylum*, 282.
97. Porter, "Funny Numbers."
98. Joseph P. Lovering, *S. Weir Mitchell* (New York: Twayne Publishers, 1971).
99. And infamous for his mistreatment of Charlotte Perkins, who chronicled her plight in the thinly fictionalized, now classic short story "The Yellow Wallpaper." Charlotte Perkins Gilman, "The Yellow Wallpaper," *New England Magazine* 11, no. 5 (1892): 647–57.
100. S. Weir Mitchell, "Address before the Fiftieth Annual Meeting of the American Medico-Psychological Association, Held in Philadelphia, May 16th, 1894," *Journal of Nervous and Mental Disease* 19, no. 7 (1894): 414.
101. Ibid.
102. Ibid., 422.
103. Ibid., 414.
104. Ibid., 426.
105. Ibid., 422.
106. "Words Fitly Spoken," *Medical Surgical Reporter*, 70, no. 22 (1894): 789; "Editorial Notes," *Cincinnati Lancet and Clinic*, 1894, no. 24 (1894): 669.
107. Quoted in Shorter, *A History of Psychiatry*, 68.
108. Quoted in Robert Whitaker, *Mad in America: Bad Science, Bad Medicine, and the Enduring Mistreatment of the Mentally Ill* (New York: Basic Books, 2003), 37.
109. Grob, *Mental Illness and American Society*, 61.
110. Walter Channing, "Some Remarks on the Address Delivered to the American Medico-Psychological Association, by S. Weir Mitchell, May 16, 1894," *American Journal of Psychiatry* 51, no. 2 (1894): 171.
111. Ibid., 172.
112. Ibid.
113. "The Study of Mind," *American Journal of Psychiatry* 17, no. 3 (1861): 235.
114. Tyler, "Tests of Insanity," 141.
115. Association of Medical Superintendents of American Institutions for the Insane (AMSAII), "Proceedings of the Association of Medical Superintendents," *American Journal of Insanity* 30, no. 2 (1873): 185.
116. Henry P. Stearns, "Some Notes on the Present State of Psychiatry," *American Journal of Psychiatry* 48, no. 1 (1891): 1–2.

CHAPTER TWO

1. "Guiteau," *American Journal of Psychiatry* 39, no. 2 (1882): 208–27.
2. John Charles Bucknill, "The Plea of Insanity in the Case of Charles Julius Guiteau," *American Journal of Psychiatry* 39, no. 2 (1882): 183.
3. "Guiteau," 209.
4. Bucknill, "The Plea of Insanity," 191.
5. Frederick A. Fenning, *The Trial of Guiteau* (Minneapolis: University of Minnesota Press, 1933), 136.
6. Quoted in Bucknill, "The Plea of Insanity," 185.
7. In his book on the trial, historian Charles Rosenberg argues that at stake was not only a dispute between superintendents and neurologists, but also a generational divide *within* psychiatry between the older superintendents and younger psychiatrists sympathetic to laboratory methods. See Charles E. Rosenberg, *The Trial of the Assassin Guiteau: Psychiatry and the Law in the Gilded Age* (Chicago: University of Chicago Press, 1995).

8. Quoted in Fenning, *The Trial of Guiteau*, 132.
9. Rosenberg, *The Trial of the Assassin Guiteau*.
10. Edward C. Spitzka, "Reform in the Scientific Study of Psychiatry," *Journal of Nervous and Mental Disease* 5, no. 2 (1878): 209.
11. Candice Millard, *Destiny of the Republic: A Tale of Madness, Medicine and the Murder of a President* (New York: Anchor Books, 2012), 278.
12. Quoted in Rosenberg, *The Trial of the Assassin Guiteau*, 97.
13. "Case of Guiteau," *American Journal of Psychiatry* 39, no. 2 (1882): 207.
14. Hoch, "On the Clinical Study," 283.
15. E. Stanley Abbot, "The Criteria of Insanity and the Problems of Psychiatry," *American Journal of Psychiatry* 59, no. 1 (1902): 2.
16. Adolf Meyer, *The Collected Papers of Adolf Meyer: Psychiatry*, vol. 2, ed. Eunice E. Winters (Baltimore, MD: Johns Hopkins University Press, 1951), 4.
17. S. D. Lamb, *Pathologist of the Mind: Adolf Meyer and the Origins of American Psychiatry* (Baltimore, MD: Johns Hopkins University Press, 2014), 46.
18. Adolf Meyer, "Presidential Address: Thirty-Five Years of Psychiatry in the United States and Our Present Outlook," *American Journal of Psychiatry* 85, no. 1 (1928): 25.
19. In his novel *Arrowsmith*, Sinclair Lewis offers a social commentary on American medicine in the 1920s by recounting the exploits of a fictional doctor, Martin Arrowsmith, whose career intersects with the major institutions of medicine of the period. See Sinclair Lewis, *Arrowsmith* (New York: Signet Classics, 2008). Meyer's career traces an equivalent route through psychiatry. The historian Edward Shorter (*A History of Psychiatry*, 92) echoes this sentiment, describing Meyer as "a kind of Johnny Appleseed through the landscape of American psychiatry."
20. Lamb, *Pathologist of the Mind*; Noll, *American Madness*.
21. Elmer Ernest Southard, "Proceedings of the Seventy-Second Annual Meeting of the American Medico-Psychological Association," *American Journal of Psychiatry* 73, no. 1 (1916): 107.
22. Adolf Meyer, *Psychobiology: A Science of Man* (Springfield, IL: Charles C. Thomas, 1957), 8.
23. Ibid., 8.
24. Quoted in Adolf Meyer and Edward Bradford Titchener, *Defining American Psychology: The Correspondence between Adolf Meyer and Edward Bradford Titchener*, ed. Ruth Leys and Rand B. Evan (Baltimore, MD: Johns Hopkins University Press, 1990), 451.
25. Adolf Meyer, "The Aims and Meaning of Psychiatric Diagnosis," *American Journal of Psychiatry* 74, no. 2 (1917): 166.
26. Meyer, *Psychobiology*, 207.
27. Lamb, *Pathologist of the Mind*.
28. Louis Menand, *The Metaphysical Club* (New York: Farrar, Straus & Giroux, 2001).
29. Dewey, *The Quest for Certainty*.
30. John Dewey, *Democracy and Education* (New York: Macmillan, 1916), 49; William James, "Pragmatism's Conception of Truth," *Journal of Philosophy, Psychology and Scientific Methods* 4, no. 6 (1907): 142.
31. Meyer, *Psychobiology*, 47.
32. William James, *The Principles of Psychology* (New York: Henry Holt and Co., 1890), 488.
33. Quoted in Meyer and Titchener, *Defining American Psychology*, 146.
34. William James, *Pragmatism: A New Name for Some Old Ways of Thinking* (New York: Longmans, Green & Co., 1907), 34.
35. Lamb, *Pathologist of the Mind*.

36. John Harley Warner, *Against the Spirit of System: The French Impulse in Nineteenth-Century American Medicine* (Princeton, NJ: Princeton University Press, 1998).

37. Meyer, *Collected Papers*, 18.

38. Wherever he went, Meyer instituted reforms in recordkeeping. For example, at Worcester, he created a system by which each individual would be assigned a single flexible case folder. This change allowed for the rapid reconstruction of each patient's entire history requisite for case-based reasoning. Previously, information on any given individual was dispersed through handwritten entries in large bound volumes that ran over 500 pages, making it impossible to efficiently reconstruct patient histories. Grob, *The State and the Mentally Ill*, 294.

39. Quoted in Gerald M. Grob, *The Inner World of American Psychiatry, 1890–1940: Selected Correspondence* (New Brunswick, NJ: Rutgers University Press, 1985), 33–34.

40. Meyer, *Collected Papers*, 135.

41. Meyer, *Psychobiology*, 207.

42. Quoted in Salmon, "Presidential Address," 4; Adolf Meyer, "The Role of the Mental Factors in Psychiatry," *American Journal of Psychiatry* 65, no. 1 (1908): 43.

43. Meyer, "The Role of the Mental Factors," 43.

44. Lamb, *Pathologist of the Mind*.

45. Meyer, "The Role of the Mental Factors," 44.

46. Meyer, *Psychobiology*, 118.

47. Meyer, *Collected Papers*, 177.

48. Ibid., 115.

49. Ibid., 39.

50. Meyer, "Presidential Address," 26.

51. Meyer, *Collected Papers*, 81.

52. Many have shared the assessment by Noll (*American Madness*, 39) that Meyer wrote in a "ruminative, tangential, and elusive (some of his contemporaries would say evasive) manner."

53. Ruth Leys, "Types of One: Adolf Meyer's Life Chart and the Representation of Individuality," *Representations* 34 (1991): 1–28.

54. Ibid., 13.

55. Clarence B. Farrar, "The Making of Psychiatric Records," *American Journal of Psychiatry* 62, no. 3 (1906): 485.

56. Charles Sanders Peirce, *The Essential Peirce*, ed. Nathan Houser and Christine J. W. Kloesel (Bloomington: Indiana University Press, 1992), 139.

57. Meyer, *Psychobiology*, 6.

58. Jonathan Sadowsky, "Beyond the Metaphor of the Pendulum: Electroconvulsive Therapy, Psychoanalysis, and the Styles of American Psychiatry," *Journal of the History of Medicine and Allied Sciences* 61, no. 1 (2006): 1–25.

59. For example, see S. Nassir Ghaemi, "Adolf Meyer: Psychiatric Anarchist," *Philosophy, Psychiatry, & Psychology* 14, no. 4 (2007): 341–45.

60. Albert M. Barrett, "The Broadened Interests of Psychiatry," *American Journal of Psychiatry* 79, no. 1 (1922): 7.

61. Lewellys F. Barker, "On the Importance of Pathological and Bacteriological Laboratories in Connection with Hospitals for the Insane," *American Journal of Psychiatry* 57, no. 3 (1901): 515.

62. Ibid.

63. Grob, *Mental Illness and American Society*, 188.

64. See Ludwik Fleck, *Genesis and Development of a Scientific Fact* (Chicago: University of Chicago Press, 1979).

65. Meyer, *Collected Papers*, 120.

66. Gerald Adler Blumer, "Presidential Address," *American Journal of Psychiatry* 60, no. 1 (1903): 3.

67. James Thomas Searcy, "Have We a Specialty?," *American Journal of Psychiatry* 70, no. 1 (1913): 263–72.

68. Barrett, "The Broadened Interests of Psychiatry," 13.

69. Bernard Sachs, "Advances in Neurology and Their Relation to Psychiatry," *American Journal of Psychiatry* 54, no. 1 (1897): 19.

70. Jacob Kasanin, "The Problem of Research in Mental Hospitals," *American Journal of Psychiatry* 92, no. 2 (1935): 401.

71. David Rosner, *A Once Charitable Enterprise: Hospitals and Healthcare in Brooklyn and New York, 1895–1915* (New York: Cambridge University Press, 1982).

72. Lunbeck, *The Psychiatric Persuasion*, 22.

73. Henry C. Eyman, "Presidential Address," *American Journal of Psychiatry* 77, no. 1 (1920): 4.

74. Grob, *The Inner World of American Psychiatry*, 12.

75. This macabre psychiatric history is described in Andrew Scull's book *Madhouse: A Tragic Tale of Megalomania and Modern Medicine* (2007) and Noll's *American Madness* (194–213).

76. Quoted in Grob, *The Inner World of American Psychiatry*, 119.

77. Quoted in ibid., 114.

78. Valenstein, *Great and Desperate Cures*.

79. Scull, *Madness in Civilization*, 316.

80. Lunbeck, *The Psychiatric Persuasion*.

81. Salmon, "Presidential Address," 3.

82. H. W. Mitchell, "Presidential Address," *American Journal of Psychiatry* 80, no. 1 (1923): 5.

83. Ibid., 6.

84. Lewellys F. Barker, "Psychiatry and Public Health," *American Journal of Psychiatry* 81, no. 1 (1924): 14.

85. John C. Whitehorn and Gregory Zilboorg, "Present Trends in American Psychiatric Research," *American Journal of Psychiatry* 90, no. 2 (1933): 311.

86. Barrett, "The Broadened Interests of Psychiatry," 9.

87. William Healy, "The Newer Psychiatry: Its Field—Training for It," *American Journal of Psychiatry* 82, no. 3 (1926): 392.

88. Eric Caplan, *Mind Games: American Culture and the Birth of Psychotherapy* (Berkeley: University of California Press, 2001); Eugene Taylor, *Shadow Culture: Psychology and Spirituality in America* (Washington, DC: Counterpoint, 1999).

89. Meyer, *Collected Papers*, 586.

90. Meyer, *Psychobiology*, 158.

91. See chapter 3 for a fuller discussion on the content of psychoanalytic theory.

92. This is a reference to Thomas Henry Huxley, who defined science as "organized common sense" (Lamb, *Pathologist of the Mind*, 35), a notion squared with American pragmatism.

93. Adolf Meyer, "Scope and Teaching of Psychobiology," *Academic Medicine* 10, no. 2 (1935): 94–95.

94. Charles P. Bancroft, "Presidential Address: Hopeful and Discouraging Aspects of the Psychiatric Outlook," *American Journal of Psychiatry* 65, no. 1 (1908): 16.

95. E. Stanley Abbot, "What Is Mental Hygiene? A Definition and an Outline," *American Journal of Psychiatry* 81, no. 2 (1924): 264.
96. Meyer, "Presidential Address," 12.
97. Clifford Beers, *A Mind That Found Itself: An Autobiography* (New York: Longmans, Green, and Co., 1908).
98. Barrett, "The Broadened Interests of Psychiatry," 13.
99. N. D. Jewson, "The Disappearance of the Sick-Man from Medical Cosmology 1870–1970," *Sociology* 10 (1976): 225–44.
100. William A. White, "Presidential Address," *American Journal of Psychiatry* 82, no. 1 (1925): 9–10.
101. Abbott, *The System of Professions*, 23.
102. Daniel J. Kevles, *In the Name of Eugenics: Genetics and the Uses of Human Heredity* (Cambridge, MA: Harvard University Press, 1995); William H. Tucker, *The Science and Politics of Racial Research* (Urbana: University of Illinois Press, 1994).
103. James W. Trent Jr., *Inventing the Feeble Mind: A History of Mental Retardation in the United States* (Berkeley: University of California Press, 1994).
104. Alexandra Minna Stern, *Eugenic Nation: Faults and Frontiers of Better Breeding in Modern America* (Berkeley: University of California Press, 2005), 102–3.
105. By 1940, thirty states had enacted statutes that provided for the sterilization of individuals confined to state institutions. Between 1907 and 1925, states performed 6,244 sterilizations. Edwin Black, *War against the Weak: Eugenics and America's Campaign to Create a Master Race* (New York: Basic Books, 2003), 122.
106. Henry J. Berkley, "General Pathology of Mental Diseases," *American Journal of Psychiatry* 56, no. 3 (1900): 459; Barker, "Psychiatry and Public Health," 24.
107. Bancroft, "Presidential Address," 12.
108. Abraham Myerson, "Psychiatric Family Studies," *American Journal of Psychiatry* 73, no. 3 (1917): 360.
109. Vernon L. Briggs, "Environmental Origin of Mental Disease in Certain Families," *American Journal of Psychiatry* 73, no. 2 (1916): 223.
110. Sanger Brown, "Applied Eugenics," *American Journal of Psychiatry* 71, no. 2 (1914): 272.
111. Ian Robert Dowbiggin, *Keeping America Sane: Psychiatry and Eugenics in the United States and Canada, 1880–1940* (Ithaca, NY: Cornell University Press, 1997).
112. Madison Bentley and Edmund Vincent Cowdry, *The Problem of Mental Disorder: A Study* (New York: McGraw-Hill, 1934), v.
113. Ibid., 2.
114. Ibid.
115. Ibid., 3.
116. Ibid., 378.
117. Ibid., 51.
118. Henry B. Elkind and Carl R. Doering, "The Application of Statistical Method to the Study of Mental Disease," *American Journal of Psychiatry* 84, no. 5 (1928): 798.
119. Kasanin, "The Problem of Research," 397.
120. Whitehorn and Zilboorg, "Present Trends," 303.
121. Elkind and Doering, "The Application," 797.
122. Gosline, "A Physiological and Anatomical Approach," 235.
123. Bonnie Ellen Blustein, "'A Hollow Square of Psychological Science': American Neurologists and Psychiatrists in Conflict," in *Madhouses, Mad Doctors, and Madmen*, 241–70.
124. Noll, *American Madness*, 277.

125. See Shorter, *A History of Psychiatry*, 87–93.

126. Ghaemi, "Adolf Meyer."

127. Lamb, *Pathologist of the Mind*.

128. Emile Durkheim, *Suicide: A Study in Sociology* (New York: Free Press, [1897] 1951).

CHAPTER THREE

1. Richard Skues, "Clark Revisited: Reappraising Freud in America," in *After Freud Left: A Century of Psychoanalysis in America*, ed. John Burnham (Chicago: University of Chicago Press, 2012), 49–84.

2. Peter Gay, *Freud: A Life for Our Time* (New York: W. W. Norton, 2006).

3. Saul Rosenzweig, *Freud, Jung, and Hall the King-Maker: The Historic Expedition to America* (St. Louis, MO: Rana House, 1992).

4. Nathan G. Hale, *Freud and the Americans* (New York: Oxford University Press, 1971), 5.

5. Rosenzweig, *Freud, Jung, and Hall the King-Maker*.

6. Quoted in Ernest Jones, *The Life and Work of Sigmund Freud: Years of Maturity, 1901–1919* (New York: Basic Books, 1953), 60.

7. George C. Ham, "Reintegration of Psychoanalysis into Teaching," *American Journal of Psychiatry* 117, no. 10 (1961): 877.

8. Iago Galdston, "Psychiatry without Freud," *AMA Archives of Neurology & Psychiatry* 66, no. 1 (1951): 69.

9. Harry Stack Sullivan, *Conceptions of Modern Psychiatry* (London: Tavistock Publication, 1953), x.

10. Elkind and Doering, "The Application," 793.

11. Zilboorg, *A History of Medical Psychology*.

12. John Forrester, *Dispatches from the Freud Wars: Psychoanalysis and Its Passions* (Cambridge, MA: Harvard University Press, 1997).

13. See Shorter, *A History of Psychiatry*; Jeffrey A. Lieberman and Ogi Ogas, *Shrinks: The Untold Story of Psychiatry* (New York: Little, Brown, 2015).

14. Lisa Appignanesi, *Mad, Bad, and Sad: A History of Women and the Mind Doctors* (New York: W. W. Norton, 2009), 194.

15. For accessible histories of psychoanalytic thought, see George Makari, *Revolution in Mind: The Creation of Psychoanalysis* (New York: HarperCollins, 2008); Stephen A. Mitchell and Margaret J. Black, *Freud and Beyond: A History of Modern Psychoanalytic Thought* (New York: Basic Books, 1995).

16. John Harley Warner, "The Fall and Rise of Professional Mystery: Epistemology, Authority, and the Emergence of Laboratory Medicine in Nineteenth-Century America," in *The Laboratory Revolution in Medicine*, ed. Andrew Cunningham and Perry Williams (New York: Cambridge University Press, 2002), 110–41.

17. Caplan, *Mind Games*.

18. Taylor, *Shadow Culture*.

19. Eli Zaretsky, *Secrets of the Soul: A Social and Cultural History of Psychoanalysis* (New York: Vintage Books, 2005).

20. Hale's two volumes, *Freud and the Americans* and *The Rise and Crisis of Psychoanalysis in the United States* (Oxford University Press, 1995), together provide the most comprehensive history of psychoanalysis in the United States. My account draws extensively from them.

21. Allan V. Horwitz, *Creating Mental Illness* (Chicago: University of Chicago Press, 2002), 46–48.

22. Hale, *Freud and the Americans*, 480.

23. Hale, *The Rise and Crisis of Psychoanalysis*, 13.

24. Sigmund Freud, *Civilization and Its Discontents* (New York: W. W. Norton, 1961).

25. Barker, "Psychiatry and Public Health," 23–24.

26. Eli Zaretsky, "Charisma or Rationalization? Domesticity and Psychoanalysis in the United States in the 1950s," *Critical Inquiry* 26, no. 2 (2000): 332.

27. Makari, *Revolution in Mind*, 474.

28. William C. Menninger, *Psychiatry in a Troubled World: Yesterday's War and Today's Challenge* (New York: Macmillan, 1948), 600.

29. Zaretsky, "Charisma or Rationalization?," 335.

30. David Mechanic, *Mental Health and Social Policy: The Emergence of Managed Care*, 4th ed. (New York: Allyn & Bacon 1999), 93.

31. Maxwell Gitelson, "Psychoanalyst, USA, 1955," *American Journal of Psychiatry* 112, no. 9 (1956): 700.

32. Menninger, *Psychiatry in a Troubled World*, vii.

33. Quoted in Hale, *The Rise and Crisis of Psychoanalysis*, 7.

34. Hale, *Freud and the Americans*.

35. Rudolph M. Loewenstein, "Ego Development and Psychoanalytic Technique," *American Journal of Psychiatry* 107, no. 8 (1951): 617.

36. Mitchell and Black, *Freud and Beyond*, 26.

37. See Martin S. Bergmann, *The Hartmann Era* (New York: Other Press, 2000).

38. Heinz Hartmann, *Ego Psychology and the Problem of Adaptation* (New York: International University Press, 1958), 7.

39. This understanding of defense mechanisms shares similarities with the prior period's understanding of habit, making it amenable to those steeped in psychobiology.

40. Robert S. Wallerstein, "The Growth and Transformation of American Ego Psychology," *Journal of the American Psychoanalytic Association* 50, no. 1 (2002): 135–68.

41. Josef Breuer and Sigmund Freud, *Studies on Hysteria* (New York: Basic Books, 2000), 305.

42. Kenneth P. Starkey, "The Lengthening Hour: Time and the Demise of Psychoanalysis as Therapy," *Social Science & Medicine* 20, no. 9 (1985): 939.

43. Hartmann, *Ego Psychology*, 31.

44. Zaretsky, "Charisma or Rationalization?"

45. Franz Alexander, "Psychoanalysis Comes of Age," *Psychoanalytic Quarterly* 7 (1938): 300.

46. White, "Presidential Address," 9.

47. Franz Alexander, "Current Problems in Dynamic Psychotherapy in Its Relationship to Psychoanalysis," *American Journal of Psychiatry* 116, no. 4 (1959): 322.

48. John Burnham, ed., *After Freud Left: A Century of Psychoanalysis in America* (Chicago: University of Chicago Press, 2012).

49. Like psychoanalysis, psychodynamic psychiatry stresses the dynamic forces between conscious and unconscious elements of the mind, exploring how these forces relate to early childhood experiences. However, it does not embrace the tenets and conceptual foundations of Freudian thought to the same degree as psychoanalytic psychiatry. Psychodynamic treatment is more eclectic, more flexible, and typically of shorter duration.

50. Karl A. Menninger, *The Human Mind* (New York: A. A. Knopf, 1930), 12, 20.

51. Ibid., 263.

52. Ibid., 264, 266.

53. Ibid., 369.

54. Gitelson, "Psychoanalyst, USA, 1955."

55. Ibid., 701.
56. Anne Sealey, "The Strange Case of the Freudian Case History: The Role of Long Case Histories in the Development of Psychoanalysis," *History of the Human Sciences* 24, no. 1 (2011): 37; Carol Berkenkotter, *Patient Tales: Case Histories and the Uses of Narrative in Psychiatry* (Columbia: University of South Carolina Press, 2008), 100.
57. Luhrmann, *Of Two Minds*, 71.
58. Trigant Burrow, "The Need of an Analytic Psychiatry," *American Journal of Psychiatry* 83, no. 3 (1927): 493.
59. Carlo Ginzburg and Anna Davin, "Morelli, Freud and Sherlock Holmes: Clues and Scientific Method," *History Workshop* 9, no. 1 (1980): 11.
60. Meyer, *Collected Papers*, 617.
61. Menninger, *The Human Mind*, 363–64.
62. A. A. Brill, *Basic Principles of Psychoanalysis* (Garden City, NY: Doubleday & Company, 1949), 41.
63. Psychoanalysts elevated time to a central concern, displaying "a faith in the efficacy of the long-term" to effect a character change in patients. Starkey, "The Lengthening Hour," 942.
64. Otto Fenichel, *Problems of Psychoanalytic Technique*, trans. David Brunswick (Albany, NY: Psychoanalytic Quarterly, 1941), 15.
65. Ibid., 29, 36.
66. Menninger, *The Human Mind*, 352.
67. Charles P. Oberndorf, "Psychiatry and Psychoanalysis," *American Journal of Psychiatry* 82, no. 4 (1926): 606; Brill, *Basic Principles*, 15.
68. Mariana Craciun, "The Cultural Work of Office Charisma: Maintaining Professional Power in Psychotherapy," *Theory and Society* 45, no. 4 (2016): 371.
69. Rudolph M. Loewenstein, "The Problem of Interpretation," *Psychoanalytic Quarterly* 20, no. 10 (1951): 1–14.
70. Ibid., 2.
71. Ibid., 5.
72. Ibid., 4.
73. Ibid., 8.
74. Ibid., 3.
75. Ibid., 5.
76. Ibid.
77. Abbott notes that professions must attain a proper level of abstraction into order to stabilize their jurisdiction. Overabstraction risks attenuating a profession's jurisdiction, diluting its cognitive core and leaving it susceptible to incursions; underabstraction risks reducing professional knowledge to that of a craft-skill unworthy of professional privileges. For more discussion, see Abbott, *The System of Professions*, 98–110.
78. Loewenstein, "The Problem of Interpretation," 5.
79. Ibid.
80. Franz Alexander, "Psychoanalysis in Western Culture," *American Journal of Psychiatry* 112, no. 9 (1956): 694.
81. Fenichel, *Problems of Psychoanalytic Technique*, 53.
82. Loewenstein, "Ego Development and Psychoanalytic Technique," 618.
83. Alexander, "Psychoanalysis in Western Culture," 501.
84. Monika Krause and Michael Guggenheim, "The Couch as a Laboratory? The Spaces of Psychoanalytic Knowledge-Production between Research, Diagnosis and Treatment," *European Journal of Sociology* 54, no. 2 (2013): 187–210.

85. Craciun, "The Cultural Work of Office Charisma."

86. "Psychotherapists produce an array of metaphors to describe the therapeutic encounter—it is a dance, a duel, a drama, an attempt to listen with a different ear, to listen for what is under the surface or behind the words; it is peeling the onion, unraveling the psyche, piercing the armor of the character; it is an attempt to see the translation of motive into action in which every action serves the self." Luhrmann, *Of Two Minds*, 57.

87. Fenichel, *Problems of Psychoanalytic Technique*, 1.

88. Janet Malcolm, *Psychoanalysis: The Impossible Profession* (New York: Vintage Books, 1982), 48.

89. Edward A. Strecker, "The Practice of Psychiatry," *Archives of Neurology & Psychiatry* 31, no. 2 (1934): 412.

90. Abraham Myerson, "The Attitude of Neurologists, Psychiatrists and Psychologists Towards Psychoanalysis," *American Journal of Psychiatry* 96, no. 3 (1939): 638.

91. Michael P. Farrell, *Collaborative Circles: Friendship Dynamics and Creative Work* (Chicago: University of Chicago Press, 2003).

92. Gay, *Freud*, 492.

93. Sigmund Freud, *The Question of Lay Analysis: Conversations with an Impartial Person*, trans. J. Strachey (New York: Norton, 1969), 61.

94. Ibid., 62.

95. Ibid., 83; quoted in Robert S. Wallerstein, *Lay Analysis: Life Inside the Controversy* (New York: Taylor & Francis, 2013).

96. Freud, *The Question of Lay Analysis*, 96.

97. Zaretsky, "Charisma or Rationalization?," 341.

98. Leland E. Hinsie, "The Relationship of Psychoanalysis to Psychiatry," *American Journal of Psychiatry* 91, no. 5 (1935): 1114.

99. Alexander, "Psychoanalysis Comes of Age," 299.

100. Ibid., 303.

101. Ibid.

102. Menninger, *Psychiatry in a Troubled World*, 121.

103. Gregory Zilboorg, "The Changing Concept of Man in Present-Day Psychiatry," *American Journal of Psychiatry* 111, no. 6 (1954): 445.

104. Leo H. Bartemeier, "Presidential Address," *American Journal of Psychiatry* 109, no. 1 (1952): 1.

105. Hale, *The Rise and Crisis of Psychoanalysis*.

106. Grob, *From Asylum to Community*, 257.

107. Barton, *History and Influence*.

108. Hale, *The Rise and Crisis of Psychoanalysis*, 246.

109. Burnham, *After Freud Left*; John J. Leveille, "Jurisdictional Competition and the Psychoanalytic Dominance of American Psychiatry," *Journal of Historical Sociology* 15, no. 2 (2012): 252–80.

110. Shorter, *A History of Psychiatry*, 171.

111. Barton, *History and Influence*.

112. Hinsie, "The Relationship of Psychoanalysis to Psychiatry," 1114.

113. Kenneth E. Appel, "Presidential Address: The Challenge of Psychiatry," *American Journal of Psychiatry* 111, no. 1 (1954): 9.

114. Israel S. Wechsler, "Critical Consideration of the Status of Neurology," *AMA Archives of Neurology & Psychiatry* 81, no. 1 (1959): 2.

115. Charles E. Goshen, "New Interdisciplinary Trends in Psychiatry," *American Journal of Psychiatry* 117, no. 10 (1961): 916.

116. Rose Laub Coser, *Training in Ambiguity: Learning through Doing in a Mental Hospital* (New York: Free Press, 1979), 6.

117. Scull, *Madness in Civilization*, 339.

118. Walter Freeman, *The Psychiatrist: Personalities and Patterns* (New York: Grune & Stratton, 1968), 150.

119. John B. McKinlay and Lisa D. Marceau, "The End of the Golden Age of Doctoring," *International Journal of Health Services* 3, no. 2 (2002): 379–416.

120. Philip J. Hilts, *Protecting America's Health: The FDA, Business, and One Hundred Years of Regulation* (New York: Alfred A. Knopf, 2003).

121. Zaretsky, *Secrets of the Soul*, 301.

122. Starkey, "The Lengthening Hour."

123. Makari, *Revolution in Mind*, 439.

124. Jurgen Ruesch, "The Trouble with Psychiatric Research," *AMA Archives of Neurology & Psychiatry* 77, no. 1 (1957): 94; Jacques Gottlieb, "The Responsibility of Public Mental Hospitals in Psychiatric Research," *American Journal of Psychiatry* 109, no. 11 (1953): 803.

125. Leo Kanner, "Gobbledygook in Psychiatric Writing," *American Journal of Psychiatry* 108, no. 6 (1951): 475.

126. Karl Popper, *Conjectures and Refutations* (New York: Basic Books, 1962).

127. Adolf Grünbaum, *The Foundations of Psychoanalysis: A Philosophical Critique* (Berkeley: University of California Press, 1984).

128. Ibid., 129.

129. Ibid., 161.

130. Ibid., 14. Psychologist and Freud critic Hans Eysenck has been making a similar argument for decades. See Hans J. Eysenck, "The Effects of Psychotherapy: An Evaluation," *Journal of Consulting Psychology* 16, no. 5 (1952): 319–24; Eysenck, *Decline and Fall of the Freudian Empire* (New York: Viking, 1985).

131. Burrow, "The Need of an Analytic Psychiatry," 496.

132. Leon Tec, "The Double-Blind Study Deserves Its Name," *American Journal of Psychiatry* 123, no. 2 (1966): 234.

133. Donald Light, "The Impact of Medical School on Future Psychiatrists," *American Journal of Psychiatry* 132, no. 6 (1975): 607.

134. Kenneth Godfrey, "The Responsibilities of Psychiatry to Medicine: A Debate," *American Journal of Psychiatry* 130, no. 2 (1973): 224.

135. Alan Gregg, "A Critique of Psychiatry," *American Journal of Psychiatry* 101, no. 3 (1944): 285.

136. Charles E. Rosenberg, "The Tyranny of Diagnosis: Specific Entities and Individual Experience," *Milbank Quarterly* 80, no. 2 (2002): 237–60.

137. Menninger, *The Human Mind*, 150–51.

138. Roy Grinker Sr., "The Sciences of Psychiatry: Fields, Fences and Riders," *American Journal of Psychiatry* 122, no. 4 (1965): 369.

139. Roy Grinker Sr., "Emerging Concepts of Mental Illness and Models of Treatment: The Medical Point of View," *American Journal of Psychiatry* 125, no. 7 (1969): 867.

140. David L. Rosenhan, "On Being Sane in Insane Places," *Science* 179, no. 4070 (1973): 250–58.

141. Ibid., 251.

142. Ibid., 257.

143. Seymour S. Kety, "The Academic Lecture: The Heuristic Aspect of Psychiatry," *American Journal of Psychiatry* 118, no. 5 (1961): 388.

144. Roy Grinker Sr., "Psychiatry Rides Madly in All Directions," *Archives of General Psychiatry* 10, no. 3 (1964): 236; Lorrin M. Koran, "Controversy in Medicine and Psychiatry," *American Journal of Psychiatry* 132, no. 10 (1975): 1064.

145. Ames Fischer and Morton R. Weinstein, "Mental Hospitals, Prestige, and the Image of Enlightenment," *Archives of General Psychiatry* 25, no. 1 (1971): 41.

146. John P. Spiegel, "Presidential Address: Psychiatry—A High-Risk Profession," *American Journal of Psychiatry* 132, no. 7 (1975): 693.

147. Joseph G. Kepecs, "Psychoanalysis Today: A Rather Lonely Island," *Archives of General Psychiatry* 18, no. 2 (1968): 164.

148. Ibid., 167.

149. Fischer and Weinstein, "Mental Hospitals," 41.

150. Grinker, "Psychiatry Rides Madly," 334.

151. Judd Marmor, "The Future of Psychoanalytic Therapy," *American Journal of Psychiatry* 130, no. 11 (1973): 1198.

152. George W. Albee, "Emerging Concepts of Mental Illness and Models of Treatment: The Psychological Point of View," *American Journal of Psychiatry* 125, no. 7 (1969): 871.

153. The treatment at Chestnut Lodge received a more sympathetic portrayal in the semi-autobiographical novel *I Never Promised You a Rose Garden*, by Joanne Greenberg (New York: Holt McDougal, 1964).

154. Alfred H. Stanton and Morris S. Schwartz, *The Mental Hospital: A Study of Institutional Participation in Psychiatric Illness & Treatment* (New York: Basic Books, 1954), v.

155. Ibid., 199.

156. Ibid.

157. John Gulton Malcolm, "Treatment Choices and Informed Consent in Psychiatry: Implications of the Osheroff Case for the Profession," *Journal of Psychiatry and Law* 14, nos. 1–2 (1986): 9–107.

158. Quoted in Malcolm, "Treatment Choices," 21.

159. *Osheroff v. Chestnut Lodge Inc.*, 62 Md. App. 519, 490 A. 2d 720 (Court of Special Appeals of Maryland, 1985), 5.

160. Ibid., 6, 12.

161. Ibid., 3.

162. Malcolm, "Treatment Choices."

163. Gerald L. Klerman, "The Psychiatric Patient's Right to Effective Treatment: Implications of *Osheroff v. Chestnut Lodge*," *American Journal of Psychiatry* 147, no. 4 (1990): 409–18.

164. Alan A. Stone, "Law, Science, and Psychiatric Malpractice: A Response," *American Journal of Psychiatry* 147, no. 4 (1990): 419–27.

165. Ibid., 420.

166. Ibid., 421.

167. Klerman, "The Psychiatric Patient's Right," 417.

168. Stone, "Law, Science," 425.

169. Perry C. Talkington, "The Presidential Address: A Time for Action," *American Journal of Psychiatry* 130, no. 7 (1973): 745.

170. Arthur, "Social Psychiatry," 846.

171. James M. Jasper, *Getting Your Way: Strategic Dilemmas in the Real World* (Chicago: University of Chicago Press, 2006), 141.

172. Abbott, *The System of Professions*; Friedson, *Professionalism*.
173. H. Jamous and B. Peloille, "Professions or Self-Perpetuating System; Changes in the French University-Hospital System," in *Professions and Professionalisation*, ed. J. A. Jackson (Cambridge: Cambridge University Press, 1970), 113.
174. Kate Schechter, *Illusions of a Future: Psychoanalysis and the Biopolitics of Desire* (Durham, NC: Duke University Press, 2014).
175. Warner, "Fall and Rise."

CHAPTER FOUR

1. Group for the Advancement of Psychiatry (GAP), "The Position of Psychiatrists in the Field of International Relations," in *Published Reports: Special Volume—Reports #1–#34 and Symposium #1* (New York: Group for the Advancement of Psychiatry, 1950), 557.
2. E. Fuller Torrey, *American Psychosis: How the Federal Government Destroyed the Mental Illness Treatment System* (New York: Oxford University Press, 2013), 12.
3. Walter Freeman and James Winston Watts, *Psychosurgery in the Treatment of Mental Disorders and Intractable Pain*, 2nd ed. (Springfield, IL: C. C. Thomas, 1950), 55.
4. Ibid., 56.
5. Shorter, *A History of Psychiatry*, 227; Pressman, *Last Resort*, 340.
6. Jack El-Hai, *The Lobotomist: A Maverick Medical Genius and His Tragic Quest to Rid the World of Mental Illness* (Hoboken, NJ: Wiley, 2007).
7. Pressman, *Last Resort*.
8. Freeman and Watts, *Psychosurgery in the Treatment of Mental Disorders*, 203.
9. W. Horsley Gantt, "Objectivity in Psychiatry," *American Journal of Psychiatry* 114, no. 11 (1958): 1046.
10. Karl M. Bowman and Milton Rose, "Do Our Medical Colleagues Know What to Expect from Psychotherapy?," *American Journal of Psychiatry* 111, no. 6 (1954): 404.
11. Eli Ginzberg, "Notes on American Psychiatry by a Social Scientist," *American Journal of Psychiatry* 106, no. 12 (1950): 937.
12. Grob, *From Asylum to Community*, 3.
13. Grob, *Mental Institutions in America*, 60.
14. Grob, *From Asylum to Community*, 72.
15. Appel, "Presidential Address," 13.
16. Beam, *Gracefully Insane*.
17. Kenneth F. Appel, "Notes from the President," *American Journal of Psychiatry* 110, no. 10 (1954): 788.
18. Valenstein, *Great and Desperate Cures*.
19. Kenneth A. Smith, Howard T. Fiedler, and Charles R. Yhost, "Clinical Notes: Thorazine," *American Journal of Psychiatry* 111, no. 8 (1955): 620.
20. Milton Rose and Mary Ann Esser, "The Impact of Recent Research Developments on Private Practice," *American Journal of Psychiatry* 117, no. 5 (1960): 431.
21. John C. Whitehorn, "American Psychiatry," *American Journal of Psychiatry* 114, no. 2 (1957): 109–10.
22. Albert Q. Maisel, "Bedlam, 1946," *Life Magazine* 20, no. 18 (May 6, 1946): 102–18.
23. Ibid., 102.
24. Ibid.
25. Ibid., 103.
26. Harold Orlansky, "An American Death Camp," *Politics* (Summer 1948): 162.
27. Frank Leon Wright, *Out of Sight, Out of Mind: A Graphic Picture of Present-Day Institutional Care of the Mentally Ill in America, Based on More Than Two Thousand Eye-Witness*

Reports (Washington, DC: National Mental Health Foundation, 1947); Mary Jane Ward, *The Snake Pit* (New York: Random House, 1946).

28. Albert Deutsch, *The Shame of the States* (New York: Harcourt, Brace, 1948), 184.

29. Ibid., 28.

30. Ibid., 96.

31. For example, see Ivan Belknap, *Human Problems of a State Mental Hospital* (New York: McGraw-Hill, 1956); Henry Warren Dunham and Samuel Kirson Weinberg, *The Culture of the State Mental Hospital* (Detroit, MI: Wayne State University Press, 1960); Stanton and Schwartz, *The Mental Hospital*; Goffman, *Asylums*.

32. Ironically, Goffman's research was conducted in a mental hospital often singled out as one of the nation's finest. Michael E. Staub, *Madness Is Civilization: When the Diagnosis Was Social, 1948–1980* (Chicago: University of Chicago Press, 2011), 85.

33. Goffman, *Asylums*.

34. Peter Sedgwick, *Psycho Politics* (Chicago: Pluto Press, 1982), 44.

35. Erving Goffman, "The Insanity of Place," in *Relations in Public* (New York: Harper & Row Publishers, 1971), 336.

36. Mike Gorman, *Every Other Bed* (New York: World Publishing Company, 1956), 10.

37. Deutsch, *The Shame of the States*, 145.

38. Ibid., 179.

39. Matthew Ross, "Community Psychiatry as an Opportunity for Medical Leadership," *Archives of General Psychiatry* 3, no. 5 (1960): 52.

40. Paul Lerman, *Deinstitutionalization and the Welfare State* (New Brunswick, NJ: Rutgers University Press, 1982).

41. Jackie L. Goldstein and Marc Godemont, "The Legend and Lessons of Geel, Belgium: A 1500-Year-Old Legend, a 21st-Century Model," *Community Mental Health Journal* 39, no. 5 (2003): 441–58.

42. See Pliny Earle, "Gheel," *American Journal of Psychiatry* 8, no. 1 (1851): 67–78; T. Parigot, "The Lunatic Colony at Gheel," *The Lancet* 70, no. 1779 (1857): 351; W. J. Morton, "The Town of Gheel, in Belgium, and Its Insane; Or, Occupation and Reasonable Liberty for Lunatics," *Journal of Nervous and Mental Disease* 8, no. 1 (1881): 102–23; Herman Ostrander, "The Colony System of Caring for the Insane," *American Journal of Psychiatry* 56, no. 3 (1900): 443–55; Paul Masoin, "An Account of the Care of the Insane in Belgium, and Particularly Those in the Colony of Gheel," *Journal of Nervous and Mental Disease* 31, no. 9 (1904): 561–76.

43. Galt, "The Farm of St. Anne."

44. Nana Tuntiya, "Free-Air Treatment for Mental Patients: The Deinstitutionalization Debate of the Nineteenth Century," *Sociological Perspectives* 50, no. 3 (2007): 469–87.

45. Burrow, "The Need of an Analytic Psychiatry," 488.

46. Edward Strecker, "The President's Message: The Leaven of Psychiatry in War and in Peace," *American Journal of Psychiatry* 100, no. 6 (1944): 1–2.

47. Grob, *From Asylum to Community*.

48. Catherine Fussinger, "'Therapeutic Community,' Psychiatry's Reformers and Anti-psychiatrists: Reconsidering Changes in the Field of Psychiatry after World War II," *History of Psychiatry* 22, no. 2 (2011): 146.

49. Menninger, *Psychiatry in a Troubled World*, viii.

50. Albert Deutsch, *The Story of GAP* (New York: Group for the Advancement of Psychiatry, 1959), 7.

51. Grob, *From Asylum to Community*, 28.

52. Group for the Advancement of Psychiatry (GAP), "The Social Responsibility of Psychiatry, A Statement of Orientation," in *Published Reports: Special Volume*, 5.

53. Ibid., 1.

54. Ibid., 4.

55. Ibid., 5.

56. Ibid.

57. Mechanic, *Mental Health and Social Policy*.

58. Robert H. Felix, *Mental Illness: Progress and Prospects* (New York: Columbia University Press, 1967), 3.

59. Ibid., 67–68.

60. Staub, *Madness Is Civilization*, 35.

61. Felix, *Mental Illness*, 75.

62. Gorman, *Every Other Bed*, 14.

63. Harry R. Brickman, Donald A. Schwartz, and S. Mark Doran, "The Psychoanalyst as Community Psychiatrist," *American Journal of Psychiatry* 122, no. 10 (1966): 1081.

64. GAP, "The Social Responsibility of Psychiatry," 4.

65. This "continuum model of mental illness" (Grob, *From Asylum to Community*, 7) holds that there is a continuum between normality and pathology when it comes to mental distress. This contrasts with a discrete conceptualization of mental illness that holds that it represents a distinct break from normality.

66. The work of psychoanalyst Harry Stack Sullivan, considered "the sociologist's psychiatrist," was significant in this regard. See Alan Sica, "Plague of Polypragmasy," *Contemporary Sociology* 43, no. 4 (2014): 453–57.

67. American Psychiatric Association, "Position Statement on Psychiatrists' Relationships with Nonmedical Mental Health Professionals," *American Journal of Psychiatry* 130, no. 3 (1973): 386.

68. Portia Bell Hume, "Community Psychiatry, Social Psychiatry, and Community Mental Health Work: Some Inter-Professional Relationships in Psychiatry and Social Work," *American Journal of Psychiatry* 121, no. 4 (1964): 343.

69. Fredrick C. Redlich and Daniel X. Freedman, *The Theory and Practice of Psychiatry* (New York: Basic Books, 1966), 80.

70. Staub, *Madness Is Civilization*, 4.

71. Psychiatric discourse was not just linked to progressive politics. It had more ambiguous effects when it came to left/right politics. For example, psychiatric discourse was used to dismiss black activists as suffering from "protest psychosis" (Metzl, *The Protest Psychosis*) and to pathologize gay rights activists as mentally ill (Tom Waidzunas, *The Straight Line: How the Fringe Science of Ex-Gay Therapy Reoriented Sexuality* [Minneapolis: University of Minnesota Press, 2015]).

72. Hume, "Community Psychiatry," 342.

73. David F. Musto, "Whatever Happened to Community Mental Health?," *Psychiatric Annals* 7, no. 10 (1977): 67.

74. Avrohm Jacobson, "A Critical Look at the Community Psychiatric Clinic," *American Journal of Psychiatry* 124, no. 4 (1967): 14; Ralph W. Gerard, "The Academic Lecture: The Biological Roots of Psychiatry," *American Journal of Psychiatry* 112, no. 2 (1955): 81.

75. Karl A. Menninger, *The Vital Balance: The Life Process in Mental Health and Illness* (New York: Viking Press, 1963), 358; Walter E. Barton, "Presidential Address: Psychiatry in Transition," *American Journal of Psychiatry* 119, no. 1 (1962): 13.

76. Ross, "Community Psychiatry," 59.

77. Ibid., 51.
78. Henry Warren Dunham, "Community Psychiatry: The Newest Therapeutic Bandwagon," *Archives of General Psychiatry* 12, no. 3 (1965): 306.
79. Ibid., 307.
80. J. A. Wheldon, "Letter to the Editor: The APA and Politics," *American Journal of Psychiatry* 128, no. 2 (1971): 237.
81. Grinker, "Psychiatry Rides Madly," 228.
82. Leo H. Bartemeier, "The Future of Psychiatry: The Report of the Joint Commission on Mental Health and Illness," *American Journal of Psychiatry* 118, no. 11 (1962): 973.
83. A. R. Foley and David S. Sanders, "Theoretical Considerations for the Development of the Community Mental Health Center Concept," *American Journal of Psychiatry* 122, no. 9 (1966): 987–88.
84. Thorazine is often overstated as a cause of deinstitutionalization, and one should scrupulously avoid accounts that focus solely on medication as *the* relevant cause. Still, psychiatrists did in fact often point to Thorazine as important in shifting the expectations for community-based care.
85. David Healy, *The Antidepressant Era* (Cambridge, MA: Harvard University Press, 1997).
86. Paul H. Hoch, "Drugs and Psychotherapy," *American Journal of Psychiatry* 116, no. 4 (1959): 305; Bartemeier, "The Future of Psychiatry," 977.
87. John F. Kennedy, "Message from the President of the United States Relative to Mental Illness and Mental Retardation," *American Journal of Psychiatry* 120, no. 8 (1964): 730.
88. Lerman, *Deinstitutionalization and the Welfare State*.
89. For example, see Leo Srole, Thomas S. Langer, Stanley T. Mitchell, Marvin K. Opler, and Thomas A. C. Rennie, *Mental Health in the Metropolis: The Midtown Manhattan Study*, vol. 1 (New York: McGraw-Hill, 1962).
90. Joint Commission on Mental Health and Illness, *Action for Mental Health: Final Report of the JCMIH* (New York: Basic Books, 1961), 52, xviii.
91. Ibid., v.
92. Ibid., 190, xiv.
93. Robert H. Felix, "Presidential Address: Psychiatrist, Medicinae Doctor," *American Journal of Psychiatry* 118, no. 1 (1961): 3.
94. Robert H. Felix, "A Model for Comprehensive Mental Health Centers," *American Journal of Public Health and the Nation's Health* 54, no. 12 (1964): 1967.
95. Ibid., 1964.
96. Felix, *Mental Illness*, 75.
97. Franklin D. Chu, Sharlin Trotter, and Ralph Nader, *The Madness Establishment: Ralph Nader's Study Group Report on the National Institute of Mental Health* (New York: Grossman Publishers, 1974).
98. Ibid., 10.
99. Ibid., 49, xiii.
100. Ibid., 8.
101. Henry A. Foley and Steven Samuel Sharfstein, *Madness and Government: Who Cares for the Mentally Ill?* (Washington, DC: American Psychiatric Press, 1983), 102.
102. Torrey, *American Psychosis*.
103. Chu, Trotter, and Nader, *The Madness Establishment*, xii.
104. Ibid., 203.
105. Shorter, *A History of Psychiatry*, 280.

106. Lerman, *Deinstitutionalization and the Welfare State*, 52.

107. Torrey, *American Psychosis*.

108. Lerman, *Deinstitutionalization and the Welfare State*, 13.

109. Susan Meyers Chandler, *Competing Realities: The Contested Terrain of Mental Health Advocacy* (New York: Praeger, 1990).

110. Shorter, *A History of Psychiatry*, 277.

111. Chandler, *Competing Realities*.

112. Stanley F. Yolles, "Community Mental Health: Issues and Policies," *American Journal of Psychiatry* 122, no. 9 (1966): 980.

113. David L. Sackett, "The Arrogance of Preventive Medicine," *Canadian Medical Association Journal* 167, no. 4 (2002): 363–64.

114. Foley and Sanders, "Theoretical Considerations," 986.

115. Kennedy, "Message from the President," 728; Felix, "Presidential Address," 3.

116. Sue Estroff, *Making It Crazy: An Ethnography of Psychiatric Clients in an American Community* (Berkeley: University of California Press, 1981), 253.

117. Howard P. Rome, "The Presidential Address: Psychiatry and Social Change Circa 1966," *American Journal of Psychiatry* 123, no. 1 (1966): 2.

118. Ross, "Community Psychiatry," 52.

119. Jacobson, "A Critical Look," 19.

120. Anthony F. Panzetta, "The Concept of Community: The Short-Circuit of the Mental Health Movement," *Archives of General Psychiatry* 25, no. 4 (1971): 291; Musto, "Whatever Happened," 55.

121. Norman W. Bell and John P. Spiegel, "Social Psychiatry: Vagaries of a Term," *Archives of General Psychiatry* 14, no. 4 (1966): 343.

122. Grob, *From Asylum to Community*.

123. American Psychiatric Association, "Position Statement," 845.

124. Ibid., 846.

125. Ross, "Community Psychiatry," 57.

126. Morton Hunt, *The Story of Psychology* (New York: Anchor Books, 2007).

127. Hunt, *The Story of Psychology*; Leveille, "Jurisdictional Competition."

128. Grob, *From Asylum to Community*; Rose, *Governing the Soul*.

129. Grob, *From Asylum to Community*, 112–13.

130. Erving Goffman, *Stigma: Notes on the Management of Spoiled Identity* (New York: J. Aronson, 1974); Thomas J. Scheff, *Being Mentally Ill: A Sociological Theory*, 3rd ed. (New York: Aldine de Gruyter, 1999).

131. Sedgwick, *Psycho Politics*.

132. Grob, *From Asylum to Community*, 280; Staub, *Madness Is Civilization*, 105.

133. Thomas S. Szasz, *The Myth of Mental Illness: Foundations of a Theory of Personal Conduct* (New York: Hoeber-Harper, 1961), 1.

134. Thomas S. Szasz, "The Myth of Mental Illness," *American Psychologist* 15, no. 2 (1960): 113–18.

135. Szasz, *The Myth of Mental Illness*, 34. Szasz's criticisms subscribe to a traditional and limited notion of illness. To be considered real, diseases must possess a demonstrable pathology at the physical, cellular, or molecular level.

136. Ibid., 4, 77.

137. Thomas S. Szasz, *The Manufacture of Madness: A Comparative Study of the Inquisition and the Mental Health Movement* (New York: Harper & Row, 1970).

138. This argument anticipated subsequent critiques of psychiatry that focused on social control and medicalization (e.g., Scheff, *Being Mentally Ill*; Irving Kenneth Zola,

"Medicine as an Institution of Social Control," *Sociological Review* 20, no. 4 [1972]: 487–504; Peter Conrad, "The Discovery of Hyperkinesis: Notes on the Medicalization of Deviant Behavior," *Social Problems* 23, no. 1 [1975]: 12–21).

139. Szasz, *The Myth of Mental Illness*, 9.

140. Frederick C. Thorne, "An Analysis of Szasz's 'Myth of Mental Illness,'" *American Journal of Psychiatry* 123, no. 6 (1966): 656.

141. Henry A. Davidson, "The New War on Psychiatry," *American Journal of Psychiatry* 121, no. 6 (1964): 531.

142. Ibid., 528–29.

143. Harvey J. Tompkins, "The Presidential Address: The Physician in Contemporary Society," *American Journal of Psychiatry* 124, no. 1 (1967): 40.

144. John P. Spiegel, "Presidential Address: Psychiatry—A High-Risk Profession," *American Journal of Psychiatry* 132, no. 7 (1975): 694.

145. Perry C. Talkington, "The Presidential Address: A Time for Action," *American Journal of Psychiatry* 130, no. 7 (1973): 745.

146. Spiegel, "Presidential Address," 694.

147. E. Fuller Torrey, *The Death of Psychiatry* (Philadelphia: Chilton Book Company, 1974), 3, 193.

148. Torrey, *The Death of Psychiatry*, 145.

149. Sedgwick, *Psycho Politics*, 213.

150. Chu, Trotter, and Nader, *The Madness Establishment*, 207.

151. In scholarly discourse, the concept of "historical consciousness" is used in many different ways. I use it to signify that psychiatrists in the 1960s and 1970s began to engage in a more conscious assessment and interpretation of the profession's history and felt a greater compulsion to situate both the present and future in relation to this history. In this sense, "historical consciousness" is similar to the traditional Marxist idea of class consciousness, or awareness of one's place in a system of class struggle. More than just an assessment of the past, historical consciousness "uses this knowledge as an element in shaping the thoughts and actions that will determine the future" (Theodor Schieder, "The Role of Historical Consciousness in Political Action," *History and Theory* 17, no. 4 [1978]: 1).

152. For example, in 1922, Albert M. Barrett observed, "The history of psychiatry has shown how such tendencies easily lead to drifting speculations and the formulation of theories that have not always been firmly moored to scientific facts." Barrett, "The Broadened Interests of Psychiatry," 9.

153. For example, see Franz Alexander, "Current Problems in Dynamic Psychotherapy in Its Relationship to Psychoanalysis," *American Journal of Psychiatry* 116, no. 4 (1959): 322–25.

154. William F. Knoff, "Psychiatric History in Psychiatric Education: Report of a Survey," *American Journal of Psychiatry* 119, no. 6 (1962): 515–19.

155. David F. Musto, "History and the Psychiatrist," *American Journal of Psychiatry*, 135, suppl. (1978): 22.

156. Historian Charles Rosenberg states, "Psychiatrists are more likely than other medical specialists to take an interest in the history of the subdiscipline, there may even be a kind of truth in the hostile whimsy that such historical interest reflects the fact that psychiatrists practice medicine as it was practiced a century or more ago." Charles E. Rosenberg, "The Crisis in Psychiatric Legitimacy: Reflections on Psychiatry, Medicine and Public Policy," in *Explaining Epidemics and Other Studies in the History of Medicine* (New York: Cambridge University Press, 1992), 254.

157. Redlich and Freedman, *The Theory and Practice of Psychiatry*, 28.

158. Darold A. Treffert, "Psychiatry Revolves as It Evolves," *Archives of General Psychiatry* 17, no. 1 (1967): 74.
159. Fischer and Weinstein, "Mental Hospitals," 41.
160. Bell and Spiegel, "Social Psychiatry," 343.

CHAPTER FIVE

1. For a detailed analysis of this controversy and the history of psychiatry and homosexuality, see Ronald Bayer, *Homosexuality and American Psychiatry: The Politics of Diagnosis* (Princeton, NJ: Princeton University Press, 1987); Waidzunas, *The Straight Line*.
2. Jack Drescher and Joseph P. Merlino, eds., *American Psychiatry and Homosexuality: An Oral History* (Binghamton, NY: Taylor & Francis), xvii.
3. Robert J. Stoller, Judd Marmor, Irving Bieber, Ronald Gold, Charles W. Socarides, Richard Green, and Robert L. Spitzer, "A Symposium: Should Homosexuality Be in the APA Nomenclature?," *American Journal of Psychiatry* 130, no. 11 (1973): 1212.
4. "The Changing View of Homosexuality," *New York Times*, February 28, 1971, L47.
5. Ibid.
6. Quoted in Bayer, *Homosexuality and American Psychiatry*, 106.
7. Quoted in David L. Scasta, "John E. Fryer, MD, and the Dr. H. Anonymous Episode," *Journal of Gay & Lesbian Psychotherapy* 6, no. 4 (2003): 83.
8. Quoted in Scasta, "John E. Fryer," 80–81.
9. Quoted in Robert L. Spitzer and Irving Bieber, "The A.P.A. Ruling on Homosexuality," *New York Times*, December 23, 1973, E5.
10. Stoller et al., "A Symposium," 1216.
11. Ibid., 1210.
12. Bayer, *Homosexuality and American Psychiatry*.
13. Psychoanalysts would take longer to come around; the American Psychoanalytic Association (APsaA) would not formally change its position on homosexuality until 1991.
14. Franklin Kameny, "Victory! We Have Been Cured," in *Gay Is Good: The Life and Letters of Gay Rights Pioneer Franklin Kameny*, ed. Michael G. Long (Syracuse, NY: Syracuse University Press, 2014), 269.
15. Alfred M. Freedman, "Presidential Address: Creating the Future," *American Journal of Psychiatry* 131, no. 7 (1974): 753.
16. Irving Philips, Herbert C. Modlin, Irving N. Berlin, Leon Eisenberg, Howard P. Rome, and Raymond W. Waggoner, "The Psychiatrist, the APA, and Social Issues: A Symposium," *American Journal of Psychiatry* 128, no. 6 (1971): 681.
17. Bertram S. Brown, "The Life of Psychiatry," *American Journal of Psychiatry*, 133, no. 5 (1976): 489.
18. Samuel B. Guze, "The Need for Toughmindedness in Psychiatric Thinking," *Southern Medical Journal* 63, no. 6 (1970): 662.
19. Geoffrey C. Bowker and Susan Leigh Star, *Sorting Things Out: Classification and Its Consequences* (Cambridge, MA: MIT Press, 1999).
20. Stefan Timmermans and Steven Epstein, "A World of Standards but Not a Standard World: Toward a Sociology of Standards and Standardization," *Annual Review of Sociology* 36 (2010): 69–89.
21. Borrowing an idea from James Scott's (1999, 80) research on high-modern state power, I treat these nosological reforms as a "project of legibility." Scott focuses on the various techniques that simplify and rationalize complex human behavior to render society legible and enable the state to exercise control over a population. In

my analysis, standardizing classification makes mental disorders more legible and thus seemingly more tractable.

22. Drawing on the work of the philosopher of science Thomas Kuhn, both psychiatrists (see Allen Frances, "A Warning Sign on the Road to DSM-V: Beware of Its Unintended Consequences," *Psychiatric Times* 26, no. 8 [2009]: 1-4; Mitchell Wilson, "DSM-III and the Transformation of American Psychiatry: A History," *American Journal of Psychiatry* 150, no. 3 [1993]) and outside observers (see Hannah S. Decker, *The Making of DSM-III* [New York: Oxford University Press, 2013]; Michael Strand, "Where Do Classifications Come From? The DSM-III, the Transformation of American Psychiatry, and the Problem of Origins in the Sociology of Knowledge," *Theory and Society* 40, no. 3 [2011]: 273–313) deem DSM-III to be a paradigm shift, a revolutionary change in the basic concepts and intellectual framework in a scientific field.

23. Chu, Trotter, and Nader, *The Madness Establishment*, xxi.

24. Alan A. Stone, "Response to the Presidential Address," *American Journal of Psychiatry* 136, no. 8 (1979): 1020.

25. Melvin Sabshin, "The Anti-Community Mental Health Movement," *American Journal of Psychiatry* 125, no. 8 (1969): 1006.

26. Ben Bursten, "Psychiatry and the Rhetoric of Models," *American Journal of Psychiatry* 136, no. 5 (1979): 661.

27. Donald Light, *Becoming Psychiatrists* (New York: W. W. Norton & Co., 1980), xi.

28. Jules H. Masserman, "Presidential Address: The Future of Psychiatry as a Scientific and Humanitarian Discipline in a Changing World," *American Journal of Psychiatry* 136, no. 8 (1979): 1016.

29. Nancy C. Andreasen, *The Broken Brain* (New York: HarperCollins, 1984), viii.

30. Masserman, "Presidential Address," 1016; Manfred Braun, "The Responsibilities of Psychiatry to Medicine: A Debate," *American Journal of Psychiatry* 130, no. 2 (1973): 225.

31. Bursten, "Psychiatry and the Rhetoric of Models," 664.

32. Kermit H. Gruberg, "The Responsibilities of Psychiatry to Medicine: A Debate," *American Journal of Psychiatry* 130, no. 2 (1973): 226.

33. Lamb, *Pathologist of the Mind*.

34. Francis J. Braceland, "Kraepelin, His System and His Influence," *American Journal of Psychiatry* 113, no. 10 (1957): 871.

35. Roger K. Blashfield, "Feighner et al., Invisible Colleges, and the Matthew Effect," *Schizophrenia Bulletin* 8, no. 1 (1982): 1–6.

36. Decker, *The Making of DSM-III*.

37. Paul Hoff, "Emil Kraepelin and Forensic Psychiatry," *International Journal of Law and Psychiatry* 21, no. 4 (1998): 350.

38. Blashfield, "Feighner et al."

39. Gerald Grob, "The Origins of American Psychiatric Epidemiology," *American Journal of Public Health* 75, no. 3 (1985): 229–36.

40. Robert Evan Kendell, *The Role of Diagnosis in Psychiatry* (New York: Blackwell Oxford, 1975), vii.

41. Basil Jackson, "The Revised Diagnostic and Statistical Manual of the American Psychiatric Association," *American Journal of Psychiatry* 127, no. 1 (1970): 66.

42. Arnold M. Ludwig and Ekkehard Othmer, "The Medical Basis of Psychiatry," *American Journal of Psychiatry* 134, no. 10 (1977): 1088.

43. John P. Feighner, Eli Robins, Samuel B. Guze, Robert A. Woodruff, George Winokur, and Rodrigo Munoz, "Diagnostic Criteria for Use in Psychiatric Research," *Archives of General Psychiatry* 26, no. 1 (1972): 57–63.

44. John P. Feighner, "Nosology: A Voice for a Systematic Data-Oriented Approach," *American Journal of Psychiatry* 136, no. 9 (1979): 1173–74.
45. Horwitz, *Creating Mental Illness.*
46. Decker, *The Making of DSM-III,* 86.
47. Robert Evan Kendell, John E. Cooper, A. J. Gourlay, J. R. M. Copeland, Lawrence Sharpe, and Barry J. Gurland, "Diagnostic Criteria of American and British Psychiatrists," *Archives of General Psychiatry* 25, no. 2 (1971): 123–30.
48. Robert L. Spitzer, "On Pseudoscience in Science, Logic in Remission, and Psychiatric Diagnosis," *Journal of Abnormal Psychology* 84, no. 5 (1975): 442–52.
49. Alison Snyder, "Robert L. Spitzer," *The Lancet* 387, no. 10017 (2016): 428.
50. Robert L. Spitzer, Jean Endicott, and Eli Robins, "Research Diagnostic Criteria: Rationale and Reliability," *Archives of General Psychiatry* 35, no. 6 (1978): 773–82.
51. Allen Frances. "Robert Spitzer: The Most Influential Psychiatrist of His Time," *The Lancet Psychiatry* 3, no. 2 (2016): 110–11.
52. Robert Spitzer, interview with author, March 15, 2011.
53. Ibid.
54. Decker, *The Making of DSM-III,* 108.
55. Prior to DSM-III, the psychiatric research enterprise "remained highly idiosyncratic, and the science surrounding psychiatric disorders floundered." Jason Schnittker, *The Diagnostic System: Why the Classification of Psychiatric Disorders Is Necessary, Difficult, and Never Settled* (New York: Columbia University Press, 2017), 31.
56. Ibid., 23.
57. Rick Mayes and Allan V. Horwitz, "DSM-III and the Revolution in the Classification of Mental illness," *Journal of the History of the Behavioral Sciences* 41, no. 3 (2005): 249–67.
58. Healy, *The Antidepressant Era,* 234.
59. Horwitz, *Creating Mental Illness.*
60. Ronald Bayer and Robert L. Spitzer, "Neurosis, Psychodynamics, and DSM-III: A History of the Controversy," *Archives of General Psychiatry* 42, no. 2 (1985): 187.
61. Robert L. Spitzer, Janet B. Williams, and Andrew E. Skodol, "DSM-III: The Major Achievements and an Overview," *American Journal of Psychiatry* 137, no. 2 (1980): 154.
62. Robert L. Spitzer and Michael Sheehy, "DSM-III: A Classification System in Development," *Psychiatric Annals* 6, no. 9 (1976): 109.
63. Spitzer, interview with author.
64. Bayer and Spitzer, "Neurosis, Psychodynamics, and DSM-III."
65. American Psychiatric Association, *Diagnostic and Statistical Manual of Mental Disorders,* 3rd ed. (Washington, DC: American Psychiatric Publishing, 1980), 6.
66. Dominic Murphy, *Psychiatry in the Scientific Image* (Cambridge, MA: MIT Press, 2012).
67. DSM critic David Healy (*The Antidepressant Era,* 233) called DSM-III "a Trojan horse by which [Neo-Kraepelinians] effected entry into the citadel of psychoanalysis."
68. Allen Frances and Arnold M. Cooper, "Descriptive and Dynamic Psychiatry: A Perspective on DSM-III," *American Journal of Psychiatry* 138, no. 9 (1981): 1202.
69. Francis X. Clines, "Neuroses Disappear as Nomenclature Changes," *New York Times,* November 21, 1978, B8.
70. Gerald L. Klerman, George E. Vaillant, Robert L. Spitzer, and Robert Michels, "A Debate on DSM-III," *American Journal of Psychiatry* 141, no. 4 (1984): 539.
71. Ibid., 550.
72. Ibid.

73. Ibid., 552–53.
74. For example, see David Faust and Richard A. Miner, "The Empiricist and His New Clothes: DSM-III in Perspective," *American Journal of Psychiatry* 143, no. 8 (1986): 962–67; Edwin R. Wallace, "What Is 'Truth'? Some Philosophical Contributions to Psychiatric Issues," *American Journal of Psychiatry* 145, no. 2 (1988): 137–47.
75. Robert O. Pasnau, "Psychiatry in Medicine: Medicine in Psychiatry," *American Journal of Psychiatry* 144, no. 8 (1987): 975–80.
76. Melvin Sabshin, "Turning Points in Twentieth-Century American Psychiatry," *American Journal of Psychiatry* 147, no. 10 (1990): 1272.
77. Metzl, *Prozac on the Couch*.
78. Hugh J. Parry, Mitchell B. Balter, Glen D. Mellinger, Ira H. Cisin, and Dean I. Manheimer, "National Patterns of Psychotherapeutic Drug Use," *Archives of General Psychiatry* 28, no. 6 (1973): 769–83.
79. Peter R. Breggin and Ginger R. Breggin, *Talking Back to Prozac: What Doctors Aren't Telling You About Today's Most Controversial Drug* (New York: St. Martin's Press, 1995), 1–2.
80. See Peter D. Kramer, *Listening to Prozac* (New York: Fourth Estate, 1994).
81. For example, see Elizabeth Wurtzel, *Prozac Nation: Young and Depressed in America* (New York: Houghton Mifflin, 1994).
82. Kramer, *Listening to Prozac*, x.
83. David Healy, *The Antidepressant Era*; Christopher Lane, *Shyness: How Normal Behavior Became a Sickness* (New Haven, CT: Yale University Press, 2007).
84. Joseph J. Schildkraut, "The Catecholamine Hypothesis of Affective Disorders: A Review of Supporting Evidence," *American Journal of Psychiatry* 122, no. 5 (1965): 509–22.
85. These shortcomings include the following: although some depressed patients have low levels of serotonin and norepinephrine, the majority do not; some depressed patients actually have abnormally high levels of serotonin and norepinephrine; some patients with no history of depression at all have low levels of these amines; despite immediate chemical changes the drugs induced, there is a delay in the onset of symptom relief; there are drugs that alleviate depression despite the fact that they have little or no effect on either serotonin or norepinephrine; and other drugs that raise serotonin and norepinephrine levels, such as amphetamines and cocaine, do not alleviate depression. See Robert M. Hirschfeld, "History and Evolution of the Monoamine Hypothesis of Depression," *Journal of Clinical Psychiatry* 61, suppl. 6 (2000): 4–6; Joanna Moncrieff, *The Myth of the Chemical Cure: A Critique of Psychiatric Drug Treatment* (New York: Palgrave Macmillan, 2009); Elliot S. Valenstein, *Blaming the Brain: The Truth about Drugs and Mental Health* (New York: Free Press, 2002).
86. Steven E. Hyman and Eric Jonathan Nestler, *The Molecular Foundations of Psychiatry* (Washington, DC: American Psychiatric Press, 1993), xvi.
87. Andreasen, *The Broken Brain*, viii.
88. Ibid., 8.
89. Ibid., 221.
90. Russell G. Vasile and Thomas G. Gutheil, "The Psychiatrist as Medical Backup: Ambiguity in the Delegation of Clinical Responsibility," *American Journal of Psychiatry* 136, no. 10 (1979): 1293.
91. See Ronald Pies, "Nuances, Narratives, and the 'Chemical Imbalance' Debate," *Psychiatric Times* 31, no. 4 (2014): 5; Steven S. Sharfstein, "Big Pharma and American Psychiatry," *Journal of Nervous and Mental Disease* 196, no. 4 (2008): 265–66.

92. For example, when SmithKline Beecham developed Paxil, it encountered a crowded antidepressant market. Rather than struggling to penetrate this market, it promoted Paxil as a specific treatment for another disorder, social anxiety disorder, in a sense creating a new market that it could dominate (Lane, *Shyness*).

93. Dorothy Nelkin and M. Susan Lindee, *The DNA Mystique: The Gene as a Cultural Icon* (Ann Arbor: University of Michigan Press, 2004).

94. Herbert Pardes, Charles A. Kaufmann, Harold Alan Pincus, and Anne West, "Genetics and Psychiatry: Past Discoveries, Current Dilemmas, and Future Directions," *American Journal of Psychiatry* 146, no. 4 (1989): 435.

95. Herbert Pardes, "Defending Humanistic Values," *American Journal of Psychiatry* 147, no. 9 (1990): 1115.

96. Thomas R. Insel and Remi Quirion, "Psychiatry as a Clinical Neuroscience Discipline," *JAMA* 294, no. 17 (2005): 2221–24.

97. Pardes, "Defending Humanistic Values," 1113.

98. Schnittker, *The Diagnostic System*, 33–34.

99. Gary J. Tucker, "Putting DSM-IV in Perspective," *American Journal of Psychiatry* 155, no. 2 (1998): 159–61.

100. Paula J. Caplan, *They Say You're Crazy: How the World's Most Powerful Psychiatrists Decide Who's Normal* (Reading, MA: Addison-Wesley, 1995), xx.

101. Roger K. Blashfield et al., "The Cycle of Classification: DSM-I through DSM-5," *Annual Review of Clinical Psychology* 10 (2014): 32.

102. Benedict Carey, "Psychiatrists Revise the Book of Human Troubles," *New York Times*, December 18, 2008, A1.

103. Ethan Watters, *Crazy Like Us: The Globalization of the American Psyche* (New York: Simon and Schuster, 2010).

104. Mitchell Wilson, "DSM-III and the Transformation of American Psychiatry," 408.

105. Spitzer, interview with author.

106. Donald G. Langsley, "Presidential Address: Today's Teachers and Tomorrow's Psychiatrists," *American Journal of Psychiatry* 138, no. 8 (1981): 1013.

107. Jerome C. Wakefield, "Diagnosing DSM-IV—Part 1: DSM-IV and the Concept of Disorder," *Behavioral Research and Therapy* 35, no. 7 (1997): 637.

108. David Reiss, Robert Plomin, and E. Mavis Hetherington. "Genetics and Psychiatry: An Unheralded Window on the Environment," *American Journal of Psychiatry* 148, no. 3 (1991): 283–91.

109. Ibid., 290.

110. For example, Stuart A. Kirk and Herb Kutchins, *The Selling of DSM: The Rhetoric of Science in Psychiatry* (Piscataway, NJ: Aldine, 1992).

111. Robert L. Spitzer, Janet B. Williams, and Andrew E. Skodol, "DSM-III: The Major Achievements and an Overview," *American Journal of Psychiatry* 137, no. 2 (1980): 151–64.

112. Kendler, "Toward a Philosophical Structure for Psychiatry," 434–35.

113. Kenneth S. Kendler, "Reflections on the Relationship Between Psychiatric Genetics and Psychiatric Nosology," *American Journal of Psychiatry* 163, no. 7 (2006): 145. For example, prominent candidate genes for schizophrenia, the most biological seeming of mental disorders, have been shown to be no more associated with the disorder than would be expected by chance. Emma C. Johnson, Richard Border, Whitney E. Melroy-Greif, Christiaan A. de Leeuw, Marissa A. Ehringer, and Matthew C. Keller, "No Evidence That Schizophrenia Candidate Genes Are More Associated with Schizophrenia Than Noncandidate Genes," *Biological Psychiatry* 82, no. 10 (2017): 702–8.

114. Michael J. Gandal, Jillian R. Haney, Neelroop N. Parikshak, Virpi Leppa, Gokul Ra-maswami, Chris Hartl, Andrew J. Schork, et al., "Shared Molecular Neuropathol-ogy across Major Psychiatric Disorders Parallels Polygenic Overlap," *Science* 359, no. 6376 (2018): 693–97.

115. First and Zimmerman, "Including Laboratory Tests," 2041.

116. Peter Conrad, "Medicalization and Social Control," *Annual Review of Sociology* 18 (1992): 209–32.

117. For an example of diagnostic expansion, take the case of Post-Traumatic Stress Dis-order (PTSD). Since its inclusion in DSM-III, the PTSD category has expanded. Sub-sequent editions of DSM-III have lowered the bar for what is considered a traumatic event—from an external evaluation of an event "outside the range of usual human experience" that would be objectively distressing to anyone to a subjective interpreta-tion based on the patient's response. Psychiatrists have also broadened what it means to "experience" trauma, expanding it from direct involvement to include witnessing or receiving information about a traumatic event.

118. Blashfield et al., "The Cycle of Classification."

119. Lane, *Shyness*; Allan V. Horwitz and Jerome C. Wakefield, *The Loss of Sadness: How Psychiatry Transformed Normal Sorrow into Depressive Disorder* (New York: Oxford Uni-versity Press, 2007); Anne E. Figert, "The Three Faces of PMS: The Professional, Gen-dered, and Scientific Structuring of a Psychiatric Disorder," *Social Problems* 42, no. 1 (1995): 56–73; Conrad, "The Discovery of Hyperkinesis," 12–21.

120. Horwitz and Wakefield, "The Epidemic in Mental Illness," 19–23.

121. Mark Olfson, Steven C. Marcus, and Harold Alan Pincus, "Trends in Office-Based Psychiatric Practice," *American Journal of Psychiatry* 156, no. 3 (1999): 451–57.

122. Ramin Mojtabai and Mark Olfson, "National Trends in Psychotherapy by Office-Based Psychiatrists," *Archives of General Psychiatry* 65, no. 8 (2008): 962–70.

123. Tami Mark, Katharine Levit, and Jeffrey Buck, "Datapoints: Psychotropic Drug Pre-scriptions by Medical Specialty," *Psychiatric Services* 60, no. 9 (2009): 1167.

124. Irving Kirsch and Guy Sapirstein, "Listening to Prozac but Hearing Placebo: A Meta-Analysis of Antidepressant Medication," *Prevention & Treatment* 1, no. 2 (1998): Arti-cle 2a; Irving Kirsch et al., "The Emperor's New Drugs: An Analysis of Antidepressant Medication Data Submitted to the US Food and Drug Administration," *Prevention & Treatment* 5, no. 1 (2002): Article 23a; Irving Kirsch et al., "Initial Severity and Antidepressant Benefits: A Meta-Analysis of Data Submitted to the Food and Drug Administration," *PLoS Medicine* 5, no. 2 (2008): 260–68.

125. See Healy, *The Antidepressant Era*; Moncrieff, *The Myth of the Chemical Cure*.

126. The debate over the efficacy of antidepressants is unsettled (see Peter Kramer, *Or-dinarily Well: The Case for Antidepressants* [New York: Farrar, Straus & Giroux, 2016], for a summary of the arguments offered by advocates of SSRIs; and Kirsch, *The Emperor's New Drugs* [New York: Basic Books, 2010] for a summary of critics' po-sitions). Some meta-analyses seem to demonstrate efficacy (Robert D. Gibbons et al., "Benefits from Antidepressants: Synthesis of 6-Week Patient-Level Outcomes from Double-Blind Placebo-Controlled Randomized Trials of Fluoxetine and Ven-lafaxine," *Archives of General Psychiatry* 69, no. 6 [2012]: 572–79; Jay C. Fournier et al., "Differential Change in Specific Depressive Symptoms During Antidepressant Medication or Cognitive Therapy," *Behaviour Research and Therapy* 51, no. 7 [2013]: 392–98; Fredrik Hieronymus et al., "Consistent Superiority of Selective Serotonin Reuptake Inhibitors over Placebo in Reducing Depressed Mood in Patients with Ma-jor Depression," *Molecular Psychiatry* 21, no. 4 [2016]: 523–30; Juan Undurraga and

Ross J. Baldessarini, "Randomized, Placebo-Controlled Trials of Antidepressants for Acute Major Depression: Thirty-Year Meta-Analytic Review," *Neuropsychopharmacology* 37 [2012]: 851–64), while others suggest that there are little to no benefits beyond that of a placebo (Kirsch and Sapirstein, "Listening to Prozac"; Kirsch et al., "The Emperor's New Drugs"; Kirsch et al., "Initial Severity"). Much of the debate hinges on competing conceptualizations as to what constitutes a significant improvement. Most research on antidepressants uses the Hamilton Depression Rating Scale, which is derived from the DSM criteria for major depressive disorder (MDD). Each item on the questionnaire is weighted 3 to 5 points, for a total of 53 points possible. Typically, a score over 20 indicates depression. Advocates of SSRIs accept *statistical* significance as an indicator of efficacy—usually operationalized as a 3-point change. Critics argue that statistical significance is not equivalent to *clinical* significance, and advocate a higher bar (e.g., a 7-point change). The FDA accepts the lower bar of statistical significance. However, recently in the UK, the National Institute for Health and Care Excellence (NICE), which establishes treatment guidelines for the National Health Service (NHS), has adopted the higher bar. As a result, the NHS discourages the use of antidepressants as a first-line treatment for depression.

Critics of antidepressants make two additional arguments. First, they argue that the body of publicly available research on antidepressants is biased and skewed because pharmaceutical companies only publish research favorable to their interests. Negative findings go unpublished. Thus, meta-analyses are biased in favor of efficacy. It is hard to assess this argument. However, when Kirsch was able to obtain unpublished studies from the FDA, he found that even for severe depression the difference between antidepressant drugs and placebos was not clinically significant, based on the standards set by the National Health Service in the UK (Kirsch et al., "Initial Severity"). Second, critics insist that the side effects of antidepressants have been intentionally understated by pharmaceutical companies, thereby warping the cost-benefit analysis of their use. A 2009 study by Sidney H. Kennedy and Sakina Rizvi found that up to 60% of patients experience some sort of sexual dysfunction when treated with SSRIs, and a 2016 study by Golder et al. revealed that pharmaceutical companies underreport their side effects, omitting 40% of all side effects from their published materials. See Sidney H. Kennedy and Sakina Rizvi, "Sexual Dysfunction, Depression and the Impact of Antidepressants," *Journal of Clinical Psychopharmacology* 29, no. 2 (2009): 157–64; Su Golder et al., "Reporting of Adverse Events in Published and Unpublished Studies of Health Care Interventions: A Systematic Review," *PLoS Medicine* 13, no. 9 (2016): 1–22.

The controversy over antidepressants is difficult to navigate. The truth, as usual, is somewhere in the muddled middle. From it, I draw three conclusions relevant for this chapter. First, there has been a concerted effort on the part of pharmaceutical companies to exaggerate the safety and efficacy of antidepressants. How much and to what degree remains unknown. Second, because the efficacy of SSRIs is by no means as clear as it has been sold, the embrace of medication management as the primary service provided by psychiatry is professionally problematic. Finally, with regard to the ongoing issue of ignorance in psychiatry, this uncertainty suggests that ignorance of the basic mechanisms of mental distress cannot be deflected by appeals to evidently superior treatments.

127. David J. Kupfer, Michael B. First, and Darrel A. Regier, *A Research Agenda for DSM-V* (Washington, DC: American Psychiatric Publishing, 2002).

128. Ibid., xv.

129. Ibid., xviii.

130. Darrel A. Regier, William E. Narrow, Emily A. Kuhl, and David J. Kupfer, *The Conceptual Evolution of DSM-5* (Washington, DC: American Psychiatric Publishing, 2011), 14.

131. Helena C. Kraemer, Patrick E. Shrout, and Maritza Rubio-Stipec, "Developing the Diagnostic and Statistical Manual V: What Will 'Statistical' Mean in DSM-V?," *Social Psychiatry and Psychiatric Epidemiology* 42, no. 4 (2007): 263.

132. Kenneth S. Kendler, "An Historical Framework for Psychiatric Nosology," *Psychological Medicine* 39, no. 12 (2009): 1938.

133. "Although we are highly adept at making models of the world," notes Kathryn Schutz, author of *Being Wrong*, "we are distinctly less adept at realizing that we have made them." Kathryn Schutz, *Being Wrong: Adventures in the Margin of Error* (New York: Ecco, 2011), 99.

134. Allen Frances, "The Most Influential Psychiatrist of Our Time Retires Undefeated," *Psychiatric Times* 28, no. 2 (2011): 41.

135. Katharine A. Phillips, Michael B. First, and Harold A, Pincus, *Advancing DSM: Dilemmas in Psychiatric Diagnosis* (Washington, DC: American Psychiatric Publishing, 2003), xii.

136. Anonymous, DSM-5 Task Force member, interview with author, May 16, 2012.

137. Anonymous, DSM-5 Task Force member, interview with author, October 19, 2011.

138. Marsha F. Lopez, Wilson M. Compton, Bridget F. Grant, and James P. Breiling, "Dimensional Approaches in Diagnostic Classification: A Critical Appraisal," *International Journal of Methods in Psychiatric Research* 16, no. 1 (2007): S6; John E. Helzer, "A Proposal for Incorporating Clinically Relevant Dimensions into DSM-5," in *The Conceptual Evolution of DSM-5*, ed. Darrel A. Regier, William E. Narrow, Emily A. Kuhl, and David Kupfer (Washington, DC: American Psychiatric Publishing, 2001), 85.

139. Anonymous, DSM-5 Task Force member, interview with author, October 6, 2011.

140. Anonymous, DSM-5 Task Force member, interview with author, April 4, 2012.

141. Anonymous, DSM-5 Task Force member, interview with author, June 6, 2013.

142. Schnittker, *The Diagnostic System*, 220–21.

143. Anonymous, DSM-5 work group member, interview with author, June 14, 2011.

144. Anonymous, DSM-5 work group member, interview with author, May 17, 2012.

145. Regier et al., *The Conceptual Evolution of DSM-5*, xxvii.

146. Owen Whooley, "Measuring Mental Disorders: The Failed Commensuration Project of DSM-5," *Social Science & Medicine* 166 (October 2016): 33–40.

147. Allen Frances and Robert Spitzer, "Letter to the APA Board of Trustees, July 7, 2009," https://www.scribd.com/document/17172432/Letter-to-APA-Board-of-Trustees-July-7-2009-From-Allen-Frances-and-Robert-Spitzer (accessed October 12, 2010).

148. Alan F. Schatzberg, James H. Scully Jr., David J. Kupfer, and Darrel A. Regier, "Setting the Record Straight: A Response to Dr. Frances' Commentary on DSM-V," *Psychiatric Times* 26, no. 8 (2009): 1–3.

149. Allen Frances, "A Warning Sign on the Road to DSM-V: Beware of Its Unintended Consequences," *Psychiatric Times* 26, no. 8 (2009): 4.

150. Allen Frances, "DSM-V Badly Off Track," *Psychiatric Times*, June 26, 2009, http://www.psychiatrictimes.com/articles/dsm-v-badly-track (accessed October 10, 2012).

151. Anonymous, psychiatrist and DSM-5 critic, interview with author, February 8, 2012.

152. Frances, "DSM-V Badly Off Track."

153. Allen Frances, "Alert to the Research Community—Be Prepared to Weigh In on DSM-V," *Psychiatric Times*, January 10, 2010, http://www.psychiatrictimes.com/articles/alert-research-community%E2%80%94be-prepared-weigh-dsm-v-0 (accessed

October 10, 2012); Allen Frances, "Psychiatry Should Stay Comfortable in Its Own Skin," *Psychology Today*, June 2, 2011, https://www.psychologytoday.com/blog/dsm5 -in-distress/201106/psychiatry-should-stay-comfortable-in-its-own-skin (accessed October 10, 2012); Allen Frances, "Whither DSM-V?," *British Journal of Psychiatry* 195, no. 5 (2009): 391–92.

154. Frances, "Psychiatry Should Stay Comfortable in Its Own Skin."

155. Anonymous, psychiatrist and DSM-5 critic, interview with author, December 8, 2010.

156. Anonymous, psychiatrist and DSM-5 critic, interview with author, March 23, 2011.

157. Anonymous, psychiatrist and DSM-5 critic, interview with author, December 17, 2010.

158. Anonymous, psychiatrist and DSM-5 critic, interview with author, March 4, 2011.

159. Kenneth S. Kendler and Michael B. First, "Alternative Futures for the DSM Revision Process: Iteration v. Paradigm Shift," *British Journal of Psychiatry*, 197, no. 4 (2010): 263.

160. Ibid.

161. Kendler, "An Historical Framework," 1939.

162. Kenneth S. Kendler, "A History of the DSM-5 Scientific Review Committee," *Psychological Medicine* 43, no. 9 (2013): 1793.

163. Ibid., 1799.

164. Rachel Cooper, "Why Is the Diagnostic and Statistical Manual of Mental Disorders So Hard to Revise? Path-Dependence and 'Lock-In' in Classification," *Studies in History and Philosophy of Biological and Biomedical Sciences* 51 (June 2015): 1–10.

165. Robert L. Spitzer, Janet B. Williams, and Jean Endicott, "Standards for DSM-5 Reliability," *American Journal of Psychiatry* 169, no. 5 (2012): 537–37.

166. Deborah Blacker and Ming T. Tsuang, "Contested Boundaries of Bipolar Disorder and the Limits of Categorical Diagnosis in Psychiatry," *American Journal of Psychiatry* 149, no. 11 (1992): 1481.

167. Another effect of the DSM-III paradigm shift was to shift the locus of psychiatric expertise from clinicians to researchers (Schnittker, *Diagnostic System*, 55).

168. Anonymous, psychiatrist and DSM-5 critic, interview with author, February 8, 2012.

169. American Psychiatric Association, *Diagnostic and Statistical Manual of Mental Disorders*, 5th ed. (Washington, DC: American Psychiatric Publishing, 2013), 5 (italics added).

170. Ibid., 7.

171. Ibid., 5–6, 12–13.

172. Dilip Jeste, "A Message from APA President Dilip Jeste, M.D., on DSM-5," *Psychiatric News*, December 1, 2012, http://www.psychnews.org/files/DSM-message.pdf (accessed December 10, 2012).

173. Thomas Insel, "Transforming Diagnosis," NIMH, April 29, 2013, http://www.nimh .nih.gov/about/director/2013/transforming-diagnosis.shtml (accessed May 15, 2013).

174. Thomas R. Insel, Bruce N. Cuthbert, Marjorie A. Garvey, Robert K. Heinssen, Daniel S. Pine, Kevin J. Quinn, Charles A. Sanislow, and Philip S. Wang, "Research Domain Criteria (RDoC): Toward a New Classification Framework for Research on Mental Disorders," *American Journal of Psychiatry* 167, no. 7 (2010): 749.

175. Owen Whooley, "Nosological Reflections: The Failure of DSM-5, the Emergence of RDoC, and the Decontextualization of Mental Distress," *Society and Mental Health* 4, no. 2 (2014): 92–110.

176. Daniel S. Pine and Robert Freedman, "Imaging a Brighter Future," *American Journal of Psychiatry* 168, no. 9 (2011): 885.

177. Carol North and Sean Yutzy, *Goodwin and Guze's Psychiatric Diagnosis* (New York: Oxford University Press, 2010), xxvi.

178. Gold and Gold, *Suspicious Minds,* 11.

179. The APA has defeated most of these efforts, but at the time of this writing, five states—Idaho, Illinois, Iowa, Louisiana, and New Mexico—allow clinical psychologists to prescribe psychopharmaceutical drugs.

180. Nada L. Stotland, "Presidential Address," *American Journal of Psychiatry* 166, no. 10 (2009): 1102–3.

181. One can argue whether the actual DSM-5 proposals warranted such a designation. Diagnostic psychiatry, as articulated by the Neo-Kraepelinians, long aspired to a genetic and neurological understanding of mental disorders. Indeed, the Task Force's proposals could be seen less as a shift away from DSM-III and more as a recommitment to its promise.

182. Bowker and Star, *Sorting Things Out.*

CONCLUSION

1. Quoted in Zilboorg, *A History of Medical Psychology,* 329.

2. Scull, *Madness in Civilization,* 380.

3. Kirsch and Sapirstein, "Listening to Prozac"; Kirsch et al., "The Emperor's New Drugs"; Kirsch et al., "Initial Severity."

4. David Healy, *Let Them Eat Prozac: The Unhealthy Relationship Between the Pharmaceutical Industry and Depression* (New York: NYU Press, 2006); Art Levine, *Mental Health Inc.: How Corruption, Lax Oversight and Failed Reforms Endanger Our Most Vulnerable Citizens* (New York: Overlook Press, 2017); Kelly Patricia O'Meara, *Psyched Out: How Psychiatry Sells Mental Illness and Pushes Pills That Kill* (Bloomington, IN: Author House, 2006).

5. Richard A. Friedman, "A Dry Pipeline for Psychiatric Drugs," *New York Times,* August 19, 2013, D3.

6. In 2012, GlaxoSmithKline paid $3 billion in fines, the largest settlement ever against a drug company, one levied in part for promoting its best-selling antidepressants for unapproved uses.

7. Mark, Levit, and Buck, "Datapoints"; Ramin Mojtabai, "Increase in Antidepressant Medication in the US Adult Population between 1990 and 2003," *Psychotherapy and Psychosomatics* 77, no. 2 (2008): 83–92.

8. Fernando Vidal, "Brainhood, Anthropological Figure of Modernity," *History of the Human Sciences* 22, no. 1 (2009): 6; Eric Racine, Ofek Bar-Ilan, and Judy Illes, "fMRI in the Public Eye," *Nature Reviews Neuroscience* 6, no. 2 (2005): 159–64.

9. Nikolas Rose and Joelle M. Abi-Rached, *Neuro: The New Brain Sciences and the Management of the Mind* (Princeton, NJ: Princeton University Press, 2013), 9.

10. Rachel Hershenberg and Marvin R. Goldfried, "Implications of RDoC for the Research and Practice of Psychotherapy," *Behavior Therapy* 46, no. 2 (2015): 156.

11. International Neuroethics Society, "BRAIN Initiative, 2013," http://www.neuroethicssociety.org/brain-initiative (accessed December 12, 2015).

12. Benedict Carey, "Blazing Trails in Brain Science," *New York Times,* February 3, 2014, https://www.nytimes.com/2014/02/04/science/blazing-trails-in-brain-science.html?_r=1 (accessed November 16, 2015).

13. John C. Markowitz, "There's Such a Thing as Too Much Neuroscience," *New York Times,* October 15, 2016, A21.

14. Alison Abbott, "US Mental-Health Chief: Psychiatry Must Get Serious About Mathematics," *Nature,* October 26, 2016, http://www.nature.com/news/us-mental-health-chief-psychiatry-must-get-serious-about-mathematics-1.20893?cookies=accepted.

15. National Institute of Mental Health, "National Institute of Mental Health: Strategic Plan for Research, 2015," https://www.nimh.nih.gov/about/strategic-planning -reports/nimh_strategicplanforresearch_508compliant_corrected_final_149979.pdf (accessed May 14, 2017).

16. Allen Frances, "Can Congress Cure the Disorder in Mental Health?," *Huffington Post*, August 3, 2013, http://www.huffingtonpost.com/allen-frances/can-congress-cure -the-dis_b_3331570.html (accessed September 17, 2016); Marvin R. Goldfried, "On Possible Consequences of National Institute of Mental Health Funding for Psychotherapy Research and Training," *Professional Psychology: Research and Practice* 47, no. 1 (2016): 77–83.

17. Sara Naomi Shostak, *Exposed Science: Genes, the Environment, and the Politics of Population Health* (Berkeley: University of California Press, 2013), 5.

18. Shitij Kapur, Anthony G. Phillips, and Thomas Insel, "Why Has It Taken So Long for Biological Psychiatry to Develop Clinical Tests and What to Do About It?," *Molecular Psychiatry* 17, no. 12 (2012): 1174.

19. Insel, "Transforming Diagnosis."

20. Pressman, *Last Resort*, 438.

21. Andrew Abbott, "Varieties of Ignorance," *American Sociologist* 41, no. 2 (2010): 174.

22. To be fair, an appreciation of ignorance, or uncertainty, has not been entirely absent from the sociology of the professions. Sociologists have examined the means by which professionals, mostly physicians, manage uncertainty at the level of practice. They observe the uncertainty rife in clinical practice and reveal how doctors negotiate it. For example, see Charles L. Bosk, *Forgive and Remember: Managing Medical Failure* (Chicago: University of Chicago Press, 1979); Renee C. Fox, *Experiment Perilous: Physicians and Patients Facing the Unknown* (New York: Transaction Publishers, 1959); Donald Light, "Uncertainty and Control in Professional Training," *Journal of Health and Social Behavior* 20, no. 4 (1979): 310–22.

23. Gross, "The Unknown in Process"; McGoey, "The Logic of Strategic Ignorance"; Proctor, *Cancer Wars*.

24. Abbott, *The System of Professions*; Freidson, *Professionalism*.

25. Warner, "Fall and Rise."

26. Freidson, *Profession of Medicine*, 3.

27. As Robert Merton observes, "The specification of ignorance amounts to problem-finding as a prelude to problem-solving." Merton, "Three Fragments," 10.

28. Coser, *Training in Ambiguity*, 8.

29. Borup et al., "The Sociology of Expectations"; Brown and Michael, "A Sociology of Expectations."

30. Hedgecoe and Martin, "The Drugs Don't Work"; Selin, "The Sociology of the Future."

31. Nik Brown. "Hope against Hype-Accountability in Biopasts, Presents and Futures," *Science & Technology Studies* 16, no. 2 (2003): 6.

32. Scull, *Madness in Civilization*, 409.

33. Charlotte Linde, *Working the Past: Narrative and Institutional Memory* (New York: Oxford University Press, 2009).

34. Zerubavel, *Time Maps*, 99.

35. These practices have been identified and explored by scholars of collective memory. See Maurice Halbwachs, *On Collective Memory* (Chicago: University of Chicago Press, 1992); Jeffrey K. Olick and Joyce Robbins, "Social Memory Studies: From 'Collective Memory' to the Historical Sociology of Mnemonic Practices," *Annual Review of Sociology* 24 (1998): 105–40; Barry Schwartz, "Memory as a Cultural System:

Abraham Lincoln in World War II," *American Sociological Review* 61, no. 5 (1996): 908–27.

36. Niklas Luhmann, "The Modernity of Science," *New German Critique*, 61 (Winter 1994): 10.

37. Ann Mische, "Projects and Possibilities: Researching Futures in Action," *Sociological Forum* 24, no. 3 (2009): 694–704; Iddo Tavory and Nina Eliasoph, "Coordinating Futures: Toward a Theory of Anticipation," *American Journal of Sociology* 118, no. 4 (2013): 908–42.

38. Gail A. Hornstein and Susan Leigh Star, "Universality Biases: How Theories about Human Nature Succeed," *Philosophy of the Social Sciences* 20, no. 4 (1990): 430.

39. Whooley, *Knowledge in the Time of Cholera*.

40. Eviatar Zerubavel, *Social Mindscapes: An Invitation to Cognitive Sociology* (Cambridge, MA: Harvard University Press, 1999), 22.

41. This is an instance in which the selection of this particular case could misconstrue the general approach to ignorance among professions. Psychiatry's atypical history affords certain opportunities for insight, while foregoing others. Such is the trade-off of research choices.

42. Thomas F. Gieryn, *Cultural Boundaries of Science: Credibility on the Line* (Chicago: University of Chicago Press, 1999).

43. Bowker and Star, *Sorting Things Out*, 5–6.

44. Starr, *The Social Transformation*.

45. Bruno Latour, *Science in Action: How to Follow Scientists and Engineers through Society* (Cambridge, MA: Harvard University Press, 1987), 78.

46. Jasper, *Getting Your Way*, 141.

47. Although psychiatry has improved on these measures since the acme of antipsychiatry sentiment in the 1970s, recent Gallup data from 2016 shows psychiatrists trailing physicians by nearly 30 points when it comes to whether respondents perceive the profession as having "high" or "very high" standards of honesty and ethics (38% to 65%). They also rate lower than nurses (84%), pharmacists (77%), and even dentists (59%). See Gallup, "Honesty/Ethics in Professions, 2016," http://www.gallup.com/poll/1654/honesty-ethics-professions.aspx (accessed May 15, 2017).

48. Janis L. Cutler, Sharon L. Alspector, Kelli J. Harding, Leslie L. Wright, and Mark J. Graham, "Medical Students' Perceptions of Psychiatry as a Career Choice," *Academic Psychiatry* 30, no. 2 (2006): 144–49; C. J. Jos and John Waite, "Medical Students' Perception of Psychiatry," *American Journal of Psychiatry* 142, no. 5 (1985): 660–61; Fredrick S. Sierles and Michael Alan Taylor, "Decline of U.S. Medical Student Career Choice of Psychiatry and What to Do About It," *American Journal of Psychiatry* 152, no. 10 (1995): 1416–26.

49. Howard S. Becker, "The Power of Inertia," *Qualitative Sociology* 18, no. 3 (1995): 301–9. Psychologists call this the "status quo bias." See William Samuelson and Richard Zeckhauser, "Status Quo Bias in Decision Making," *Journal of Risk and Uncertainty* 1, no. 1 (1988): 7–59.

50. Max Weber, *Economy and Society: An Outline of Interpretive Sociology*, vol. 1, ed. Guenther Ross and Claus Wittich (Berkeley: University of California Press, 1978), 326.

51. Zilboorg, *A History of Medical Psychology*.

52. Ibid., 324.

53. Pressman, *Last Resort*, 438.

54. Shorter, *A History of Psychiatry*, 326.

55. Foucault, *Madness and Civilization*.

56. Ibid., xxviii.
57. Goffman, "The Insanity of Place," 356.
58. Scheff, *Being Mentally Ill.*
59. Rosenberg, "Contested Boundaries," 409.
60. Ibid., 411.
61. Joint Commission on Mental Health and Illness, *Action for Mental Health*, 58.
62. Ibid. (italics in original).
63. Arlie Hochschild, *Strangers in Their Own Land: Anger and Mourning on the American Right* (New York: New Press, 2016), 5.
64. Dinesh Bhugra and Kwame McKenzie, "Expressed Emotion across Cultures," *Advances in Psychiatric Treatment* 9, no. 5 (2003): 342–48; Ronald L. Butzlaff and Jill M Hooley, "Expressed Emotion and Psychiatric Relapse: A Meta-Analysis," *Archives of General Psychiatry* 55, no. 6 (1998): 547–52; Jill M. Hooley, "Expressed Emotion and Relapse of Psychopathology," *Annual Review of Clinical Psychology* 3 (2007):·329–52; Harriet P. Lefley, "Expressed Emotion: Conceptual, Clinical, and Social Policy Issues," *Psychiatric Services* 43, no. 6 (1992): 591–98.
65. Bruce G. Link et al., "Public Conceptions of Mental Illness: Labels, Causes, Dangerousness, and Social Distance," *American Journal of Public Health* 89, no. 9 (1999): 1328–33; Jack K. Martin et al., "The Construction of Fear: Americans' Preferences for Social Distance from Children and Adolescents with Mental Health Problems," *Journal of Health and Social Behavior* 48, no. 1 (2007): 50–67; Andrew R. Payton and Peggy A. Thoits, "Medicalization, Direct-to-Consumer Advertising, and Mental Illness Stigma," *Society and Mental Health* 1, no. 1 (2011): 55–70; Jo C. Phelan, "Geneticization of Deviant Behavior and Consequences for Stigma: The Case of Mental Illness," *Journal of Health and Social Behavior* 46, no. 4 (2005): 307–22; Jason Schnittker, "An Uncertain Revolution: Why the Rise of a Genetic Model of Mental Illness Has Not Increased Tolerance," *Social Science & Medicine* 67, no. 9 (2008): 1370–81.
66. Otto F. Wahl, *Media Madness: Public Images of Mental Illness* (New Brunswick, NJ: Rutgers University Press, 1997).
67. Jonathan Metzl and Kenneth MacLeish, "Mental Illness, Mass Shootings, and the Politics of American Firearms," *American Journal of Public Health* 105, no. 2 (2015): 240–49.
68. Sarah L. Desmarais et al., "Community Violence Perpetration and Victimization Among Adults with Mental Illnesses," *American Journal of Public Health* 104, no. 12 (2014): 2342–49; Karen Hughes et al., "Prevalence and Risk of Violence Against Adults with Disabilities: A Systematic Review and Meta-Analysis of Observational Studies," *The Lancet* 379 (9826): 1621–29.
69. Jenny Gold, "A Dearth of Psychiatric Hospital Beds for California Patients in Crisis," *NPR*, April 14, 2016, http://www.npr.org/sections/health-shots/2016/04/14/474210027/a -dearth-of-psychiatric-hospital-beds-for-california-patients-in-crisis?utm_source=twitter .com&utm_medium=social&utm_campaign=npr&utm_term=nprnews&utm_content =20160414 (accessed September 27, 2016).
70. National Alliance on Mental Health, "Mental Health by the Numbers," https://www .nami.org/Learn-More/Mental-Health-By-the-Numbers (accessed February 15, 2018).
71. E. Fuller Torrey, *Nowhere to Go: The Tragic Odyssey of the Homeless Mentally Ill* (New York: Harper & Row, 1988).
72. Treatment Advocacy Center, "Serious Mental Illness (SMI) Prevalence in Jails and Prisons, September 2016," http://www.treatmentadvocacycenter.org/storage/docu ments/backgrounders/smi-in-jails-and-prisons.pdf (accessed May 3, 2017).

73. Ibid.

74. Kimberly Kindy, "Fatal Police Shootings in 2015 Approaching 400 Nationwide," *Washington Post* (May 30, 2015), https://www.washingtonpost.com/national/fatal-police-shootings-in-2015-approaching-400-nationwide/2015/05/30/d322256a-058e-11e5-a428-c984eb077d4e_story.html?utm_term=.aad386020a75 (accessed June 9, 2017); Treatment Advocacy Center, "Overlooked and Undercounted: The Role of Mental Illness in Fatal Law Enforcement Encounters, December 2015," http://www.treatmentadvocacycenter.org/storage/documents/overlooked-in-the-undercounted.pdf (accessed June 9, 2017).

75. Rachel Aviv, "Your Son Is Deceased," *New Yorker* (February 2, 2015), http://www.newyorker.com/magazine/2015/02/02/son-deceased (accessed February 15, 2015); Laurel Wamsley, "After Inmate with Schizophrenia Dies in Shower, Fla. Prosecutor Finds No Wrongdoing," *NPR* (March 19, 2017), http://www.npr.org/sections/thetwo-way/2017/03/19/520743255/after-schizophrenic-inmate-dies-in-a-shower-florida-prosecutor-finds-no-wrongdoi (accessed March 20, 2017).

76. Goffman, *Stigma*.

BIBLIOGRAPHY

Note: Bibliography includes important secondary materials used in the formulation of the book's analysis. For all other citations, see chapter endnotes.

Abend, Gabriel. 2006. "Styles of Styles of Sociological Thought: Sociologies, Epistemologies, and the Mexican and US Quests for Truth." *Sociological Theory* 24 (1): 1–41.

Abbott, Andrew. 1988. *The System of Professions: An Essay on the Division of Expert Labor.* Chicago: University of Chicago Press.

———. 2001. *Chaos of Disciplines.* Chicago: University of Chicago Press.

———. 2010. "Varieties of Ignorance." *American Sociologist* 41 (2): 174–89.

Ackerknecht, Erwin H. 1968. *A Short History of Psychiatry.* Translated by Sula Wolff. New York: Hafner Publishing Company.

Andreasen, Nancy C. 1984. *The Broken Brain.* New York: HarperCollins.

Appignanesi. Lisa. 2009. *Mad, Bad, and Sad: A History of Women and the Mind Doctors.* New York: W. W. Norton.

Barton, Walter E. 1987. *The History and Influence of the American Psychiatric Association.* Arlington, VA: American Psychiatric Publishing.

Bayer, Ronald. 1987. *Homosexuality and American Psychiatry: The Politics of Diagnosis.* Princeton, NJ: Princeton University Press.

Bayer, Ronald, and Robert L. Spitzer. 1985. "Neurosis, Psychodynamics, and DSM-III: A History of the Controversy." *Archives of General Psychiatry* 42 (2): 187–96.

Beam, Alex. 2009. *Gracefully Insane: The Rise and Fall of America's Premier Mental Hospital.* New York: Public Affairs.

Becker, Howard S. 1995. "The Power of Inertia." *Qualitative Sociology* 18 (3): 301–9.

Bergmann, Martin S. 2000. *The Hartmann Era.* New York: Other Press.

Berkenkotter, Carol. 2008. *Patient Tales: Case Histories and the Uses of Narrative in Psychiatry.* Columbia: University of South Carolina Press.

Bhugra, Dinesh, and Kwame McKenzie. 2003. "Expressed Emotion across Cultures." *Advances in Psychiatric Treatment* 9 (5): 342–48.

Biehl, Joao. 2005. *Vita: Life in a Zone of Social Abandonment.* Berkeley: University of California Press.

Black, Edwin. 2003. *War against the Weak: Eugenics and America's Campaign to Create a Master Race.* New York: Basic Books.

Blashfield, Roger K. 1982. "Feighner et al., Invisible Colleges, and the Matthew Effect." *Schizophrenia Bulletin* 8 (1): 1–6.

Blashfield, Roger K., Jared W. Keeley, Elizabeth H. Flanagan, and Shannon R. Miles. 2014. "The Cycle of Classification: DSM-I through DSM-5." *Annual Review of Clinical Psychology* 10: 25–51.

Blustein, Bonnie Ellen. 1981. "'A Hollow Square of Psychological Science': American Neurologists and Psychiatrists in Conflict." In *Madhouses, Mad-Doctors, and Madmen*, edited by Andrew Scull, 241–70. Princeton, NJ: Princeton University Press.

Borup, Mads, Nik Brown, Kornelia Konrad, and Harro van Lente. 2006. "The Sociology of Expectations in Science and Technology." *Technology Analysis & Strategic Management* 18 (3–4): 285–98.

Bosk, Charles L. 1979. *Forgive and Remember: Managing Medical Failure*. Chicago: University of Chicago Press.

Bowker, Geoffrey C., and Susan Leigh Star. 1999. *Sorting Things Out: Classification and Its Consequences*. Cambridge, MA: MIT Press.

Breggin, Peter R., and Ginger R. Breggin. 1995. *Talking Back to Prozac: What Doctors Aren't Telling You About Today's Most Controversial Drug*. New York: St. Martin's Press.

Brown, Nik. 2003. "Hope against Hype—Accountability in Biopasts, Presents and Futures." *Science & Technology Studies* 16 (2): 3–21.

Brown, Nik, and Mike Michael. 2003. "A Sociology of Expectations: Retrospecting Prospects and Prospecting Retrospects." *Technology Analysis & Strategic Management* 15 (1): 3–18.

Brown, Nik, and Brian Rappert. 2017. *Contested Futures: A Sociology of Prospective Techno-Science*. London: Taylor & Francis.

Brown, Thomas J. 1998. *Dorothea Dix: New England Reformer*. Cambridge, MA: Harvard University Press.

Burnham, John, ed. 2012. *After Freud Left: A Century of Psychoanalysis in America*. Chicago: University of Chicago Press.

Busfield, Joan 1996. *Men, Women and Madness: Understanding Gender and Mental Disorder*. London: Macmillan.

Butzlaff, Ronald L., and Jill M. Hooley. 1998. "Expressed Emotion and Psychiatric Relapse: A Meta-Analysis." *Archives of General Psychiatry* 55 (6): 547–52.

Caplan, Eric. 2001. *Mind Games: American Culture and the Birth of Psychotherapy*. Berkeley: University of California Press.

Caplan, Paula J. 1995. *They Say You're Crazy: How the World's Most Powerful Psychiatrists Decide Who's Normal*. Reading, MA: Addison-Wesley.

Carlson, Eric T. 1958. "The Influence of Phrenology on Early American Psychiatric Thought." *American Journal of Psychiatry* 115 (6): 535–38.

Chandler, Susan Meyers. 1990. *Competing Realities: The Contested Terrain of Mental Health Advocacy*. New York: Praeger.

Chesler, Phyllis. 1973. *Women & Madness*. New York: Avon Books.

Conrad, Peter. 1975. "The Discovery of Hyperkinesis: Notes on the Medicalization of Deviant Behavior." *Social Problems* 23 (1): 12–21.

———. 1992. "Medicalization and Social Control." *Annual Review of Sociology* 18: 209–32.

———. 2007. *The Medicalization of Society: On the Transformation of Human Conditions into Treatable Disorders*. Baltimore, MD: Johns Hopkins University Press.

Cooper, Rachel. 2015. "Why Is the Diagnostic and Statistical Manual of Mental Disorders So Hard to Revise? Path-Dependence and 'Lock-In' in Classification." *Studies in History and Philosophy of Science Part C: Studies in History and Philosophy of Biological and Biomedical Sciences* 51: 1–10.

Coser, Rose Laub. 1979. *Training in Ambiguity: Learning through Doing in a Mental Hospital*. New York: Free Press.

Craciun, Mariana. 2016. "The Cultural Work of Office Charisma: Maintaining Professional Power in Psychotherapy." *Theory and Society* 45 (4): 361–83.

Cusanus, Nicolas. 2007. *Of Learned Ignorance*. Eugene, OR: Wipf & Stock Publishers.

Dain, Norman. 1964. *Concepts of Insanity in the United States, 1789–1865*. New Brunswick, NJ: Rutgers University Press.

Decker, Hannah S. 2007. "How Kraepelinian Was Kraepelin? How Kraepelinian Are the Neo-Kraepelinians?—from Emil Kraepelin to DSM-III." *History of Psychiatry* 18 (3): 337–60.

———. 2013. *The Making of DSM-III*. New York: Oxford University Press.

Deutsch, Albert. 1936. "The Cult of Curability, Its Rise and Decline: A Page from Psychiatric History." *American Journal of Psychiatry* 92 (6): 1261–80.

———. 1948. *The Shame of the States*. New York: Harcourt, Brace.

———. 1959. *The Story of GAP*. New York: Group for the Advancement of Psychiatry.

Dewey, John. 1916. *Democracy and Education*. New York: Macmillan.

———. 1929. *The Quest for Certainty: A Study of the Relation of Knowledge and Action*. New York: Minton, Balch & Co.

Douglas, Mary. 1986. *How Institutions Think*. Syracuse, NY: Syracuse University Press.

Dowbiggin, Ian Robert. 1997. *Keeping America Sane: Psychiatry and Eugenics in the United States and Canada, 1880–1940*. Ithaca, NY: Cornell University Press.

Drescher, Jack, and Joseph P. Merlino, eds. 2012. *American Psychiatry and Homosexuality: An Oral History*. Binghamton, NY: Taylor & Francis.

Dunham, Henry Warren, and Samuel Kirson Weinberg. 1960. *The Culture of the State Mental Hospital*. Detroit, MI: Wayne State University Press.

Durkheim, Emile. [1897] 1951. *Suicide: A Study in Sociology*. New York: Free Press.

Dwyer, Ellen. 1987. *Homes for the Mad: Life Inside Two Nineteenth-Century Asylums*. New Brunswick, NJ: Rutgers University Press.

El-Hai, Jack. 2007. *The Lobotomist: A Maverick Medical Genius and His Tragic Quest to Rid the World of Mental Illness*. Hoboken, NJ: Wiley.

Emirbayer, Mustafa, and Ann Mische. 1998. "What Is Agency?" *American Journal of Sociology* 103 (4): 962–1023.

Engel, Jonathan. 2008. *American Therapy: The Rise of Psychotherapy in the United States*. New York: Gotham Books.

Eysenck, Hans Jurgen. 1985. *Decline and Fall of the Freudian Empire*. New York: Viking.

Farrell, Michael P. 2003. *Collaborative Circles: Friendship Dynamics and Creative Work*. Chicago: University of Chicago Press.

Figert, Anne E. 1995. "The Three Faces of PMS: The Professional, Gendered, and Scientific Structuring of a Psychiatric Disorder." *Social Problems* 42 (1): 56–73.

Firestein, Stuart. 2012. *Ignorance: How It Drives Science*. New York: Oxford University Press.

Fleck, Ludwik. 1979. *Genesis and Development of a Scientific Fact*. Chicago: University of Chicago Press.

Foley, Henry A., and Steven Samuel Sharfstein. 1983. *Madness and Government: Who Cares for the Mentally Ill?* Washington, DC: American Psychiatric Press.

Forrester, John. 1997. *Dispatches from the Freud Wars: Psychoanalysis and Its Passions*. Cambridge, MA: Harvard University Press.

Fortun, Mike. 2008. *Promising Genomics: Iceland and deCODE Genetics in a World of Speculation*. Berkeley: University of California Press.

Foucault, Michel. 1988. *Madness and Civilization: A History of Insanity in the Age of Reason*. New York: Vintage Books.

———. 2006. *Psychiatric Power: Lectures at the Collège de France, 1973–1974*. New York: St. Martin's Press.

———. 2013. *History of Madness*. Translated by Jean Khalfa. New York: Routledge.

Fournier, Jay C., Robert J. DeRubeis, Steven D. Hollon, Robert Gallop, Richard C. Shelton, and Jay D. Amsterdam. 2013. "Differential Change in Specific Depressive Symptoms During Antidepressant Medication or Cognitive Therapy." *Behaviour Research and Therapy* 51 (7): 392–98.

Fox, Renee C. 1959. *Experiment Perilous: Physicians and Patients Facing the Unknown*. New York: Transaction Publishers.

Freidson, Eliot. 1986. *Professional Powers: A Study of the Institutionalization of Formal Knowledge*. Chicago: University of Chicago Press.

———. 1988. *Profession of Medicine: A Study of the Sociology of Applied Knowledge*. Chicago: University of Chicago Press.

———. 2001. *Professionalism: The Third Logic*. Chicago: University of Chicago Press.

Frickel, Scott, Sahra Gibbon, Jeff Howard, Gwen Ottinger, and David Hess. 2009. "Undone Science: Charting Social Movement and Civil Society Challenges to Research Agenda Setting." *Science, Technology & Human Values* 35 (4): 444–73.

Frickel, Scott, and M. Bess Vincent. 2011. "Katrina's Contamination: Regulatory Knowledge Gaps in the Making and Unmaking of Environmental Contention." In *Dynamics of Disaster: Lessons on Risk, Response, and Recovery*, edited by Barbara Allen and Rachel Dowty Beech, 11–28. New York: Routledge.

Friedman, Richard A. 2013. "A Dry Pipeline for Psychiatric Drugs." *New York Times*, August 19, D3.

———. 2015. "Psychiatry's Identity Crisis." *New York Times*, July 17, SR5.

Fussinger, Catherine. 2011. "'Therapeutic Community,' Psychiatry's Reformers and Antipsychiatrists: Reconsidering Changes in the Field of Psychiatry after World War II." *History of Psychiatry* 22 (2): 146–63.

Gamwell, Lynn, and Nancy Tomes. 1995. *Madness in America: Cultural and Medical Perceptions of Mental Illness before 1914*. Ithaca, NY: Cornell University Press.

Gay, Peter. 2006. *Freud: A Life for Our Time*. New York: W. W. Norton.

Ghaemi, S. Nassir. 2007. "Adolf Meyer: Psychiatric Anarchist." *Philosophy, Psychiatry, & Psychology* 14 (4): 341–45.

Gibbons, Robert D., Kwan Hur, C. Hendricks Brown, John M. Davis, and J. John Mann. 2012. "Benefits from Antidepressants: Synthesis of 6-Week Patient-Level Outcomes from Double-Blind Placebo-Controlled Randomized Trials of Fluoxetine and Venlafaxine." *Archives of General Psychiatry* 69 (6): 572–79.

Gieryn, Thomas F. 1999. *Cultural Boundaries of Science: Credibility on the Line*. Chicago: University of Chicago Press.

Ginzburg, Carlo, and Anna Davin. 1980. "Morelli, Freud and Sherlock Holmes: Clues and Scientific Method." *History Workshop* 9 (1): 5–36.

Goffman, Erving. 1962. *Asylums: Essays on the Social Situation of Mental Patients and Other Inmates*. Chicago: Aldine Publishing.

———. 1971. "The Insanity of Place." In *Relations in Public*, 335–90. New York: Harper & Row Publishers.

———. 1974. *Stigma: Notes on the Management of Spoiled Identity*. New York: J. Aronson.

Gold, Joel, and Ian Gold. 2015. *Suspicious Minds: How Culture Shapes Madness*. New York: Free Press.

Golder, Su, Yoon K. Loke, Kath Wright, and Gill Norman. 2016. "Reporting of Adverse Events in Published and Unpublished Studies of Health Care Interventions: A Systematic Review." *PLoS Medicine* 13 (9): 1–22.

Gollaher, David. 1995. *Voice for the Mad: The Life of Dorothea Dix*. New York: Free Press.

Goodheart, Lawrence B. 2003. *Mad Yankees: The Hartford Retreat for the Insane and Nineteenth-Century Psychiatry.* Amherst, MA: University of Massachusetts Press.

Greenberg, Gary. 2013. *The Book of Woe: The DSM and the Unmaking of Psychiatry.* New York: Blue Rider Press.

Greenberg, Joanne. 1964. *I Never Promised You a Rose Garden.* New York: Holt McDougal.

Grob, Gerald N. 1966. *The State and the Mentally Ill: A History of Worcester State Hospital in Massachusetts, 1830–1920.* Durham: University of North Carolina Press.

———. 1983. *Mental Illness and American Society, 1875–1940.* Princeton, NJ: Princeton University Press.

———. 1985a. *The Inner World of American Psychiatry, 1890–1940: Selected Correspondence.* New Brunswick, NJ: Rutgers University Press.

———. 1985b. "The Origins of American Psychiatric Epidemiology." *American Journal of Public Health* 75 (3): 229–36.

———. 1991. *From Asylum to Community: Mental Health Policy in Modern America.* Princeton, NJ: Princeton University Press.

———. 1998. "Psychiatry's Holy Grail: The Search for the Mechanisms of Mental Diseases." *Bulletin of the History of Medicine* 72 (2): 189–219.

———. 2008. *Mental Institutions in America: Social Policy to 1875.* New Brunswick, NJ: Transaction Publishers.

Gross, Matthias. 2007. "The Unknown in Process: Dynamic Connections of Ignorance, Non-Knowledge and Related Concepts." *Current Sociology* 55 (5): 742–59.

———. 2010. *Ignorance and Surprise: Science, Society, and Ecological Design.* Cambridge, MA: MIT Press.

Gross, Matthias, and Linsey McGoey. 2015. *Routledge International Handbook of Ignorance Studies.* New York: Taylor & Francis.

Gross, Neil. 2009. "A Pragmatist Theory of Social Mechanisms." *American Sociological Review* 74 (3): 358–79.

Hacking, Ian. 1985. "Styles of Scientific Reasoning." In *Post-Analytic Philosophy*, edited by John Rajchman and Cornel West, 145–65. New York: Columbia University Press.

———. 2002. *Mad Travelers: Reflections on the Reality of Transient Mental Illnesses.* Cambridge, MA: Harvard University Press.

Halbwachs, Maurice. 1992. *On Collective Memory.* Chicago: University of Chicago Press.

Hale, Nathan G. 1971. *Freud and the Americans.* New York: Oxford University Press.

———. 1995. *The Rise and Crisis of Psychoanalysis in the United States: Freud and the Americans, 1917–1985.* New York: Oxford University Press.

Halpin, Michael. 2016. "The DSM and Professional Practice Research, Clinical, and Institutional Perspectives." *Journal of Health and Social Behavior* 57 (2): 153–67.

Halttunen, Karen. 1982. *Confidence Men and Painted Women: A Study of Middle-Class Culture in America, 1830–1870.* New Haven, CT: Yale University Press.

Haydu, Jeffrey. 1998. "Making Use of the Past: Time Periods as Cases to Compare and as Sequences of Problem Solving." *American Journal of Sociology* 104 (2): 339–71.

Healy, David. 1997. *The Antidepressant Era.* Cambridge, MA: Harvard University Press.

———. 2006. *Let Them Eat Prozac: The Unhealthy Relationship Between the Pharmaceutical Industry and Depression.* New York: NYU Press.

Hedgecoe, Adam M. 2003. "Terminology and the Construction of Scientific Disciplines: The Case of Pharmacogenomics." *Science, Technology, & Human Values* 28 (4): 513–37.

Hedgecoe, Adam, and Paul Martin. 2003. "The Drugs Don't Work: Expectations and the Shaping of Pharmacogenetics." *Social Studies of Science* 33 (3): 327–64.

Hieronymus, Fredrik, Johan Fredrik Emilsson, Staffan Nilsson, and Elias Eriksson. 2016. "Consistent Superiority of Selective Serotonin Reuptake Inhibitors over Placebo in Reducing Depressed Mood in Patients with Major Depression." *Molecular Psychiatry* 21 (4): 523–30.

Hilgartner, Stephen. 2000. *Science on Stage: Expert Advice as Public Drama*. Stanford, CA: Stanford University Press.

Hilts, Philip J. 2003. *Protecting America's Health: The FDA, Business, and One Hundred Years of Regulation*. New York: Alfred A. Knopf.

Hirschfeld, Robert M. 2000. "History and Evolution of the Monoamine Hypothesis of Depression." *Journal of Clinical Psychiatry* 61 (suppl. 6): 4–6.

Hochschild, Arlie. 2016. *Strangers in Their Own Land: Anger and Mourning on the American Right*. New York: New Press.

Hoff, Paul. 1998. "Emil Kraepelin and Forensic Psychiatry." *International Journal of Law and Psychiatry* 21 (4): 343–53.

Hooley, Jill M. 2007. "Expressed Emotion and Relapse of Psychopathology." *Annual Review of Clinical Psychology* 3: 329–52.

Hornstein, Gail A., and Susan Leigh Star. 1990. "Universality Biases: How Theories about Human Nature Succeed." *Philosophy of the Social Sciences* 20 (4): 421–36.

Horwitz, Allan V. 2002. *Creating Mental Illness*. Chicago: University of Chicago Press.

Horwitz, Allan V., and Jerome C. Wakefield. 2006. "The Epidemic in Mental Illness: Clinical Fact or Survey Artifact?" *contexts* 5 (1): 19–23.

———. 2007. *The Loss of Sadness: How Psychiatry Transformed Normal Sorrow into Depressive Disorder*. New York: Oxford University Press.

Howe, Daniel Walker. 2007. *What Hath God Wrought: The Transformation of America, 1815–1848*. New York: Oxford University Press.

Hughes, Karen, Mark A. Bellis, Lisa Jones, Sara Wood, Geoff Bates, Lindsay Eckley, Ellie McCoy, Christopher Mikton, Tom Shakespeare, and Alana Officer. 2012. "Prevalence and Risk of Violence Against Adults with Disabilities: A Systematic Review and Meta-Analysis of Observational Studies." *The Lancet* 379 (9826): 1621–29.

Hunt, Morton. 2007. *The Story of Psychology*. New York: Anchor Books.

James, William. 1890. *The Principles of Psychology*. New York: Henry Holt and Co.

———. 1907. "Pragmatism's Conception of Truth." *Journal of Philosophy, Psychology and Scientific Methods* 4 (6): 141–55.

Jasper, James M. 2006. *Getting Your Way: Strategic Dilemmas in the Real World*. Chicago: University of Chicago Press.

Jewson, N. D. 1976. "The Disappearance of the Sick-Man from Medical Cosmology, 1870–1970." *Sociology* 10 (2): 225–44.

Joyce, Kelly A. 2008. *Magnetic Appeal: MRI and the Myth of Transparency*. Ithaca, NY: Cornell University Press.

Kameny, Franklin. 2014. "Victory! We Have Been Cured." In *Gay Is Good: The Life and Letters of Gay Rights Pioneer Franklin Kameny*, edited by Michael G. Long, 269–87. Syracuse, NY: Syracuse University Press.

Katz, Jack. 1979. "Concerted Ignorance: The Social Construction of Cover-Up." *Urban Life* 8 (3): 295–316.

Kelman, Steven. 1987. "The Political Foundations of American Statistical Policy." In *The Politics of Statistics*, edited by William Alonso and Paul Starr, 275–302. New York: Russell Sage Foundation.

Kempner, Joanna, Jon F. Merz, and Charles L. Bosk. 2011. "Forbidden Knowledge: Public Controversy and the Production of Nonknowledge." *Sociological Forum* 26 (3): 475–500.

Kennedy, Sidney H., and Sakina Rizvi. 2009. "Sexual Dysfunction, Depression, and the Impact of Antidepressants." *Journal of Clinical Psychopharmacology* 29 (2): 157–64.

Kevles, Daniel J. 1995. *In the Name of Eugenics: Genetics and the Uses of Human Heredity.* Cambridge, MA: Harvard University Press.

Kirk, Stuart A., and Herb Kutchins. 1992. *The Selling of DSM: The Rhetoric of Science in Psychiatry.* Piscataway, NJ: Aldine.

Kirsch, Irving. 2010. *The Emperor's New Drugs: Exploding the Antidepressant Myth.* New York: Basic Books.

Kirsch, Irving, Brett J. Deacon, Tania B. Huedo-Medina, Alan Scoboria, Thomas J. Moore, and Blair T. Johnson. 2008. "Initial Severity and Antidepressant Benefits: A Meta-Analysis of Data Submitted to the Food and Drug Administration." *PLoS Medicine* 5 (2): 260–68.

Kirsch, Irving, Thomas J. Moore, Alan Scoboria, and Sarah S. Nicholls. 2002. "The Emperor's New Drugs: An Analysis of Antidepressant Medication Data Submitted to the US Food and Drug Administration." *Prevention & Treatment* 5 (1): 23a.

Kirsch, Irving, and Guy Sapirstein. 1998. "Listening to Prozac but Hearing Placebo: A Meta-Analysis of Antidepressant Medication." *Prevention & Treatment* 1 (2): 2a.

Knorr-Cetina, Karin. 1999. *Epistemic Cultures: How the Sciences Make Knowledge.* Cambridge, MA: Harvard University Press.

Kramer, Peter D. 1994. *Listening to Prozac.* New York: Fourth Estate.

———. 2016. *Ordinarily Well: The Case for Antidepressants.* New York: Farrar, Straus & Giroux.

Krause, Monika, and Michael Guggenheim. 2013. "The Couch as a Laboratory? The Spaces of Psychoanalytic Knowledge-Production Between Research, Diagnosis and Treatment." *European Journal of Sociology* 54 (2): 187–210.

Kuhn, Thomas S. 1996. *The Structure of Scientific Revolutions,* 3rd ed. Chicago: University of Chicago Press.

Lamb, S. D. 2014. *Pathologist of the Mind: Adolf Meyer and the Origins of American Psychiatry.* Baltimore, MD: Johns Hopkins University Press.

Lane, Christopher. 2007. *Shyness: How Normal Behavior Became a Sickness.* New Haven, CT: Yale University Press.

Latour, Bruno. 1987. *Science in Action: How to Follow Scientists and Engineers through Society.* Cambridge, MA: Harvard University Press.

———. 1988. *The Pasteurization of France.* Cambridge, MA: Harvard University Press.

Lefley, Harriet P. 1992. "Expressed Emotion: Conceptual, Clinical, and Social Policy Issues." *Psychiatric Services* 43 (6): 591–98.

Lerman, Paul. 1982. *Deinstitutionalization and the Welfare State.* New Brunswick, NJ: Rutgers University Press.

Leveille, J. J. 2002. "Jurisdictional Competition and the Psychoanalytic Dominance of American Psychiatry." *Journal of Historical Sociology* 15 (2): 252–80.

Levine, Art. 2017. *Mental Health Inc.: How Corruption, Lax Oversight and Failed Reforms Endanger Our Most Vulnerable Citizens.* New York: Overlook Press.

Lewis, Sinclair. 2008. *Arrowsmith.* New York: Signet Classics.

Leys, Ruth. 1991. "Types of One: Adolf Meyer's Life Chart and the Representation of Individuality." *Representations* 34: 1–28.

Lieberman, Jeffrey A., and Ogi Ogas. 2015. *Shrinks: The Untold Story of Psychiatry.* New York: Little, Brown.

Light, Donald. 1979. "Uncertainty and Control in Professional Training." *Journal of Health and Social Behavior* 20 (4): 310–22.

———. 1980. *Becoming Psychiatrists.* New York: W. W. Norton & Co.

Linde, Charlotte. 2009. *Working the Past: Narrative and Institutional Memory*. New York: Oxford University Press.

Link, Bruce G., Jo C. Phelan, Michaeline Bresnahan, Ann Stueve, and Bernice A. Pescosolido. 1999. "Public Conceptions of Mental Illness: Labels, Causes, Dangerousness, and Social Distance." *American Journal of Public Health* 89 (9): 1328–33.

Lovering, Joseph P. 1971. *S. Weir Mitchell*. New York: Twayne Publishers.

Luhmann, Niklas. 1994. "The Modernity of Science." *New German Critique* 61 (Winter): 9–23.

Luhrmann, Tracy M. 2001. *Of Two Minds: An Anthropologist Looks at American Psychiatry*. New York: Vintage Books.

Lunbeck, Elizabeth. 1996. *The Psychiatric Persuasion: Knowledge, Gender, and Power in Modern America*. Princeton, NJ: Princeton University Press.

———. 2014. *The Americanization of Narcissism*. Cambridge, MA: Harvard University Press.

Makari, George. 2008. *Revolution in Mind: The Creation of Psychoanalysis*. New York: HarperCollins.

———. 2015. *Soul Machine: The Invention of the Modern Mind*. New York: W. W. Norton.

Malcolm, Janet. 1982. *Psychoanalysis: The Impossible Profession*. New York: Vintage Books.

Mallard, Grégoire, and Andrew Lakoff. 2012. "How Claims to Know the Future Are Used to Understand the Present." In *Social Knowledge in the Making*, edited by Neil Gross, Charles Camic, and Michèle Lamont, 339–77. Chicago: University of Chicago Press.

Mark, Tami, L. Katharine Levit, and Jeffrey Buck. 2009. "Datapoints: Psychotropic Drug Prescriptions by Medical Specialty." *Psychiatric Services* 60 (9): 1167.

Martin, Jack K., Bernice A. Pescosolido, Sigrun Olafsdottir, and Jane D. McLeod. 2007. "The Construction of Fear: Americans' Preferences for Social Distance from Children and Adolescents with Mental Health Problems." *Journal of Health and Social Behavior* 48 (1): 50–67.

Martin, Paul A. 1999. "Genes as Drugs: The Social Shaping of Gene Therapy and the Reconstruction of Genetic Disease." *Sociology of Health & Illness* 21 (5): 517–38.

Mayes, Rick, and Allan V. Horwitz. 2005. "DSM-III and the Revolution in the Classification of Mental Illness." *Journal of the History of the Behavioral Sciences* 41 (3): 249–67.

McCandless, Peter. 1996. *Moonlight, Magnolias & Madness: Insanity in South Carolina from the Colonial Period to the Progressive Era*. Durham: University of North Carolina Press.

McGoey, Linsey. 2012. "The Logic of Strategic Ignorance." *British Journal of Sociology* 63 (3): 533–76.

Mechanic, David. 1999. *Mental Health and Social Policy: The Emergence of Managed Care*, 4th ed. New York: Allyn & Bacon.

Menand, Louis. 2001. *The Metaphysical Club*. New York: Farrar, Straus & Giroux.

Menninger, Roy W., and John Case Nemiah. 2000. *American Psychiatry after World War II (1944–1994)*. Washington, DC: American Psychiatric Press.

Menninger, William C. 1948. *Psychiatry in a Troubled World: Yesterday's War and Today's Challenge*. New York: Macmillan.

Merton, Robert K. 1987. "Three Fragments from A Sociologist's Notebooks: Establishing the Phenomenon, Specified Ignorance, and Strategic Research Materials." *Annual Review of Sociology* 13 (1): 1–29.

Metzl, Jonathan. 2003. *Prozac on the Couch: Prescribing Gender in the Era of Wonder Drugs*. Durham, NC: Duke University Press.

———. 2010. *The Protest Psychosis: How Schizophrenia Became a Black Disease*. Boston: Beacon Press.

Metzl, Jonathan, and Kenneth MacLeish. 2015. "Mental Illness, Mass Shootings, and the Politics of American Firearms." *American Journal of Public Health* 105 (2): 240–49.

Millard, Candice. 2012. *Destiny of the Republic: A Tale of Madness, Medicine and the Murder of a President*. New York: Anchor Books.

Mills, Charles W. 1997. *The Racial Contract*. Ithaca, NY: Cornell University Press.

Mische, Ann. 2009. "Projects and Possibilities: Researching Futures in Action." *Sociological Forum* 24 (3): 694–704.

Mitchell, Stephen A., and Margaret J. Black. 1995. *Freud and Beyond: A History of Modern Psychoanalytic Thought*. New York: Basic Books.

Mojtabai, Ramin. 2008. "Increase in Antidepressant Medication in the US Adult Population Between 1990 and 2003." *Psychotherapy and Psychosomatics* 77 (2): 83–92.

Mojtabai, Ramin, and Mark Olfson. 2008. "National Trends in Psychotherapy by Office-Based Psychiatrists." *Archives of General Psychiatry* 65 (8): 962–70.

———. 2011. "Proportion of Antidepressants Prescribed Without a Psychiatric Diagnosis Is Growing." *Health Affairs* 30 (8): 1434–42.

Moncrieff, Joanna. 2009. *The Myth of the Chemical Cure: A Critique of Psychiatric Drug Treatment*. New York: Palgrave Macmillan.

Moore, Wilbert E., and Melvin M. Tumin. 1949. "Some Social Functions of Ignorance." *American Sociological Review* 14 (6): 787–95.

Murphy, Dominic. 2012. *Psychiatry in the Scientific Image*. Cambridge, MA: MIT Press.

Nelkin, Dorothy, and M. Susan Lindee. 2004. *The DNA Mystique: The Gene as a Cultural Icon*. Ann Arbor: University of Michigan Press.

Nerlich, Brigitte, and Christopher Halliday. 2007. "Avian Flu: The Creation of Expectations in the Interplay between Science and the Media." *Sociology of Health & Illness* 29 (1): 46–65.

Noll, Richard. 2011. *American Madness*. Cambridge, MA: Harvard University Press.

North, Carol, and Sean Yutzy. 2010. *Goodwin and Guze's Psychiatric Diagnosis*. New York: Oxford University Press.

Olfson, Mark, Steven C. Marcus, and Harold Alan Pincus. 1999. "Trends in Office-Based Psychiatric Practice." *American Journal of Psychiatry* 156 (3): 451–57.

Olick, Jeffrey K., and Joyce Robbins. 1998. "Social Memory Studies: From 'Collective Memory' to the Historical Sociology of Mnemonic Practices." *Annual Review of Sociology* 24: 105–40.

O'Meara, Kelly Patricia. 2006. *Psyched Out: How Psychiatry Sells Mental Illness and Pushes Pills That Kill*. Bloomington, IN: Author House.

Payton, Andrew R., and Peggy A. Thoits. 2011. "Medicalization, Direct-to-Consumer Advertising, and Mental Illness Stigma." *Society and Mental Health* 1 (1): 55–70.

Peirce, Charles Sanders. 1992. *The Essential Peirce*. Edited by Nathan Houser and Christine J. W. Kloesel. Bloomington: Indiana University Press.

Phelan, Jo C. 2005. "Geneticization of Deviant Behavior and Consequences for Stigma: The Case of Mental Illness." *Journal of Health and Social Behavior* 46 (4): 307–22.

Pickersgill, Martyn. 2011. "'Promising' Therapies: Neuroscience, Clinical Practice, and the Treatment of Psychopathy." *Sociology of Health & Illness* 33 (3): 448–64.

Poovey, Mary. 1998. *A History of the Modern Fact: Problems of Knowledge in the Sciences of Wealth and Society*. Chicago: University of Chicago Press.

Porter, Roy. 1989. *A Social History of Madness: Stories of the Insane*. New York: E. P. Dutton.

Porter, Roy, and David Wright. 2003. *The Confinement of the Insane: International Perspectives, 1800–1965*. New York: Cambridge University Press.

Porter, Theodore M. 1996. *Trust in Numbers: The Pursuit of Objectivity in Science and Public Life*. Princeton, NJ: Princeton University Press.

———. 2012. "Funny Numbers." *Culture Unbound: Journal of Current Cultural Research* 4: 585–98.

Pressman, Jack D. 2002. *Last Resort: Psychosurgery and the Limits of Medicine*. New York: Cambridge University Press.

Proctor, Robert. 1995. *Cancer Wars: How Politics Shapes What We Know and Don't Know About Cancer*. New York: Basic Books.

Proctor, Robert, and Londa L. Schiebinger, eds. 2008. *Agnotology: The Making and Unmaking of Ignorance*. Stanford, CA: Stanford University Press.

Racine, Eric, Ofek Bar-Ilan, and Judy Illes. 2005. "fMRI in the Public Eye." *Nature Reviews Neuroscience* 6 (2): 159–64.

Rawls, John. 1999. *A Theory of Justice*. New York: Oxford University Press.

Reiss, Benjamin. 2008. *Theaters of Madness: Insane Asylums and Nineteenth-Century American Culture*. Chicago: University of Chicago Press.

Rose, Nikolas S. 1990. *Governing the Soul: The Shaping of the Private Self*. New York: Routledge.

Rose, Nikolas, and Joelle M. Abi-Rached. 2013. *Neuro: The New Brain Sciences and the Management of the Mind*. Princeton, NJ: Princeton University Press.

Rosenberg, Charles E. 1992. "The Crisis in Psychiatric Legitimacy: Reflections on Psychiatry, Medicine and Public Policy." In *Explaining Epidemics and Other Studies in the History of Medicine*, 245–57. New York: Cambridge University Press.

———. 1995. *The Trial of the Assassin Guiteau: Psychiatry and the Law in the Gilded Age*. Chicago: University of Chicago Press.

———. 2002. "The Tyranny of Diagnosis: Specific Entities and Individual Experience." *Milbank Quarterly* 80 (2): 237–60.

———. 2006. "Contested Boundaries: Psychiatry, Disease, and Diagnosis." *Perspectives in Biology and Medicine* 49 (3): 407–24.

———. 2007. *Our Present Complaint: American Medicine, Then and Now*. Baltimore, MD: Johns Hopkins University Press.

Rosenzweig, Saul. 1992. *Freud, Jung, and Hall the King-Maker: The Historic Expedition to America (1909), with G. Stanley Hall as Host and William James as Guest*. St. Louis, MO: Rana House.

Rosner, David. 1982. *A Once Charitable Enterprise: Hospitals and Healthcare in Brooklyn and New York, 1895–1915*. New York: Cambridge University Press.

Rothman, David J. 1971. *The Discovery of the Asylum: Social Order and Disorder in the New Republic*. Hawthorne, NY: Aldine de Gruyter.

Sackett, David L. 2002. "The Arrogance of Preventive Medicine." *Canadian Medical Association Journal* 167 (4): 363–64.

Sadowsky, Jonathan. 2006. "Beyond the Metaphor of the Pendulum: Electroconvulsive Therapy, Psychoanalysis, and the Styles of American Psychiatry." *Journal of the History of Medicine and Allied Sciences* 61 (1): 1–25.

Samuelson, William, and Richard Zeckhauser. 1988. "Status Quo Bias in Decision Making." *Journal of Risk and Uncertainty* 1 (1): 7–59.

Scasta, David L. 2003. "John E. Fryer, MD, and the Dr. H. Anonymous Episode." *Journal of Gay & Lesbian Psychotherapy* 6 (4): 73–84.

Schechter, Kate. 2014. *Illusions of a Future: Psychoanalysis and the Biopolitics of Desire*. Durham, NC: Duke University Press.

Scheff, Thomas J. 1999. *Being Mentally Ill: A Sociological Theory*, 3rd ed. New York: Aldine de Gruyter.

Schieder, Theodor. 1978. "The Role of Historical Consciousness in Political Action." *History and Theory* 17 (4): 1–18.

Schneck, Jerome M. 1960. *A History of Psychiatry*. Springfield, IL: Charles C. Thomas.

Schnittker, Jason. 2008. "An Uncertain Revolution: Why the Rise of a Genetic Model of Mental Illness Has Not Increased Tolerance." *Social Science & Medicine* 67 (9): 1370–81.

———. 2017. *The Diagnostic System: Why the Classification of Psychiatric Disorders Is Necessary, Difficult, and Never Settled*. New York: Columbia University Press.

Schutz, Kathryn. 2011. *Being Wrong: Adventures in the Margin of Error*. New York: Ecco.

Schwartz, Barry. 1996. "Memory as a Cultural System: Abraham Lincoln in World War II." *American Sociological Review* 61 (5): 908–27.

Scott, James C. 1999. *Seeing Like a State: How Certain Schemes to Improve the Human Condition Have Failed*. New Haven, CT: Yale University Press.

Scull, Andrew, ed. 1981. *Madhouses, Mad-Doctors, and Madmen: The Social History of Psychiatry in the Victorian Era*. Philadelphia: University of Pennsylvania Press.

———. 1984. *Decarceration: Community Treatment and the Deviant—A Radical View*. New Brunswick, NJ: Rutgers University Press.

———. 1989. *Social Order/Mental Disorder: Anglo-American Psychiatry in Historical Perspective*. Berkeley: University of California Press.

———. 2005. *The Most Solitary of Afflictions: Madness and Society in Britain, 1700–1900*. New Haven, CT: Yale University Press.

———. 2007. *Madhouse: A Tragic Tale of Megalomania and Modern Medicine*. New Haven, CT: Yale University Press.

———. 2015. *Madness in Civilization: A Cultural History of Insanity, from the Bible to Freud, from the Madhouse to Modern Medicine*. Princeton, NJ: Princeton University Press.

Sealey, Anne. 2011. "The Strange Case of the Freudian Case History: The Role of Long Case Histories in the Development of Psychoanalysis." *History of the Human Sciences* 24 (1): 36–50.

Sedgwick, Peter. 1982. *Psycho Politics*. Chicago: Pluto Press.

Selin, Cynthia. 2008. "The Sociology of the Future: Tracing Stories of Technology and Time." *Sociology Compass* 2 (6): 1878–95.

Selling, Lowell S. 1942. *Men against Madness*. New York: New York Home Library.

Shattuck, Roger. 1997. *Forbidden Knowledge: From Prometheus to Pornography*. Wilmington, MA: Mariner Books.

Shorter, Edward. 1997. *A History of Psychiatry: From the Era of the Asylum to the Age of Prozac*. New York: John Wiley & Sons.

———. 2005. *A Historical Dictionary of Psychiatry*. New York: Oxford University Press.

Shostak, Sara Naomi. 2013. *Exposed Science: Genes, the Environment, and the Politics of Population Health*. Berkeley: University of California Press.

Showalter, Elaine. 1985. *The Female Malady: Women, Madness, and English Culture, 1830–1980*. New York: Pantheon Books.

Sica, Alan. 2014. "Plague of Polypragmasy." *Contemporary Sociology* 43 (4): 453–57.

Smith, Dena T. 2014. "The Diminished Resistance to Medicalization in Psychiatry: Psychoanalysis Meets the Medical Model of Mental Illness." *Society and Mental Health* 4 (2): 75–91.

Smithson, Michael. 1985. "Toward a Social Theory of Ignorance." *Journal for the Theory of Social Behaviour* 15 (2): 151–72.

Snyder, Alison. 2016. "Robert L. Spitzer." *The Lancet* 387 (10017): 428.

Stanton, Alfred H., and M. S. Schwartz. 1954. *The Mental Hospital: A Study of Institutional Participation in Psychiatric Illness & Treatment*. New York: Basic Books.

Starkey, Kenneth P. 1985. "The Lengthening Hour: Time and the Demise of Psychoanalysis as Therapy." *Social Science & Medicine* 20 (9): 939–43.

Starr, Paul. 1982. *The Social Transformation of American Medicine*. New York: Basic Books.

Staub, Michael E. 2011. *Madness Is Civilization: When the Diagnosis Was Social, 1948–1980*. Chicago: University of Chicago Press.

Stern, Alexandra Minna. 2005. *Eugenic Nation: Faults and Frontiers of Better Breeding in Modern America*. Berkeley: University of California Press.

Strand, Michael. 2011. "Where Do Classifications Come from? The DSM-III, the Transformation of American Psychiatry, and the Problem of Origins in the Sociology of Knowledge." *Theory and Society* 40 (3): 273–313.

Szasz, Thomas S. 1960. "The Myth of Mental Illness." *American Psychologist* 15 (2): 113–18.

———. 1961. *The Myth of Mental Illness: Foundations of a Theory of Personal Conduct*. New York: Hoeber-Harper.

———. 1970. *The Manufacture of Madness: A Comparative Study of the Inquisition and the Mental Health Movement*. New York: Harper & Row.

Taleb, Nassim Nicholas. 2010. *The Black Swan: The Impact of the Highly Improbable Fragility*. New York: Random House Publishing Group.

Tavory, Iddo, and Nina Eliasoph. 2013. "Coordinating Futures: Toward a Theory of Anticipation." *American Journal of Sociology* 118 (4): 908–42.

Taylor, Eugene. 1999. *Shadow Culture: Psychology and Spirituality in America*. Washington, DC: Counterpoint.

Timmermans, Stefan, and Steven Epstein. 2010. "A World of Standards but Not a Standard World: Toward a Sociology of Standards and Standardization." *Annual Review of Sociology* 36: 69–89.

Tocqueville, Alexis de. 2004. *Democracy in America*. Translated by Arthur Goldhammer. New York: Library of America.

Tomes, Nancy. 1984. *A Generous Confidence: Thomas Story Kirkbride and the Art of Asylum-Keeping, 1840–1883*. New York: Cambridge University Press.

Torrey, E. Fuller. 1974. *The Death of Psychiatry*. Philadelphia: Chilton Book Company.

———. 1988. *Nowhere to Go: The Tragic Odyssey of the Homeless Mentally Ill*. New York: Harper & Row.

———. 2013. *American Psychosis: How the Federal Government Destroyed the Mental Illness Treatment System*. New York: Oxford University Press.

Toulmin, Stephen Edelston. 1992. *Cosmopolis: The Hidden Agenda of Modernity*. Chicago: University of Chicago Press.

Trent, James W. Jr. 1994. *Inventing the Feeble Mind: A History of Mental Retardation in the United States*. Berkeley: University of California Press.

Tuana, Nancy. 2004. "Coming to Understand: Orgasm and the Epistemology of Ignorance." *Hypatia* 19 (1): 194–232.

Tucker, William H. 1994. *The Science and Politics of Racial Research*. Urbana: University of Illinois Press.

Tuntiya, Nana. 2007. "Free-Air Treatment for Mental Patients: The Deinstitutionalization Debate of the Nineteenth Century." *Sociological Perspectives* 50 (3): 469–87.

Tyler, Kenneth, George K. York, David A. Steinberg, Michael S. Okun, Michelle Steinbach, Richard Satran, Edward J. Fine, Tara Manteghi, Thomas P. Bleck, and Jerry W. Swanson. 2003. "Part 2: History of 20th Century Neurology: Decade by Decade." *Annals of Neurology* 53 (S4): S27–S45.

Valenstein, Elliot S. 1986. *Great and Desperate Cures: The Rise and Decline of Psychosurgery and Other Radical Treatments for Mental Illness*. New York: Basic Books.

———. 2002. *Blaming the Brain: The Truth about Drugs and Mental Health*. New York: Free Press.

van Lente, Harro. 1993. *Promising Technology: The Dynamics of Expectations in Technological Developments.* Chicago: Eburon.

van Lente, Harro, and Arie Rip. 1998. "The Rise of Membrane Technology: From Rhetorics to Social Reality." *Social Studies of Science* 28 (2): 221–54.

Vidal, Fernando. 2009. "Brainhood, Anthropological Figure of Modernity." *History of the Human Sciences* 22 (1): 5–36.

Wahl, Otto F. 1997. *Media Madness: Public Images of Mental Illness.* New Brunswick, NJ: Rutgers University Press.

Waidzunas, Tom. 2015. *The Straight Line: How the Fringe Science of Ex-Gay Therapy Reoriented Sexuality.* Minneapolis: University of Minnesota Press.

Wake, Naoko. 2007. "The Military, Psychiatry, and 'Unfit' Soldiers, 1939–1942." *Journal of the History of Medicine and Allied Sciences* 62 (4): 461–94.

Wakefield, Jerome C. 1997. "Diagnosing DSM-IV—Part 1: DSM-IV and the Concept of Disorder." *Behavioral Research and Therapy* 35 (7): 633–49.

Wallace, Edwin R., and John Gach. 2008. *History of Psychiatry and Medical Psychology.* New York: Springer.

Wallerstein, Robert S. 2002. "The Growth and Transformation of American Ego Psychology." *Journal of the American Psychoanalytic Association* 50 (1): 135–68.

———. 2013. *Lay Analysis: Life Inside the Controversy.* New York: Taylor & Francis.

Warner, John Harley. 1998. *Against the Spirit of System: The French Impulse in Nineteenth-Century American Medicine.* Princeton, NJ: Princeton University Press.

———. 2002. "The Fall and Rise of Professional Mystery: Epistemology, Authority, and the Emergence of Laboratory Medicine in Nineteenth-Century America." In *The Laboratory Revolution in Medicine,* edited by Andrew Cunningham and Perry Williams, 110–41. New York: Cambridge University Press.

Watters, Ethan. 2010. *Crazy Like Us: The Globalization of the American Psyche.* New York: Simon and Schuster.

Weber, Max. 1978. *Economy and Society: An Outline of Interpretive Sociology,* vol. 1, edited by Guenther Ross and Claus Wittich. Berkeley: University of California Press.

Weiner, Dora B. 1992. "Philippe Pinel's 'Memoir on Madness' of December 11, 1794." *American Journal of Psychiatry* 149 (6): 725–32.

Whitaker, Robert. 2003. *Mad in America: Bad Science, Bad Medicine, and the Enduring Mistreatment of the Mentally Ill.* New York: Basic Books.

Whooley, Owen. 2010. "Diagnostic Ambivalence: Psychiatric Workarounds and the Diagnostic and Statistical Manual of Mental Disorders." *Sociology of Health & Illness* 32 (3): 452–69.

———. 2013. *Knowledge in the Time of Cholera: The Struggle over American Medicine in the Nineteenth Century.* Chicago: University of Chicago Press.

———. 2014. "Nosological Reflections: The Failure of DSM-5, the Emergence of RDoC, and the Decontextualization of Mental Distress." *Society and Mental Health* 4 (2): 92–110.

———. 2016. "Measuring Mental Disorders: The Failed Commensuration Project of DSM-5." *Social Science & Medicine* 166: 33–40.

Wilson, Mitchell. 1993. "DSM-III and the Transformation of American Psychiatry: A History." *American Journal of Psychiatry* 150 (3): 399–410.

Wright, Lawrence. 2013. *Going Clear: Scientology, Hollywood, and the Prison of Belief.* New York: Vintage.

Yanni, Carla. 2007. *The Architecture of Madness: Insane Asylums in the United States.* Minneapolis: University of Minnesota Press.

Zaretsky, Eli. 2000. "Charisma or Rationalization? Domesticity and Psychoanalysis in the United States in the 1950s." *Critical Inquiry* 26 (2): 328–54.

———. 2005. *Secrets of the Soul: A Social and Cultural History of Psychoanalysis.* New York: Vintage Books.

Zerubavel, Eviatar. 1999. *Social Mindscapes: An Invitation to Cognitive Sociology.* Cambridge, MA: Harvard University Press.

———. 2003. *Time Maps: Collective Memory and the Social Shape of the Past.* Chicago: University of Chicago Press.

———. 2015. "The Social Structure of Denial." In *Culture, Society, and Democracy: The Interpretive Approach,* edited by Isaac Reed and Jeffrey Alexander, 181–88. New York: Routledge.

Ziff, Katherine. 2012. *Asylum on the Hill: History of a Healing Landscape.* Athens: Ohio University Press.

Zilboorg, Gregory. 1967. *A History of Medical Psychology.* New York: W. W. Norton.

Zola, Irving Kenneth. 1972. "Medicine as an Institution of Social Control." *Sociological Review* 20 (4): 487–504.

INDEX

Page numbers in italics refer to figures.